This book is dedicated to my mother, Janice Cole Clark,
and to the memory of my father, Kempton Clark,
with thanks and appreciation
for their lifelong love and support.
They have fed my spirit and nourished my soul.

CONTENTS

Preface **vi** | Acknowledgments **viii**

PART I   **Eating Strategies for High Energy**   **1**

1 A Plan for Good Nutrition **3**

2 Healthy Choices Make Healthy Bodies **27**

3 Better Diets Begin With Breakfast **53**

4 Meals to Fight Stress and Fatigue **69**

5 Snacks for Cravings and Preexercise Energy ... **89**

6 Fueling During and After Exercise **113**

7 Eliminating Carbohydrate Confusion **137**

8 Protein and Performance **161**

PART II   **Balancing Weight and Activity**   **179**

9 Finding a Healthy Body Fat Level **181**

10 Bulking Up Without Adding Fat **203**

11 Losing Weight Without Starvation **217**

12 Eating Disorders and Food Obsessions **241**

Nancy Clark's

HUMAN KINETICS

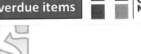

Library of Congress Cataloging-in-Publication Data

Clark, Nancy, 1951-
  [Sports nutrition guidebook]
  Nancy Clark's sports nutrition guidebook / Nancy Clark.-- 3rd ed.
    p. cm.
Includes bibliographical references and index.
  ISBN 0-7360-4602-X
  1.Athletes--Nutrition.   I. Title: Sports nutrition guidebook.   II.
Title.
  TX361.A8C54 2003
  613.2'024'796--dc21

                                        2003009149

ISBN: 0-7360-4602-X

The Web addresses cited in this text were current as of May 2003, unless otherwise noted.

Acquisitions Editor: Martin Barnard; **Developmental Editor:** Laura Pulliam; **Assistant Editor:** Alisha Jeddeloh; **Copyeditor:** Bob Replinger; **Proofreader:** Pam Johnson; **Indexer:** Robert Swanson; **Permission Manager:** Toni Harte; **Graphic Designer:** Robert Reuther; **Graphic Artist:** Sandra Meier; **Art Manager:** Dan Wendt; **Cover Designer:** Jack W. Davis; **Illustrator:** Roberto Sabas; **Printer:** Versa Press

Human Kinetics books are available at special discounts for bulk purchase. Special editions or book excerpts can also be created to specification. For details, contact the Special Sales Manager at Human Kinetics.

Printed in the United States of America   10   9   8   7   6   5   4   3

Human Kinetics
Web site: www.HumanKinetics.com

United States: Human Kinetics
P.O. Box 5076, Champaign, IL 61825-5076
800-747-4457
e-mail: humank@hkusa.com

Canada: Human Kinetics
475 Devonshire Road Unit 100, Windsor, ON N8Y 2L5
800-465-7301 (in Canada only)
e-mail: orders@hkcanada.com

Europe: Human Kinetics
107 Bradford Road, Stanningley, Leeds LS28 6AT, United Kingdom
+44 (0) 113 255 5665
e-mail: hk@hkeurope.com

Australia: Human Kinetics
57A Price Avenue, Lower Mitcham, South Australia 5062
08 8277 1555
e-mail: liaw@hkaustralia.com

New Zealand: Human Kinetics
Division of Sports Distributors NZ Ltd., P.O. Box 300 226 Albany
North Shore City, Auckland
0064 9 448 1207
e-mail: blairc@hknewz.com

PART III   Winning Recipes   265

Recipe Contributors   266

Introduction to Recipes   267

13 Breads and Breakfasts **273**

14 Pasta, Rice, and Potatoes **287**

15 Vegetables and Salads **301**

16 Chicken and Turkey **311**

17 Fish and Seafood **327**

18 Beef and Pork **337**

19 Beans and Tofu **345**

20 Beverages and Smoothies **355**

21 Snacks and Desserts **361**

Appendix A   Recommended Reading   **375**

Appendix B   For More Information   **380**

Appendix C   Selected References   **389**

Index   **396** | About the Author   **405**

PREFACE

People exercise for many reasons:

- David, a hospital administrator, exercises to relieve stress.
- Tim, a newly retired executive, is training for his first Ironman triathlon.
- Julia, an at-home mom, exercises to get her body back to her pre-pregnancy shape.
- Tricia, a high school student, hopes to earn a soccer scholarship for college.
- Janice, a grandmother, knows that she has to "use it or lose it."

For every reason that people exercise, they have a similar reason to eat well. Regardless of whether you are exercising to improve your performance, body shape, health, life span, or weight, or if you are simply active all day with kids, work, and a busy lifestyle, you'll feel better and perform better when you fuel your body optimally. To do this, you must eat the right combinations of foods at the right times. In trying to do so, questions may arise:

- What should I eat before I go to the gym?
- How can I lose weight and have energy to exercise?
- Can I eat well even if I eat out all the time?
- What about energy bars—are they better than, let's say, bananas?
- How do I carbo load for my first marathon?
- What should my kids eat before their 9:00 A.M. soccer game?
- How can I calm my sweet tooth? I'm addicted to sugar!

The purpose of *Nancy Clark's Sports Nutrition Guidebook, Third Edition* is to answer your questions about food, nutrition, and weight management. Whether you are a casual exerciser, competitive athlete, fitness fanatic, struggling dieter, parent of a youth athlete, aspiring Olympian, or just a busy person trying to survive this marathon called life, you'll learn how to have more energy, delay—or better yet, *prevent*—fatigue, and stay healthy throughout each day.

In *Nancy Clark's Sports Nutrition Guidebook, Third Edition,* I'll share with you the winning nutrition strategies I've taught my clients. As director of nutrition services at SportsMedicine Associates, one of the largest sports-injury clinics in the Boston area, I've counseled active people of all lifestyles, occupations, ages, and athletic abilities—lawyers, moms, executives, students, retired teachers, golf pros, Olympians. I've taught them how to eat well, feel great, manage their weight concerns, enjoy high energy all day long, and be at peace with food.

For most of my clients, achieving these goals means learning how to eat well on the run and when under stress. They learn how to navigate their way healthfully through grocery stores, fast-food drive-throughs, restaurants, food courts, and even their own kitchens. No longer do they associate holidays, birthday parties, and vacations with blown-diet days.

If you, like my clients, struggle with how to eat well for sports, exercise, weight control, and health, these obstacles undoubtedly hinder your intentions to eat well:

- No time to eat (to say nothing of eat *well*)
- Little energy (or interest) for preparing wholesome meals
- A stressful lifestyle

Nancy Clark's Sports Nutrition Guidebook, Third Edition offers you the practical solutions to overcoming these barriers. You'll learn how to eat wisely and well—even with your active lifestyle. I invite you to keep reading this how-to nutrition guide and learn practical eating strategies that will boost your energy, enhance your exercise program, help you lose or gain weight (if desired), protect your good health, and invest in lifelong well-being.

Eat well—and enjoy your good health and high energy.

Nancy Clark, MS, RD
Director of Nutrition Services
SportsMedicine Associates
830 Boylston Street, Suite 205
Brookline, MA 02467
www.nancyclarkrd.com

ACKNOWLEDGMENTS

I wish to offer my sincere thanks and appreciation to my loving husband John, son John Michael, and daughter Mary for bringing balance, fun, and meaning to my daily life.

I would also like to thank my running buddies Jean Smith and Katherine Farrell for their miles of support throughout this marathon called Life, and my clients, for teaching me about sports nutrition in action. Their experiences allow me to provide better help to others with nutrition concerns. I have changed their names and occupations in this book to protect their privacy. Thank you, also, to the recipe contributors for sharing their favorite food ideas, and to Laura Pulliam, Toni Harte, Martin Barnard, Rainer Martens, Sandra Meier, and the staff at Human Kinetics Publishers. And finally, a big thank you to the faithful recipe testers, Joe and Wendy Czarnicki, Joan and Rex Hawley, and Don Lawson, for being enthusiastic eaters, as well as valued neighbors.

PART I

Eating Strategies for High Energy

1

A Plan for Good Nutrition

"I know what I *should* eat. I just don't do it." This familiar statement tends to be among my clients' first words. Although food is important for fueling the body and investing in overall health, many of my clients sleep through breakfast, work through lunch, skimp on meals, and then feed themselves not-so-healthful snacks. Students, parents, business people, casual exercisers, and competitive athletes alike repeatedly express their frustrations with trying to eat high-quality diets. The stress and fatigue associated with long work hours, well-intentioned attempts to lose weight, and efforts to schedule exercise can all mean that food becomes more of a stress than one of life's pleasures.

In this chapter, you'll learn how to eat right all day long, even if you have a stressful lifestyle. Whether you work out at the health club, compete with a varsity team, aspire to be an Olympian, or simply are busy playing with your kids, you can nourish yourself with a diet that supports good health and high energy, even if you are eating on the run.

Nutrition Basics

One key to eating well is to prevent yourself from getting too hungry. When people get too hungry, they tend to care less about what they choose to eat and more about rewarding themselves with a treat because they survived yet another hectic day. By preventing hunger, you can curb your physiological desire to eat excessive treats, as well as tame your psychological desire to reward yourself with, let's say, a gorgeous chocolate brownie.

When you fuel your body appropriately, you have the mental energy you need to choose the healthful foods that support your exercise program and invest in your health. When choosing these meals and snacks, try to base your nutrition game plan on these three important keys to healthful eating:

1. **Variety.** The more different types of foods you eat, the more different types of nutrients you consume. For example, although oranges are an excellent source of vitamin C and carbohydrates, they fail to provide iron or protein. Beef offers iron and protein but not vitamin C or carbohydrates. The combination of an orange consumed for dessert after a lunchtime roast-beef sandwich may be a more powerful and health-protective combination than each food eaten alone, a concept known as synergy.

   Many Americans eat the same 10 to 15 foods each week. If you find yourself eating a repetitive menu, at least try to eat different brands of cereal topped with different fruits for breakfast, different types of sandwiches and breads for lunch, and lots of different colorful vegetables in the salad. I recommend to my clients that they target eating 3 different kinds of foods at a meal and 35 different types of foods per week. Count them!

2. **Wholesomeness.** Choose whole or lightly processed foods as often as possible. For instance, choose whole-wheat bread rather than white bread, apples rather than apple juice, baked potatoes rather than potato chips. Foods in their natural state usually have more nutritional value and fewer questionable ingredients.

3. **Moderation.** Rather than think about food as being good or bad for your health, think about moderation. Even soda pop and chips, in moderation, can fit into a nourishing diet if you balance them with healthier choices during the rest of the day. For example, you can compensate for a greasy sausage and biscuit at breakfast by selecting a low-fat turkey sandwich for lunch.

What Shape Is Your Diet?

Whereas square meals and a well-rounded diet were once the shape of good nutrition, a pyramid reflects the shape of nutrition for the 21st century. The U.S. Department of Agriculture has developed the Food Guide Pyramid model, which divides food into six groupings of varied sizes that stack into a pyramid. The pyramid supports the concept of a diet based on carbohydrate-rich foods and offers the visual message that you should eat a foundation of wholesome breads, cereals, and grains at each meal; generous amounts of fruits and vegetables; and lesser amounts of fatty animal proteins and dairy foods. Visualize two-thirds of your plate being covered by fruits, vegetables, and whole grains and one-third by protein-rich foods. The tip of the pyramid allows for a taste of refined sugars and unhealthful fats.

Unfortunately for their health, many of my clients eat a linear diet: apples, apples, apples; energy bars, energy bars, energy bars; pasta, pasta, pasta. Repetitive eating keeps life simple, minimizes decisions, and simplifies shopping, but it can result in an inadequate diet and chronic fatigue. If your diet looks more like a line than a pyramid, keep reading. You'll learn how to eat more of the best foods, eat less of the rest, and create a food plan that invests in high energy, good health, and weight management.

Shaping Your Daily Diet

When contemplating your daily food choices, keep the food pyramid in mind. You can consume the recommended intake of the vitamins,

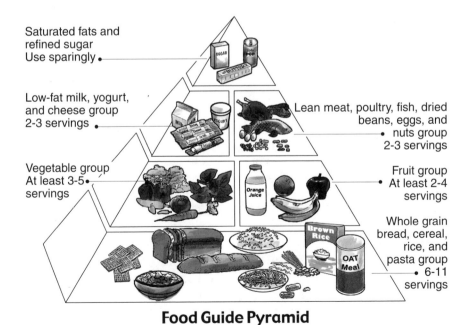

Saturated fats and refined sugar
Use sparingly

Low-fat milk, yogurt, and cheese group
2-3 servings

Lean meat, poultry, fish, dried beans, eggs, and nuts group
2-3 servings

Vegetable group
At least 3-5 servings

Fruit group
At least 2-4 servings

Whole grain bread, cereal, rice, and pasta group
6-11 servings

Food Guide Pyramid

minerals, amino acids (the building blocks of protein), and other nutrients you need for good health within 1,200 to 1,500 calories if you wisely select from a variety of wholesome foods. Because many active people consume 2,000 to 5,000 calories (depending on their age, level of activity, body size, and gender), they have the chance to consume abundant amounts of vitamins and other nutrients. For example, the high school football player who guzzled a quart of orange juice for a postexercise refresher consumed five times the recommended intake of vitamin C in this mere "snack." Dieters, on the other hand, tend to take in fewer calories, and they need to carefully select nutrient-dense foods—foods that offer the most nutritional value for the least amount of calories to reduce the risk of consuming a nutrient-deficient diet.

To help you select the nutrient-dense foods that fit your lifestyle, follow this good nutrition game plan.

Planning for Good Nutrition: Whole Grains and Starches

As illustrated by the food pyramid, wholesome breads, cereals, and other grain foods are the foundation of an optimal diet, particularly a sports diet. Unrefined grains are excellent sources of carbohydrates, fiber, and B vitamins. They fuel your muscles, protect against needless muscular fatigue, and reduce problems with constipation if they're fiber rich. And despite popular belief, the carbohydrates in grains are not fattening; excess calories are fattening. Excess calories often come from the fats (butter, mayonnaise, gravy) that accompany rolls, sandwich bread, rice, and other carbs. If weight is an issue, I recommend that you limit the fats but enjoy fiber-rich breads, cereals, and other whole grains. These foods help curb hunger and assist with weight management. Wholesome carbohydrates should be the foundation of both a weight-reduction program and a sports diet.

Grains account for about 25 percent of the energy consumed in the United States, but unfortunately for our health about 95 percent of this is from refined grains. The refining process strips grains of their bran and germ, thereby removing fiber, antioxidants, minerals, and other health-protective compounds. People who eat diets based on refined grains tend to have a higher incidence of chronic diseases, such as heart disease and adult-onset diabetes (Pereira et al., *Effect of whole grains*, 2002).

When selecting grains, go with the whole grain! Try to choose the ones that have been only lightly processed, if processed at all. For example, brown rice, whole-wheat bread, and stoned-wheat crackers offer more B vitamins, potassium, and fiber than refined white rice, white bread, and white crackers. Other whole grains include rye crackers,

Triscuits (preferably the low-fat variety), popcorn, corn tortillas, corn taco shells, whole-wheat pita bread, bulgur, and barley. When reading food labels, look for one of the following listed first in the ingredient list: whole rye, whole wheat, whole oats, brown rice, oatmeal. These whole grains offer hundreds of phytochemicals that play key roles in reducing the risk of heart disease, diabetes, and cancer.

How Much Is Enough?

If you consume about 55 to 65 percent of your calories from carbohydrates, you'll be getting adequate carbs to fully fuel your muscles. You can do this by eating at least 6 to 11 servings of wholesome grains every day. Although this may sound like an overwhelming amount of food, it's not. You simply need to understand the definition of *serving*. Serving sizes are shown here:

Grain food	Standard serving	Common portion	Number of pyramid servings
Cereal	1 oz	2-4 oz (1 bowl)	2-4
Bread	1 average slice	2 slices per sandwich	2
Bagel	1/2 small	1 large	3-4
Pasta	1/2 cup cooked	2-3 cups	4-6
Rice	1/2 cup cooked	1-2 cups	2-4

Six to 11 grain servings is only 2 to 4 servings per meal, or the equivalent of about 150 to 300 calories—not much for hungry exercisers who require 600 to 900 calories per meal. Most active people commonly eat double or even triple servings of grains at each meal.

Top Choices

Whole-grain cereals. Total, Wheaties, Cheerios, Müeslix, and Shredded Wheat are examples of whole-grain cereals. Look for the words "whole grain" on the cereal box or in the list of ingredients. See chapter 3 for more information on cereals.

Oatmeal. When cooked into a tasty hot cereal, or eaten raw as in muesli, oatmeal makes a wonderful breakfast that helps lower cholesterol and protect against heart disease. Some people even keep microwaveable packets of instant oatmeal in their desk drawers for cozy afternoon snacks. Oatmeal (either instant and regular) is a whole-grain food with a slow-to-digest carbohydrate that offers sustained energy and is perfect for a preexercise snack.

Bagels and muffins. Bagels (pumpernickel, rye, whole wheat) and low-fat muffins (bran, corn, oatmeal) are more healthful than muffins, doughnuts, buttered toast, croissants, or pastries made with white flour. Add yogurt and orange juice and you have a meal on the run that's easily available from a convenience store or cafeteria, if not from home.

Whole-grain and dark breads. When it comes to choosing bread products, remember that whole-grain breads tend to have more nutritional value than white breads. At the supermarket, select the hearty brands that have whole wheat, rye, or oatmeal listed as the first ingredient. Keep fresh multigrain bakery breads in the freezer so that you'll have a supply on hand for toast, sandwiches, or a snack. When at the sandwich shop, request the turkey with tomato on dark rye!

Stoned-wheat and whole-grain crackers. These low-fat munchies are a perfect high-carbohydrate snack for your sports diet. Be sure to choose wholesome brands of crackers with low fat content, not the ones that leave you with greasy fingers!

Popcorn. Whether popped in air or just a little canola oil, popcorn is a fun way to boost your whole-grain intake. The trick is to avoid smothering it in butter or salt. How about sprinkling it with taco seasoning mix, Italian seasonings, or a seasoned popcorn spray?

Planning for Good Nutrition: Fruits

As the food pyramid shows, fruits add to the strong foundation of carbohydrates needed for your sports diet. Fruits are rich in carbohydrates, fiber, potassium, and many vitamins, especially vitamin C. The nutrients in fruits improve healing, aid in recovery after exercise, and reduce the risk of cancer, high blood pressure, and constipation.

How Much Is Enough?

The recommended intake is at least two to four fruit servings per day. This may seem like a lot, but it often translates into only one or two pieces of fruit. When people have trouble getting fruit into their daily menus, I recommend that they simply schedule it into their breakfast routine. A tall glass of orange juice and a large banana on your cereal will cover your minimum fruit requirement for the entire day. These are among the more nutritious fruits, so you'll be getting a good start to the day.

Fruit	Standard serving	Common portion	Number of pyramid servings
Orange juice	6 oz	12 oz	2
Apple	1 medium	1 large	2
Banana	1 small	1 large	2-3
Canned fruit	1/2 cup	1 cup	2

Top Choices

If you have trouble including fruit in your diet because it is not readily available or because it spoils before you get around to eating it, the following tips will help you balance your intake better and make these foods a top priority in your good nutrition game plan.

Citrus fruits and juices. Whether it's the whole fruit or fresh, frozen, or canned juice, citrus fruits such as oranges, grapefruits, clementines, and tangerines surpass many other fruits or juices in vitamin C and potassium content.

If the hassle of peeling an orange or a grapefruit is a deterrent for you, just drink its juice. The whole fruit has slightly more nutritional value, but given the option of a quick glass of juice or nothing, juice does the job! Just eight ounces (about 250 milliliters) of orange juice provides more than the daily reference intake of 75 milligrams of vitamin C, all the potassium you might have lost in an hour-long workout, and folic acid, a B vitamin needed for building protein and red blood cells and protecting against heart disease. Orange juice also has fewer calories and more nutrients than many other juices, such as cranberry, apple, and pineapple juice.

To boost your juice intake, stock up on cans of the frozen juice concentrate, buy juice boxes for lunch or snacks, and look for cans or bottles of juice in vending machines. Better yet, stock whole oranges in your refrigerator and pack them in your gym bag.

Bananas. This low-fat, high-fiber, and high-potassium fruit is perfect for busy people, and it even comes prewrapped! Bananas are excellent for replacing potassium lost in sweat. The potassium protects against high blood pressure. To boost your banana intake, include bananas on cereal, pack one in your lunch bag for a satisfying dessert, or keep them on hand for a quick and easy energy-boosting snack. My all-time favorite combination is banana with peanut butter, stoned-wheat crackers, and a glass of low-fat milk—a well-balanced meal or snack that includes a variety of foods (fruit, protein, grains, dairy).

To prevent bananas from becoming overripe, store them in the refrigerator. The skin may turn black from the cold, but the fruit itself will be fine. Another trick is to keep banana chunks in the freezer. These frozen nuggets taste just like banana ice cream but have far fewer calories and blend nicely with milk into creamy smoothies. (See the recipe for fruit smoothies on page 357.)

Without a doubt, bananas are among the most popular sports snacks. I once saw a cyclist with two bananas safely taped to his helmet, ready to grab when he needed an energy boost.

Cantaloupe, kiwi, strawberries, and other berries. These nutrient-dense fruits are also good sources of vitamin C and potassium.

Dried fruits. Convenient and portable, dried fruits are rich in potassium and carbohydrates.

If you are eating too little fruit, be sure that the fruit you eat is nutritionally the best. The information in table 1.1 can help guide your choices.

TABLE 1.1

Comparing Fruits

Fruit	Amount	Calories	A (IU)	C (mg)	Potassium (mg)
Apple	1 medium	80	75	10	160
Apple juice	1 cup	115	0	2	300
Apricots	10 halves dried	85	2,550	1	480
Banana	1 medium	105	90	10	450
Blueberries, raw	1 cup	80	145	20	260
Cantaloupe	1 cup pieces	55	5,160	70	495
Cherries	10 sweet	50	145	5	150
Cranberry juice	1 cup	140	10	90	55
Dates	5 dried	115	20	—	270
Figs	1 medium raw	35	70	1	115
Grapefruit	1/2 medium pink	40	155	45	170
Grapefruit juice	1 cup white	95	25	95	400
Grapes	1 cup	60	90	5	175
Honeydew melon	1 cup cubes	60	70	40	460
Kiwi	1 medium	45	135	75	250
Orange, navel	1 medium	60	240	75	230
Orange juice	1 cup fresh	110	500	125	500
Peach	1 medium	35	465	5	170
Pear	1 medium	100	35	5	210
Pineapple	1 cup raw	75	35	25	175
Pineapple juice	1 cup	140	13	25	335
Prunes	5 dried	100	830	2	310
Raisins	1/3 cup	150	5	2	375
Strawberries	1 cup raw	45	40	85	245
Watermelon	1 cup	50	585	15	185

Planning for Good Nutrition: Vegetables

Like fruits, vegetables contribute important carbohydrates to the foundation of your sports diet. Vegetables are what I call nature's vitamin pills, because they are excellent sources of vitamin C, beta-carotene (the plant form of vitamin A), potassium, magnesium, and many other vitamins, minerals, and health-protective substances. In general, vegetables have a little more nutritional value than fruits. Hence, if you don't eat much fruit, you can compensate by eating more veggies. You'll get similar vitamins and minerals, if not more.

How Much Is Enough?

The recommended intake is at least three to five servings of vegetables per day. Many busy people rarely eat that much in a week! If you are vegetable challenged, the trick is to eat large portions when you do eat vegetables—a big pile rather than a standard serving.

Food	Standard serving	Suggested portion	Number of pyramid servings
Broccoli	1 small stalk	2 large stalks	3-4
Spinach	1/2 cup	10 oz box, frozen	3
Salad bar	small bowl	large bowl	3-4
Spaghetti sauce	1/2 cup	1 cup	2

Top Choices

Any vegetable is good for you. Of course, vegetables fresh from the garden are best, but they are often impossible to obtain. Frozen vegetables are a good second choice; freezing destroys little nutritional value. Overcooking is a prime nutrient destroyer, so cook fresh or frozen vegetables only until they are tender-crisp, preferably in the microwave oven, steamer, or wok.

Because canned vegetables are processed quickly, they retain many of their nutrients. Using the vegetable water for soups or stews minimizes the loss. Rinsing canned vegetables with plain water can reduce their higher sodium levels.

Dark, colorful vegetables usually have more nutritional value than paler ones. If you are struggling to improve your diet, boost your intake of colorful broccoli, spinach, green peppers, tomatoes, and carrots. They are more nutrient dense than pale lettuces, cucumbers, zucchini, mushrooms, and celery. (In no way are these pale vegetables bad for you; the colorful ones are just better.) Here's the scoop on a few of the top vegetable choices.

Broccoli, spinach, and peppers (green, red, or yellow). These low-fat, potassium-rich vegetables are loaded with vitamin C and the health-protective carotenes that are the precursors of vitamin A. One stalk (one-half cup) of steamed broccoli offers you the RDI for vitamin C, as does half a large pepper or a spinach salad. I enjoy munching on a pepper instead of an apple for a snack; it offers more vitamins and potassium and fewer calories. What a nutritional bargain!

Tomatoes and tomato sauce. In salads or on pasta or pizza, tomato products are another easy way to boost your veggie intake. They are good sources of potassium, fiber, and vitamin C (one medium-sized tomato provides half the RDI for vitamin C), carotenes (the plant form of vitamin A), and lycopene, a phytochemical that protects against certain cancers. Tomato juice and vegetable juice are additional suggestions for fast-laners who lack the time or interest to cook. They can enjoyably drink their veggies! Commercial tomato products tend to be high in sodium, however, so people with high blood pressure should limit their intake or choose the low-sodium brands.

Cruciferous vegetables (members of the cabbage family). Cabbage, broccoli, cauliflower, brussels sprouts, bok choy, collards, kale, kohlrabi, and mustard greens may protect against cancer, as may carotene-rich choices such as carrots, winter squash, and greens. Do your health a favor by focusing on these choices. You can't go wrong eating piles of these.

If you are eating too few vegetables, be sure the ones you eat are among the best. The information in table 1.2 can help guide your choices, as can the information in the salad section in chapter 4.

TABLE 1.2

Comparing Vegetables

Vegetable	Amount	Calories	A (IU)	C (mg)	Potassium (mg)
Asparagus	8 spears cooked	35	980	30	260
Beets	1/2 cup boiled	35	30	5	260
Broccoli	1 cup cooked	50	3,500	75	330
Brussels sprouts	8 medium cooked	60	1,100	100	500
Cabbage, green	1 cup cooked	30	200	35	145
Carrot	1 medium raw	30	20,250	10	230
Cauliflower	1 cup cooked	30	20	55	180
Celery	1 seven-in. stalk	5	55	5	115
Corn	1/2 cup frozen	65	180	5	120
Cucumber	1/3 medium	15	220	5	150
Green beans	1 cup cooked	45	820	15	370
Kale	1 cup cooked	40	9,600	55	300
Lettuce, iceberg	7 leaves	15	455	5	160
Lettuce, romaine	2 cups shredded	15	2,900	30	320
Mushrooms	1 cup pieces raw	20	0	2	260
Onion	1/2 cup chopped	30	0	5	125
Peas, green	1/2 cup cooked	60	530	10	135
Pepper, green	1 cup diced	30	630	90	180
Potato, baked	1 large with skin	220	0	50	1,700
Spinach	1 cup cooked	40	14,750	20	840
Squash, summer	1 cup cooked	35	520	10	345
Squash, winter	1 cup baked	80	7,200	20	890
Sweet potato	1 medium baked	120	25,000	30	400
Tomato	1 small raw	25	770	25	275
Recommended intake:			>5,000	>60	>3,500

Adapted, by permission, from the Center for Science in the Public Interest's *Nutrition Action Newsletter* © CSPI 2000.

The Nutrition Rainbow

Strive to eat a variety of colors of fruits and vegetables. Each color offers different kinds of the health-protective phytochemicals that are linked with reducing the risk of cancer and heart disease:

Color	Fruit	Vegetable
Red	Strawberries, watermelon	Red peppers, tomatoes*
Green	Kiwi, grapes, honeydew melon	Peas, beans, spinach, broccoli
Blue or purple	Blueberries, grapes, prunes	Eggplant, beets
Orange	Mango, peaches, cantaloupe	Carrots, sweet potato, pumpkin
Yellow	Pineapple, star fruit	Summer squash, corn
White	Banana, pears	Garlic, onions

*Technically, tomatoes are a fruit.

Planning for Good Nutrition: Protein-Rich Foods

Protein from animals (meats, seafood, eggs, and poultry) and plants (beans, nuts, and legumes) is also important in your daily diet, but you should not eat it in the same quantity as you do breads, grains, fruits, and vegetables. Protein-rich foods provide the amino acids you need to build and repair muscles. By eating darker meats with iron and zinc, you reduce the risk of iron-deficiency anemia.

How Much Is Enough?

You should eat two to three servings of protein-rich foods every day. Athletes tend to eat either too much or too little protein, depending on their health consciousness or lifestyle. Whereas some athletes fill up on too much meat, others choose to bypass animal proteins and neglect to replace the beef with beans.

Slabs of steak and huge hamburgers have no place in an athlete's diet, or anyone's diet. Excess protein isn't stored as bulging muscles or used for muscle fuel. But adequate amounts of protein are important for building muscles and repairing tissues. The purpose of this section is to highlight quick and easy protein choices.

Protein-rich food	Standard serving	Common portion	Number of pyramid servings
Tuna	1/3 of 6 oz can	1 whole can	3
Chicken	2 oz drumstick	6 oz breast	3
Peanut butter	2 tbsp	2-4 tbsp	1-2
Lentil soup	1 cup	1 bowl	2
Kidney beans	1/2 cup	1 cup	2

The protein rule of thumb is to include a total of 4 to 6 ounces (110 to 170 grams) of protein-rich food at lunch or at dinner, or to eat half that amount at each meal. Four ounces is much less than the portions most Americans eat: 10-ounce steaks, 6-ounce chicken breasts, 6-ounce cans of tuna. Many athletes polish off their required protein by lunchtime and continue to eat one to two times more than they need.

Other people, however, miss out on adequate protein when they eat only a salad for lunch or plain pasta or stir-fry veggies for dinner. Dieters, for example, who dine exclusively on salads and vegetables commonly neglect their protein needs. See chapter 8 for more information on protein needs, vegetarian diets, and muscle-building foods.

Top Choices

All types of protein-rich foods contain valuable amino acids. See table 1.3 for a comparison of some popular protein-rich foods.

The following choices can enhance your sports diet.

Chicken and turkey. Poultry generally has less saturated fat than red meats, so it tends to be a more heart-healthful choice. Just be sure to buy skinless chicken or discard the skin (which is high in fat) before cooking. Cooked until crispy, poultry skin can be a big temptation.

Fish. Fresh, frozen, or canned fish not only provides a lot of protein but also protects your health. The recommended target is two to three fish meals (canned or fresh) per week, with the best choices being the oilier varieties that live in cold ocean waters, such as salmon, mackerel, albacore tuna, swordfish, sardines, bluefish, and herring. But any fish is better than no fish (see chapter 2).

Lean beef. A lean roast-beef sandwich made with two thick slices of multigrain bread for carbohydrates is an excellent choice for not only protein but also iron (prevents anemia), for zinc (needed for muscle growth and repair), and for B vitamins (helps produce energy). Top round (such as you'd buy at a deli), eye of round, and round tip are among the leanest cuts of beef. A lean roast-beef sandwich is preferable in terms of heart health and nutritional value than a grilled-cheese sandwich, chicken salad, or a hamburger because of these nutrients and the lower fat content.

Peanut butter. Although peanut butter by the jar full can be a dangerous diet breaker, a few tablespoons on whole-grain bread, crackers, a bagel, or banana offers protein, vitamins, and fiber in a satisfying snack or a quick meal. Being a source of plant protein, peanut butter has no cholesterol. People who eat at least two servings of peanut butter (or peanuts) per week tend to have a lower risk of heart disease (Kris-Etherton et al. 2001). Enjoy this childhood favorite!

Canned beans. Vegetarian refried beans (tucked into a tortilla sprinkled with salsa and grated low-fat cheese and then heated in the micro-

TABLE 1.3

Comparing Protein Content

Animal proteins	Protein (grams)
Beef, roast, 4 oz cooked*	30
Chicken breast, 4 oz cooked	35
Tuna, 1 can (6.5 oz)	30-40
Egg, 1	6
Egg white, 1	3
Plant proteins	
Soy milk, 1 cup	7
Lentils, 1/2 cup	7
Baked beans, 1/2 cup	7
Peanut butter, 2 tbsp	9
Tofu, 1/4 cake (4 oz)	11
Dairy products	
Milk, yogurt, 1 cup	8
Milk powder, 1/3 cup	8
Cheese, cheddar, 1 oz	7
Cheese, American, 1 slice (2/3 oz)	6
Cottage cheese, 1/2 cup	15
Breads, cereals, grains	
Bread, 1 slice	2
Cold cereal, 1 oz	2
Oatmeal, 1/3 cup dry or 2/3 cup cooked	5
Rice, 1/3 cup dry or 1 cup cooked	4
Pasta, 2 oz dry or 1 cup cooked	8
Starchy vegetables**	
Peas, 1/2 cup cooked	2
Carrots, 1/2 cup cooked	2
Corn, 1/2 cup cooked	2
Beets, 1/2 cup cooked	2
Winter squash, 1/2 cup	2
Potato, 1 small	2

*4 oz cooked = 5-6 oz raw (approx. size of deck of cards)

**Whereas starchy vegetables contribute a little protein, most watery vegetables (and fruits) offer negligible amounts of protein. They may contribute a total of 5 to 10 grams of protein per day, depending on how much you eat.

wave oven), baked beans (on top of a baked potato), and canned garbanzo or kidney beans (added to a salad) are three easy ways to boost your intake of these plant proteins, which are also excellent sources of carbohydrates. If you tend to avoid beans because they make you flatulent, try eating them with Beano, a product available at many health-food stores and pharmacies that takes the gas out of vegetarian diets.

Tofu. Tofu is a vegetable protein that may reduce your risk of heart disease and cancer. Tofu is an easy addition to a meatless diet because you don't have to cook it. Tofu has a mild flavor, so you can easily add it to salads, chili, spaghetti sauce, lasagna, and other casseroles. Look for it in the vegetable section of your grocery store. Buy "firm" tofu for slicing or cutting into cubes, and "soft" or "silken" tofu for blending into milkshakes or dips.

Even those who don't cook can easily incorporate adequate protein into a day's diet. Buy lean roast beef, rotisserie chicken, and turkey breast at the deli counter. Open a can of tuna or salmon. Vegetarians can also add protein with little effort. Peanut butter, hummus (chickpea spread), and nuts are good sources. Protein-rich canned beans, lentils, and legumes are quick and convenient during your busy week. If you prefer to cook them yourself, simply cook them in quantity on the weekend so that you'll have enough to last through the week. Tofu is another healthful, versatile protein that you don't have to cook.

Planning for Good Nutrition: Low-Fat Dairy Products

Dairy foods such as low-fat milk, yogurt, and cheese are not only quick and easy sources of protein, but are also rich in calcium, a mineral that is particularly important for growing teens and women and men of all ages. A calcium-rich diet helps maintain strong bones, reduces the risk of osteoporosis, and protects against high blood pressure. A low-fat, dairy-rich diet may protect against weight gain and type 2 diabetes (Pereira, et al., *Dairy consumption,* 2002). Dairy foods are also rich in riboflavin, a B vitamin that helps convert food into energy.

Make no bones about it! Low-fat milk and other calcium-rich foods should be an important part of your diet throughout your lifetime. Because your bones are alive, they need calcium daily. The best choices include 1 percent or skim milk, yogurt, and low-fat cheeses (part-skim mozzarella, string cheese, lite brands of cheddar). These sources of calcium are preferable to supplements because they include many other nutrients involved in bone health, such as vitamin D and phosphorous.

Many of my clients tell me, "I don't drink milk, but I do take a calcium supplement." I remind them that calcium supplements are poor substitutes for calcium-rich dairy products. Low-fat milk and yogurt offer a full spectrum of important vitamins, minerals, and protein; a calcium supplement offers only calcium. Milk, for example, is rich in vitamin D, potassium, and phosphorous—nutrients that work in combination to help your body use calcium effectively. Milk is also one of the best sources of riboflavin, a vitamin that helps convert the food you eat into energy. Active people, who generate more energy than their sedentary counterparts, need more riboflavin. If you don't eat dairy products your riboflavin intake is also likely to be poor.

Boosting Your Calcium Intake

Here are some tips to help you boost your calcium intake to build and maintain strong bones:

- For breakfast, eat cereal with one cup of low-fat or skim milk (or soy milk).
- With crunchy cereal, like granola, use yogurt in place of milk.
- With hot cereal, cook the cereal in milk or mix in one-third cup of powdered milk.
- When grabbing a quick meal, choose pizza with low-fat mozzarella cheese or sandwiches with low-fat cheese.
- Make calcium-rich salads by adding low-fat grated cheese, cottage cheese, or tofu cubes.
- Blenderize soft tofu or plain yogurt with salad seasonings for a calcium-rich dressing. Read the labels on the tofu containers, being sure to choose the brands processed with calcium sulfate; otherwise, the tofu will be calcium poor.
- Drink low-fat, skim, or soy milk with lunch, snacks, or dinner.
- Add extra milk (instead of cream) to coffee and enjoy lattes.
- Take powdered milk to the office to replace coffee whiteners.
- Drink milk-based hot cocoa in place of coffee.
- Snack on fruit-flavored yogurt rather than ice cream.
- Enjoy frozen yogurt or pudding made with low-fat milk for a tasty low-fat calcium treat.
- Eat canned salmon or sardines with bones for an easy lunch option; serve with crackers.
- Add tofu to oriental soups or stir-fry meals.
- Chow down on dark green, leafy vegetables

Granted, taking a calcium supplement is better than consuming no calcium. But I highly recommend a nutrition consultation with a registered dietitian to ensure appropriate calcium intake. This nutrition professional can help you optimize your diet so that you get the right balance of all the nutrients you need for good health and optimal sports performance.

Children and teens need calcium for growth. Unfortunately, their favorite beverage, soda pop, commonly displaces milk from the diet and contributes to weakened bones. Adults also need calcium to maintain strong bones. Although you may stop growing by age 20, you don't reach peak bone density until age 30 to 35. The amount of calcium stored in your bones at that age is a critical factor in your susceptibility to fractures as you grow older. After age 35, bones start to thin as a normal part of aging. A calcium-rich diet, in combination with exercise, can slow this process. In the next chapter I will further discuss the serious health problem of osteoporosis.

Dairy products are not the only natural sources of calcium, but they tend to be the most concentrated and convenient sources for those who eat and run. If you exclude or limit your consumption of dairy products, you'll have difficulty consuming the recommended intake of calcium from natural foods. For example, to absorb the same amount of calcium that you would obtain from one glass of milk, you'd need to eat either 3 cups of broccoli, 8 cups of spinach, 2 1/2 cups of white beans, 6 cups of pinto beans, 6 cups of sesame seeds, or 30 cups of unfortified soy milk. The easier bet is to choose calcium-fortified foods, such as calcium-enriched soy milk, orange juice, or breakfast cereals such as Total. Table 1.4 lists a few of the more common calcium sources.

TABLE 1.4

Calcium Equivalents

The following foods all provide about 300 milligrams of calcium. Two to three choices per day, or one at each meal, will contribute to meeting your calcium needs.

Calcium-rich food	Amount
Dairy	
Milk	1 cup
Milk powder	1/3 cup dry
Yogurt	1 cup
Cheese	1.5 oz
Cottage cheese	2 cups
Frozen yogurt	1.5 cups
Pizza, cheese	2 slices
Proteins	
Soy milk, enriched	1 cup
Tofu	5 oz (1/2 cake)
Salmon, canned with bones	4 oz
Sardines, canned with bones	3 oz
Almonds	3/4 cup
Vegetables	
Broccoli, cooked	3 cups
Collard or turnip greens, cooked	1 cup
Kale or mustard greens, cooked	1 1/2 cups
Bok choy	2 cups
Calcium-fortified foods	
Total cereal	1 cup
Orange juice, calcium enriched	1 cup

How Much Is Enough?

For only 300 calories, even weight-conscious athletes can easily get the minimum three servings of low-fat dairy foods that are recommended per day.

Dairy food	Standard serving	Athlete's portion	Number of pyramid servings
Milk	8 oz	12 oz	1.5
Yogurt	8 oz	1-2 per day	1-2
Cheese on pizza	1.5 oz	3 oz (4 slices pizza)	2

Here are the calcium intakes recommended by the National Academy of Sciences. Be sure to get at least half, if not all, of your calcium requirements from food.

Age group	Optimal daily calcium (mg)	Servings of calcium-rich food
Children		
1-3 years	500	2
4-8 years	800	3
Teens		
9-18 years	1,300	4
Women		
19-50 years	1,000	3
>50 years (menopausal)	1,200-1,500	4-5
Amenorrheic athletes	1,200-1,500	4-5
Pregnant or breast feeding	1,000-1,500	4-5
Men		
19-50 years	1,000	3
>50 years	1,200	4

Top Choices

To consume the amount of calcium you need to build and maintain strong bones (1,000 to 1,500 milligrams per day), you should plan to include a calcium-rich food in each meal.

Milk and yogurt, low-fat or nonfat. These are among the richest and healthiest sources of calcium because they have most of the fat removed but retain all the calcium and protein. A glass of whole milk (3.5 percent fat) has the same amount of fat as two pats of butter, but skim milk (0 percent fat) has almost no fat. Calcium-fortified soy milk is also a fine alternative.

Plain yogurt is one of the richest food sources of calcium. Ice cream and frozen yogurt are only fair sources of calcium. I consider these foods treats that fit into the tip of the food pyramid, not basic sources of calcium. See table 1.4 for additional comparisons of calcium-rich foods.

Low-fat cheese. Because many brands of fat-free cheese tend to be unpalatable, I suggest that you defer to moderate portions of the low-fat options. They are usually tasty and add both calcium and protein to pasta, chili, and other vegetarian meals.

Dark green veggies. Broccoli, bok choy (a vegetable common in Chinese cookery), and kale are among the best vegetable sources of calcium. Spinach also contains calcium, but your body can absorb very little of it.

Milk Myths

Myths abound regarding milk for athletes. The following stories highlight common concerns and questions about milk in a sports diet.

- A high school swimmer who drank milk by the quart ("I can polish off a half gallon at dinner!") was concerned that this much milk would lead to calcium deposits. For most healthy people this is unlikely. When you consume more calcium than your body needs, your body excretes the excess.

- One football player thought that milk causes cotton mouth. It doesn't. The dryness he experienced before competition was caused by nervousness and anxiety, not milk.

- A runner had heard that milk is hard to digest and causes stomach cramping. It doesn't unless you are lactose intolerant. Low-fat milk and dairy products are comfort foods that tend to digest easily, but some people have trouble digesting milk because they lack an enzyme (lactase) that digests milk sugar (lactose). They need to find alternative calcium sources. Some lactose-intolerant people who cannot digest milk can tolerate yogurt, hard cheeses, or even small amounts of milk taken with a meal. Others enjoy Lactaid milk, a lactose-free brand available at supermarkets.

- A skier hobbled into my office on crutches, wondering if his broken bone would benefit from guzzling gallons of milk. Drinking extra milk does not hasten the healing process! Six to eight weeks and a balanced diet are the two main keys to mending broken bones.

FYI: Frozen Yogurt Information

Many of my clients eat too much frozen yogurt. If you are a fro-yo addict, this information will help you put this dietary delight into perspective.

- Frozen yogurt may be fat free, but it is not calorie free. A large serving (8 to 12 ounces, or 240 to 360 grams) can easily contribute 200 to 400 calories to your diet. With the cone and a few mix-ins, you have the calorie equivalent of a small meal but with far less nutritional value.
- Unlike regular yogurt that is a nutrient-dense food, frozen yogurt is a sugar-based food that has less calcium and protein than you might suspect. Frozen yogurt fits into the tip of the food pyramid. I consider it a sugar-based food that contains a little milk, not a milk-based food. Yes, the sugar in frozen yogurt fuels your muscles, but it can derail your good nutrition game plan.
- Gourmet frozen yogurt tends to have the same fat content as light ice cream. Be sure to read food labels to avoid being fooled!

Planning for Good Nutrition: Fats, Oils, and Sweets

Sitting on a foundation of wholesome foods, the tip of the pyramid includes some refined sugars and saturated fats. This image suggests that a diet need not be perfect (that is, with no fat or sugar) to be healthful. Fats and sugars, despite being nutrient poor, add flavor and enjoyment.

How Much Is Enough?

Some people eat too many fats, oils, and sweets from the tip of the food pyramid instead of eating a wholesome diet of grains, fruits, and vegetables from the base. If you have a junk-food diet that topples the tip, you should correct the imbalance. You can easily do so by eating more wholesome foods from the base and body of the pyramid before you get too hungry. If you are like most active people, after you get too hungry, you'll tend to choose foods low in nutrients and high in fats and sugar. You'll seek apple pie, not apples, and carrot cake, not carrots. The simple solution to the junk-food diet is to prevent hunger by first eating wholesome meals.

Certain fats, as listed in the following section, are a positive addition to a diet. These good fats need not be limited to the tip of the pyramid; you can enjoy them in reasonable amounts because they are health enhancing. Chapter 2 has more information about good fats.

Portion Distortion

Once upon a time, food was served in portions conducive to good health. Today, we are accustomed to "supersize" meals; "small" is no longer on the menu. Even cars are coming with larger cup holders—a sign that society has accepted these large portions as normal. Because we are eating more meals away from home, large food portions are becoming a major contributor to weight gain.

When eating at fast-food restaurants, in particular, we are bombarded with the value-meal promotions that emphasize how much we can get for a reasonable price. The true price is overeating, weight gain, and a nation plagued with obesity.

	Calories	Calories from fat
Burger King Whopper with cheese	795	415
Large fries	500	220
Large soda	330	0
Total:	1,625	635 (70 g)
Big Mac	590	310
Supersize fries	610	260
Vanilla triple shake	570	150
Total:	1,770	720 (80 g)
Lower fat, lower calorie choice:		
McDonald's quarter-pound hamburger	430	190
Low-fat milk	100	20
Total:	530	210 (23 g)

Nutrition information from www.mcdonalds.com and www.burgerking.com, May 2003.

Top Choices

Given that 20 to 35 percent of the calories in your diet can appropriately come from fat and about 10 percent can appropriately come from sugar, the following foods are some of the best ways to spend these calories.

Olive oil. This monounsaturated fat is associated with low risk of heart disease and cancer. Use it for salads, sautéing, and cooking.

Walnuts. Thought to be protective against heart disease, walnuts are a fine addition to salads, cooked vegetables, and even pasta meals.

Molasses. Confirming the rule that the darker the food is, the more nutrients it has, molasses is among the darkest of sugars, and it has the most nutrients. Molasses is a fair source of potassium, calcium, and iron—if you eat enough of it. For a change of taste, add a tablespoon to milk for taffy milk, mix some in yogurt, or spread it on a peanut butter sandwich.

Berry jams. Because of the seeds in raspberry, strawberry, and blackberry jams, these sweet spreads have a little fiber that somewhat boosts their healthfulness. Preferable to strained jellies, the jams offer slightly more fruit value, but you still have to count them as primarily sugar.

In the next chapter I will provide more details about the best fats, and in chapter 5 I'll discuss more about how to fit sweets appropriately into snacks and snack attacks.

Building a Strong Pyramid

Now that you have read this chapter, you know which foods are the best choices. The trick is to assemble the best foods into wholesome meals and snacks. I recommend that you try to choose from at least three out of five food groups at each meal. Here's how this might work.

Sample menu	1	2	3
1. Grain	Oatmeal	Whole-wheat wrap	Pizza crust
2. Fruit	Raisins	Apple	
3. Vegetable		Lettuce, tomato	Tomato sauce
4. Dairy	Low-fat milk	Low-fat yogurt	Cheese
5. Protein	Almonds	Turkey	

Foods made from a combination of ingredients can create a well-balanced meal in one dish. For example, vegetable pizza topped with peppers, onions, and mushrooms is far from a junk food. It offers calcium-rich dairy food (from the low-fat mozzarella); vegetables rich in potassium, beta-carotene, and vitamin C (from the tomato sauce and vegetable toppings); and carbohydrate-rich grain foods in the (preferably whole-wheat) crust. A dinner of thick-crust pizza with a foundation of carbohydrates better fits the pyramid plan than does a fried chicken dinner that is mostly protein and fat.

Shaping your diet into a strong food pyramid need not be a major task. You simply need to know how to choose more of the best foods and less of the rest. You also need to fuel your body on a regular schedule, eating every two to four hours rather than having one or two big meals per day. Having even-sized meals interspersed with snacks is conducive to preventing hunger, optimizing healthful food choices, lowering cholesterol, and preventing weight gain. The following chapters offer additional tips to help you enjoy a tasty, pleasurable, nourishing, yet simple sports diet. Read on!

What Are Vitamins and Minerals?

Vitamins are metabolic catalysts that regulate biochemical reactions within your body. Minerals are natural substances that have unique metabolic roles. For example, calcium maintains the rigid structure of bones, sodium helps control water balance, and iron transports oxygen to the muscles. Your body cannot manufacture vitamins or minerals, which is why you must obtain them through your diet. To date, 14 vitamins and 15 minerals have been discovered, each with a specific function. For example, thiamin helps convert glucose into energy, vitamin D controls the way your body uses calcium, and vitamin A is part of an eye pigment that helps you see in dim light. The trick is to get enough of a vitamin or mineral to invest in optimal health without getting too much and experiencing harmful reactions.

You need adequate vitamins and minerals to function optimally, but no scientific evidence to date proves that extra vitamins and minerals offer a competitive edge. Despite claims to the contrary, supplements will not enhance performance, increase strength or endurance, provide energy, or build muscles.

Many active people wonder if exercise increases their vitamin and mineral needs. For the most part, no. Exercising doesn't burn vitamins, just as cars don't burn spark plugs. Vitamins and minerals are catalysts that are needed for metabolic processes to occur. No evidence to date shows that vitamin supplementation improves performance in people who are adequately nourished. Also keep in mind that the more you exercise, the more you eat and the more vitamins and minerals you consume. Most athletes consume more calories, and therefore more vitamins and minerals, than inactive people with smaller appetites do. Deficiencies are more likely to occur in a sedentary person who eats very little, such as an elderly grandparent, than in an active person who eats hefty portions.

Deficiencies of vitamins and minerals do not develop overnight but over the course of months or years, such as can happen in a person with anorexia or one who eats an inadequate vegetarian diet. In fact, your body stores some vitamins in stockpiles (A, D, E, K—the fat-soluble vitamins) and others in smaller amounts (B, C—the water-soluble vitamins). Most healthy people have enough vitamin C stored in the liver to last six weeks. Hence, one day of suboptimal eating will not result in a nutritionally depleted body.

By using the Food Guide Pyramid, you can consume the vitamins and minerals you need through wholesome foods. Because many foods today (including energy bars and breakfast cereals) are highly fortified, many people consume far more vitamins and minerals than they realize and have no need to take supplemental pills. For the most part, the health-conscious people who take vitamins tend to eat well and do not need a supplement. But there is no harm in taking a simple multivitamin pill for health insurance.

Taking a simple multivitamin and mineral pill is appropriate in certain situations. The following circumstances may put individuals at risk of developing nutritional deficiencies:

- **Restricting calories.** Dieters who eat less than 1,200 to 1,500 calories daily may miss some important nutrients.
- **Allergic to certain foods.** People who can't eat certain types of foods, such as fruits or wheat, need to compensate with alternative vitamin sources to avoid deficiencies in some nutrients.
- **Lactose intolerant.** The inability to digest the milk sugar found in dairy products is a common occurrence among African American and Hispanic people. Avoiding dairy foods can result in a diet deficient in riboflavin and the mineral calcium.
- **Pregnant.** Expectant mothers require additional vitamins and iron, but they should consult with their physicians before taking a supplement.
- **Contemplating pregnancy.** Women who are thinking about becoming pregnant should be sure to have a diet rich in folic acid. They should also take a multivitamin with 400 micrograms of folacin. This B vitamin helps to prevent brain damage in the fetus at the time of conception and can help reduce the risk of some types of birth defects.
- **Total vegetarians.** People who abstain from eating any animal foods may become deficient in vitamins B-12, D, and riboflavin. Those who eat a poorly balanced vegetarian diet can also become deficient in protein, iron, and zinc.

If you are currently taking supplements and are not knowledgeable about vitamins or minerals, I recommend that you get a nutrition checkup with a registered dietitian (RD). The RD will be able to evaluate your diet and tell you not only what nutrients you are getting but also the best food sources for those you are missing. To find an RD, use the American Dietetic Association's referral network at www.eatright.org (or call 800-366-1655). You can also call the nutrition department at your local hospital or sports medicine clinic, or look in the yellow pages under dietitian or nutritionist and select a name followed by "RD."

To help you determine whether you are getting the right balance of these nutrients, the government has established the Reference Daily Intakes (RDIs) as a standard for nutrient intake. Their recommendations for vitamins and minerals exceed the average nutritional requirements to meet the needs of nearly all people, including athletes. The following table lists the 1997-2001 subgrouping of the RDIs, the Recommended Dietary Allowances (RDAs) or Adequate Intakes (AIs, used when an RDA cannot be determined for a particular nutrient), as well as the Tolerable Upper Intake Level (UL), the highest level of a daily nutrient intake that is likely to pose no health risks. Above this Upper Intake Level, there is potential for increased risk.

You can get the recommended intake of most nutrients (except possibly for iron) by eating a variety of foods from the food pyramid. This amount will not only prevent nutritional deficiencies but also reduce the risk of chronic diseases such as osteoporosis, cancer, and heart disease. If you choose to supplement your diet, be wary of taking more than the UL. When an Upper Level cannot be determined (ND), the safest bet is to consume levels close to the RDA.

(continued)

Nutrient	Daily Value (on food labels)	Recommended Dietary Allowance or Adequate Intake		Tolerable Upper Limit
		Women	**Men**	**Women & men**
Vitamin A (IU/day)	5,000 IU	2,333	3,000	10,000 IU
Vitamin C (mg/day)	60	75	90	2,000
Vitamin D (IU/day)	400 IU	200 (<age 50)	200	2,000 IU
		400 (50-70)	400	
		600 (>age 70)	600	
Vitamin E (mg/day)*	15	15	30	1,000
Vitamin K (mcg/day)	80	90	120	ND
Thiamin (mg/day)	1.5	1.1	1.2	ND
Riboflavin (mg/day)	1.7	1.1	1.3	ND
Niacin (mg/day)	20	14	16	35
B-6 (mg/day)	2	1.3	1.3	100
		1.5 (>age 50)	1.7	
Folate (mcg/day)	400	400	400	1,000
		600 (if pregnant)		
B-12 (mcg/day)	6	2.4	2.4	ND
Calcium (mg/day)	1,000	1,000	1,000	2,500
		1,200 (>age 50)	1,200	
Iron (mg/day)	18	18	8	45**
		8 (postmenopause)		
Zinc (mg/day)	15	8	11	40

ND = Not Determined

*To convert International Units (IU) into milligrams (mg), multiply IU by 0.45. That is, 400 IU of vitamin E equates to 180 mg of vitamin E.

**The Upper Limit does not apply to people who are taking an iron supplement as a short-term medical treatment for iron-deficiency anemia.

Source: Food and Nutrition Board, Institute of Medicine. *Dietary Reference Intakes.* Landover, MD: National Academy Press. 1998, 2000.

2

Healthy Choices Make Healthy Bodies

Just as the right foods can be powerfully health protective, the wrong foods can be powerfully bad for your health. That is, eating excessive portions of foods filled with saturated fats and refined sugars can contribute to obesity, heart disease, cancer, hypertension, diabetes, kidney failure, and other diseases associated with excessive eating. Eating a diet (as outlined in chapter 1) based on wholesome grains, fruits, vegetables, dried beans, lean proteins, low-fat dairy, nuts, and olive oil—in addition to an active lifestyle—invests in optimal health. Conveniently, the same wholesome foods you eat to enhance your health also enhance your athletic performance. The trick is to choose more of the best foods and less of the rest, so that you'll be able to enjoy lifelong health and high energy.

Confusion abounds about foods that are good or bad for your health. My clients repeatedly ask me, "What foods should I avoid?" My answer is that the only bad foods are foods that are moldy or poisonous (or foods to which you are allergic); all other foods can be balanced into a healthful food plan based on moderation and variety. The purpose of this chapter is to help you make wise food choices and tip the balance in your favor for lifelong good health.

Diet and Heart Health

Heart disease is the number-one killer in America. Two ways to reduce your risk of heart disease are being physically fit and eating wisely. Yet, active people often believe they are exempt from the food rules about heart-healthy eating. They assume that being physically fit protects them from heart disease. Wrong! A friend of mine, a seemingly healthy 48-year-old marathoner, died suddenly of a massive heart attack. He'd run for 2 hours 10 minutes, stopped his watch, and was later found dead in the running path. Everyone was shocked.

Unfortunately, even the most health-conscious people can find themselves confused by the constant updates and changes of heart-health information. This leaves us wondering what the real answers are to questions like the following: Is beef bad? What about eggs? Should I use butter or margarine? The answers vary from person to person, because we each have a unique genetic makeup. It won't be long before dietary recommendations will be based on genetic tests. But for today, here are my suggestions for optimizing your diet, based on the latest nutrition studies.

Know Your Number

Cholesterol is a waxy substance that accumulates in the walls of the blood vessels throughout the body, especially those in the heart, and contributes to hardening of the arteries. This buildup limits blood flow to the heart muscle and contributes to heart attacks. You consume cholesterol when you eat animal foods; cholesterol is a part of animal cells. Your body also makes cholesterol. Foods with saturated fats (butter, lard) and trans-fats (in many commercially baked goods) can increase the level of cholesterol in the blood, thereby increasing the risk of cardiovascular (cardio = heart; vascular = blood vessel) disease.

Because genetics play a large role in heart and blood vessel health, you may have a blood cholesterol that puts you at a high risk for developing cardiovascular disease even if you eat a healthy diet. One 28-year-old triathlete was shocked to discover his cholesterol was very high. He probably inherited this trait from his father and grandfather, both of whom had heart attacks in their 50s.

By knowing your cholesterol level, you can assess your risk of developing heart disease. Make an appointment with your doctor to get your blood tested for these health indicators:

- **Total cholesterol.** Your body contains different types of cholesterol, including HDL and LDL. The sum of the types of cholesterol is called your total cholesterol. The desired target level is less than 200 milligrams total cholesterol per deciliter of blood (milligrams per deciliter).

- **HDL cholesterol.** High-density lipoprotein cholesterol is the "good stuff" that carries the bad cholesterol out of the arteries. The desired target level is more than 50 milligrams HDL per deciliter.
- **LDL cholesterol.** Low-density lipoprotein cholesterol is the "bad stuff" that clogs arteries. A level greater than 160 milligrams per deciliter is associated with a higher risk of heart disease.
- **Ratio of total cholesterol to HDL.** At least 25 percent of your total blood cholesterol should be HDL. Because exercise tends to boost HDL, active people often have a higher percentage of this good cholesterol. Their total cholesterol may be higher than that of a sedentary person, but as long as 25 percent of it is HDL, these individuals have a lower risk of heart problems. The higher the HDL percentage, the better.

After you know your blood cholesterol level, you'll be better able to determine how strict you need to be with your diet. For example, if your level is far less than 200 milligrams and if your 97-year-old parents are still alive and thriving, you can be less obsessive about your eating habits than is your buddy whose cholesterol is a risky 250 milligrams and whose father suddenly died of a heart attack at age 54. Another possible blood test for people with a family history of heart disease but no obvious risk factors is a test that checks levels of homocysteine, an amino acid in the blood. High homocysteine levels are associated with a higher risk of heart disease. A third test is CRP, or C-reactive protein, a measure of inflammation. Arteries weakened by inflammation are also associated with a higher risk of heart disease. Know where you stand when it comes to heart disease.

Beef for Heart Health

Ten years ago, everyone shunned beef, believing it to be an artery clogger. Today, health experts tell us that small portions of lean beef aren't so bad after all, especially for athletes who need iron, zinc, and other important nutrients in beef. Despite popular belief, beef is not exceptionally high in cholesterol; it has a cholesterol value similar to that of chicken and fish. Cholesterol, which is a part of animal cells, was once thought to contribute to heart disease, but we now know that cholesterol is less of a culprit than saturated fat. Refer to table 2.1 for a comparison of fat and cholesterol in meat and dairy products.

Saturated fat is hard at room temperature (like the fat on uncooked steak, and different from chicken fat, which is softer and less saturated). Beef tends to have more saturated fat than chicken or fish, so that's why it has a bad reputation among health watchers. In the past decade, the healthfulness of beef and other meats has improved because farmers have learned how to raise animals that are leaner, and because butchers are trimming more of the fat from the meat at stores. Hence, you can easily fit beef (and pork and lamb) into a heart-healthy sports diet if you select lean cuts, such as eye of round, rump roast, sirloin tip, flank steak, top round, and tenderloin and eat smaller

TABLE 2.1

Fat and Cholesterol in Common Foods

Food product	Amount	Fat (g)	Cholesterol (mg)
Milk			
Skim	1 cup	0	5
2% low-fat	1 cup	5	20
Whole	1 cup	8	35
Cheese			
Cheddar	1 oz	10	30
Mozzarella, part skim	1 oz	5	15
Cottage cheese, 1% fat	1/2 cup	1	5
Ice cream			
Expensive brands			
16% fat	1/2 cup	12-18	40-50
Less expensive brands			
10% fat	1/2 cup	5-10	30-35
Low-fat	1/2 cup	3-5	10-20
Meats and fish (cooked)			
Pork, roast loin	4 oz	8	85
Beef, 90% lean hamburger	4 oz	18	95
Ham, canned lean	4 oz	6	50
Chicken, roast breast	4 oz	2	95
Tuna, canned white	4 oz	3	45
McDonald's Big Mac		34	85
McDonald's Filet-o-Fish		26	50

Nutrient data from food labels, McDonald's Corporation (www.mcdonalds.com) and J. Pennington, 1998, *Bowes & Church's Food Values of Portions Commonly Used*, 17th ed. (Philadelphia: Lippincott).

portions, limiting yourself to a piece of lean protein about the size of the palm of your hand.

Fish for Heart Health

If good health is your wish, get hooked on fish! Research indicates that fish may guard against not only heart disease but also hypertension, cancer, arthritis, and who knows what else! The omega-3 fatty acids, the special polyunsaturated fat found in fish oil, block many harmful biochemical reactions that can cause blood to clot (predisposing you to heart attack and stroke) and the heart to beat irregularly (as occurs during a heart attack). Some researchers believe that fish oils can prevent heart disease rather than merely have a beneficial effect after the onset of the disease. A comparison of the rates of death from heart disease in men in a fishing village versus men in a farming village suggests a four times lower incidence of heart disease among the men in the fishing village. They ate 10 times more fish than the farmers and had much higher blood levels of the health-protective omega-3 fats (Torres et al. 2000). A study of almost 85,000 U.S. nurses suggests women who ate fish two to four times a week had a 31 percent lower risk of heart disease compared with those who rarely ate fish (Hu et al. 2002).

The American Heart Association recommends eating at least two meals per week of oily fish to help reduce your risk of heart disease. Eating more fish for dinner not only contributes fish oil to your diet but also can displace meat meals high in saturated fat. Table 2.2 can help guide your fish choices so that you select the fish highest in omega-3 fats. Just be sure that your fish is prepared in low-fat ways—not fried or broiled in butter. If you shy away from cooking fish, simply take advantage of canned tuna (mixed with low-fat mayonnaise), salmon, and sardines.

Unfortunately, the fish highest in omega-3 fatty acids also deliver a dose of methyl mercury from industrial pollution of the oceans. Long-term consumption of mercury can potentially contribute to neurological and cardiovascular problems in adults and cause significant damage to the developing brains of infants and children. The FDA advises pregnant and breastfeeding women that they can safely eat up to 12 ounces (340 grams) of fish a week (this includes a large safety margin) but should avoid shark, swordfish, king mackerel, and tile fish and limit their tuna intake to one six-ounce can per week. These fish are long-lived and large; they accumulate mercury in their tissues

TABLE 2.2

Fish Highest in Omega-3 Fatty Acids

The simplest advice is to eat fish two to three times a week. The ideal target is an average of 1.0 gram of omega-3s a day. EPA and DHA are two types of omega-3 fats.

Fish, 6 oz cooked (8 oz raw)	Omega-3 fats (g EPA and DHA)
Salmon, Atlantic, farmed	2.0-3.6
Sardines, in sardine oil (3 oz)	2.0-3.4
Salmon, Atlantic, wild	1.8-3.1
Swordfish	0.7-3.1
Salmon, coho, farmed	3.0
Trout, rainbow, farmed	2.0
Trout, rainbow, wild	1.7
Salmon, coho, wild	1.4
Sardines, in vegetable oil (3 oz)	1.0
Halibut	0.8
Tuna, white, canned (3 oz)	0.7
Tuna, fresh	0.5
Pollock	0.4
Lobster (3 oz)	0.1-0.4
Shrimp (3 oz)	0.3

Data from the American Heart Association.

over time by eating many smaller mercury-containing fish. Very small children should be careful about eating too much fish, but the American Heart Association assures us that the benefits of eating fish for the general population far outweigh the risk of mercury poisoning.

If you are not a fish fan, and if you have heart disease, the American Heart Association suggests fish oil capsules as an alternative (Kris-Etherton, Harris, and Appel 2002). But be aware that these supplements contain only a small amount of omega-3s compared with what you would get with a fish dinner, so you might have to take several capsules to get the equivalent of one four-ounce (112-gram) serving of salmon. An alternative way to is to get a less potent type of omega-3 fat from plant sources, such as flaxseed oil, walnuts, tofu, soy nuts, canola, and olive oil.

Soy Foods for Heart Health

Soy-based foods such as tofu and soy milk contain substances called isoflavones that can block cholesterol from being made. If you have high cholesterol and substitute soy-based foods for animal foods, you can lower your LDL cholesterol, as well as triglycerides and total cholesterol, while increasing the good HDL cholesterol. The American Heart Association recommends eating 25 or more grams of soy protein per day (three to four servings) as a safe, effective way to reduce the bad LDL cholesterol. You can boost your soy intake by consuming soy milk (on cereal, in pancakes, puddings, shakes), adding tofu to spaghetti sauce, munching on soy nuts, or enjoying soy sausages, soy bacon, soy burgers, tofu dogs, and other products that make it easy to eat more soy. Because any soy is better than none, simply try to increase your intake from nothing to something—preferably a serving a day, if not more.

Eggs and Heart Health

Eggs have gotten a bad rap when it comes to healthy eating. Medical experts have told us that eating eggs is bad because a single egg has 210 milligrams of cholesterol, which just about hits the American Heart Association's recommended limit of 300 milligrams per day. But recent studies suggest that egg cholesterol may have little effect on the blood cholesterol level in many people, especially in combination with an overall low-fat diet (Ginsberg et al. 1995; Kritchevsky and Kritchevsky 2000).

To date, it is unclear whether the cholesterol that you eat affects the cholesterol in your blood, because most of the cholesterol in the blood is made in the liver. We do know that dietary fats affect the way the body disposes of cholesterol. In particular, saturated fats (such as butter and beef fat) appear to inhibit the ability of the body to get rid of the bad form of cholesterol (low-density lipoprotein, or LDL) that clogs arteries. We also know that some people respond more readily than others to a low-cholesterol diet, and that dietary recommendations need to be individualized.

So, when it comes to eggs, you should limit your intake if you have a high blood cholesterol level and a family history of heart disease. The American Heart Association recommends a limit of four egg yolks per week, including those used in cooking. Otherwise, if you have low blood cholesterol and no family history of heart disease, you may eat this highly nutritious protein source as a part of your balanced nutrition game plan. An estimated 85 percent of Americans can eat a high-cholesterol diet with no elevation of blood cholesterol.

When choosing eggs, you might want to buy brands that contain health-protective omega-3 fatty acids (100 milligrams per egg). These "designer eggs" are from chickens given a special vegetarian feed that includes canola oil and improves the fat content of the egg yolk. They also contain more vitamin E than other eggs and are a preferable choice to standard eggs for a heart-healthier diet.

Oatmeal and Soluble Fiber for Heart Health

The type of fiber found in oats (soluble fiber) and the soluble fiber in barley, lentils, split peas, and beans protect against heart disease. Find ways to include more of these foods in your diet. For example, trade in bagels for oatmeal or oat bran, and swap roast beef sandwiches for bean and barley soups. Research suggests that eating a bowlful of oatmeal (1 1/2 cups cooked) each day can help people attain lower cholesterol levels, especially when eaten as part of a low-fat diet, and especially when the person has elevated cholesterol levels to start (Expert Panel 2001).

Oat bran, available in the hot-cereal section of supermarkets and health-food stores, is similar to Cream of Wheat but has a nutty flavor. Enjoy it as a hot cereal (add chopped almonds and raisins for a nice texture contrast) or bake it into muffins. If you don't have time for cooking oatmeal at breakfast, one or two packets of instant oatmeal can be an enjoyable snack alternative.

Foods high in soluble fiber are not only a heart-healthy choice but also an excellent preexercise food. They tend to have what is called a low glycemic index. That is, they provide a sustained release of energy into the bloodstream, and they can enhance your endurance and stamina if you will be exercising longer than 60 to 90 minutes. (See chapter 7 for more information about the glycemic index.)

Morning exercisers can easily include oatmeal or—better yet, oat bran—in their daily sports diet by planning it for their preexercise snack. Simply microwave it according to the directions on the package (but prepare it with low-fat milk instead of water) while you start to read the morning newspaper, cool it off with milk to make it soupy, drink it down, read the rest of the paper, and then head out the door feeling comfortably fed and well fueled.

I'll talk more about soluble fiber in the upcoming section on fiber.

Cooking Oils for Heart Health

When it comes to selecting heart-healthy cooking fats, the rule is the softer the better. That is, soft (liquid) vegetable oils have a higher percentage of unsaturated fats compared with harder (solid) fats such as margarines and butter. Olive oil and canola oil are the two preferred fats to include in a heart-healthy diet. These oils are rich in monounsaturated fats and are considered better choices than safflower, corn, sunflower, and other polyunsaturated vegetable oils. Use olive and canola oils with salads, pesto, and pasta and when sautéing. Just be sure to use only moderate amounts if you want to lose body fat. Their calories, although preferable to the calories from butter or lard, still count and add up quickly.

Cooking with olive and canola oil is far more healthful than using butter, bacon grease, lard, salt pork, and animal fats that are solid at room temperature. If you use a significant amount of margarine and resist the advice to eat less of it, you might want to use the new margarines with stanol esters (Benecol, Take Control). A tablespoon at each meal can contribute to lower LDL (bad) cholesterol.

Hard fats not only come in the form of butter and lard but also hide as trans-fats in many commercial baked goods such as crackers, cakes, cookies, chips, popcorn, and chocolate candy. Trans-fats are made by adding hydrogen to mono- and polyunsaturated fats. This process converts them into a "partially hydrogenated" saturated fat. The bad news is that food labels do not list these trans-fats as saturated fat, so processed foods are able to claim "low saturated fat" even though they are high in trans-fats. Your best bet is to limit your intake of fast foods and commercially baked foods. Trans-fats are another reason that apples and carrots are far better for you than store-bought apple pie and carrot cake.

Nuts and Peanut Butter for Heart Health

Although many people try to stay away from nuts and peanut butter because they fear them as being fattening, surveys with more than 260,000 people indicate that eating one serving of nuts or peanut butter five times a week can reduce the risk of heart disease by 50 percent (Kris-Etherton et al. 2001), to say nothing of lowering the risk of type 2 diabetes by about 25 percent. Nuts are rich in monounsaturated fats (as well as folate, niacin, thiamin, magnesium, fiber, and other health-protective nutrients). Adding walnuts to oatmeal, peanut butter to a bagel, sliced almonds to a salad, and mixed nuts to dried fruit for trail mix are just a few simple ways to include these health-protective foods in your daily diet—to say nothing of enjoying a good old peanut butter sandwich for lunch.

The trick with nuts and peanut butter is to keep the portion within your calorie budget. The good news is that nuts are satisfying and a few will curb your hunger for a while. Dieters can successfully lose weight and keep it off when they include nuts, peanut butter, and other healthful fats as a part of their daily diet (McManus et al. 2001).

For more information about diet and heart disease, check the American Heart Association's Web site: www.americanheart.org.

Fitting Fat Into Your Diet

Both a sports diet and a heart-healthy diet limit fat to 20 to 35 percent of calorie intake. The American Heart Association advises you to eat more of the good plant and fish oils and less of the saturated animal fats. It also recommends cutting back on partially hydrogenated vegetable oils (trans-fats), and coconut and palm oils, three highly saturated vegetable oils commonly used in processed foods.

I advise athletes to aim for a 25 percent fat diet that allows space for plenty of carbohydrates to fuel their muscles. Hence, if you are an active woman who eats about 2,000 calories per day, 500 of them could appropriately come from fat:

25 percent fat × 2,000 total calories = 500 calories from fat

By rationing your intake of foods obviously high in fat (butter, margarine, mayonnaise, salad dressing, ice cream, cookies, chips), you'll end up with a diet that's about 25 percent fat.

If you have a very high cholesterol level, your physician may recommend a diet that is 20 percent fat. This restriction is for people clinically endangered by heart disease, not for healthy people who have low cholesterol levels. I talk often to food fanatics with low cholesterol who try to eliminate all fats from their diet. They burden themselves with needless restrictions; a low-fat diet need not be a no-fat diet. Some fat is appropriate for a well-balanced diet as well as for weight management.

Your weight in kilograms (1 kilogram is 2.2 pounds) is a rough estimation of the number of grams of fat you can healthfully include in your diet. For a more precise calculation, follow these three steps:

1. Estimate how many calories you need per day (see chapter 11 for instructions).

(continued)

(continued)

2. Multiply your total daily calories by 25 percent (.25) to determine the number of fat calories you can appropriately eat. For example, .25 × 2,000 calories = 500 calories from fat.

3. Divide your allotted fat calories by 9 to determine the number of grams of fat in your daily fat budget (one gram of fat is 9 calories.) For example, if you are entitled to 500 fat calories, 500 fat calories ÷ 9 calories per gram = 56 grams of fat.

The following table can help you determine your target fat intake. If you are underweight or very active, you may want more calories from fat to help boost your total calorie intake. Plan to eat more of the heart-healthy fats, such as peanut butter, nuts, and olive or canola oils.

Low Fat: What's That?

For a heart-healthy sports diet, you should limit your fat intake to about 20 to 35 percent of your total calories (20 percent if you have high cholesterol; 35 percent if you need more calories to prevent weight loss). In general, athletes can fuel their muscles better if they trade some calories from (saturated) fat for more calories from carbohydrates. Don't trade away too much fat, however, and be left with an unbalanced diet that can hurt your performance.

	Grams of fat in diet		
Calorie needs per day	20% fat	25% fat	30% fat
1,500	30	40	50
1,800	40	50	60
2,000	45	55	65
2,400	55	65	80
2,600	60	70	85

Supplements for Heart Health

Questions arise about the role of vitamin supplements to enhance heart health. Living healthfully would be much easier if we could just take a pill that would compensate for both suboptimal eating and suboptimal genetics! Here's what we know to date.

Antioxidant Vitamins

Antioxidant vitamins, such as C, E, and beta-carotene, have been touted as protectors against heart disease. But in a study with more than 20,000 people ages 40 to 80, those who took a daily mixture of 600 IU of vitamin E, 250 milligrams of vitamin C, and 20 milligrams (33,300 IU) of beta-carotene had no lower risk than those who took a placebo (Marchioli et al. 2001).

In a three-year study of overweight men with heart disease who took a daily mixture of 800 IU of vitamin E, 1,000 milligrams of vitamin C, 25 milligrams of beta-carotene, and 100 micrograms of selenium, the antioxidants did not significantly improve the health profile or protect against progression of heart disease. In fact, with men who were taking cholesterol-lowering medications (statins), the vitamin supplements interfered with the effectiveness of the medication (Brown, Zhao, Chiat, et al. 2001).

The bottom line is that you can't rely on antioxidant supplements to protect your heart health. Your best bet is to eat abundant fruits, vegetables, and whole grains; enjoy peanut butter, nuts, and fish; eat healthier fats such as olive and canola oil; and maintain a healthy weight

Are Supplements Health Insurance?

Although taking a simple multivitamin certainly will not hurt your health, the verdict is yet unclear about whether it will improve your health if you already have a good diet (and most people who take supplements eat well).

Taking a multivitamin and mineral supplement does not compensate for a high-fat, low-fiber, unbalanced diet. If you choose to take a vitamin supplement, look first at your daily foods to see if you are already consuming these vitamins through highly fortified foods, like energy bars and breakfast cereals. If not, the following guidelines can help you zero in on the best bets. Above all, think food first.

- Choose a supplement with the vitamins and minerals close to 100 percent of the Daily Values (DV). Don't expect to find 100 percent of the DV for calcium and magnesium listed on a label, because these minerals are too bulky to put in one pill.

- Don't buy supplements that contain excessive doses of vitamins and minerals, particularly minerals. High doses of one mineral can offset the benefits of another. For example, too much zinc can interfere with the absorption of copper.

- Buy a supplement before its expiration date and store it in a cool, dry place.

- Ignore claims about "natural" vitamins; they tend to be blends of natural and synthetic vitamins and offer no benefits. The exception is vitamin E, which is more potent in its natural form, but the difference is inconsequential.

- Chelated supplements offer no advantages, nor do those made without sugar or starch, nor those with the highest price tag.

- Look for "U.S.P." on the label. This indicates the manufacturer followed standards established by the U.S. Pharmacopoeia.

- Buying nationally known brands of supplements may improve the likelihood of getting what you believe you are buying. That is, sometimes a pill may only contain 100 milligrams of vitamin C, although the label states 250 milligrams. Going to www.consumerlab.com (a tester of many supplements) can help you identify quality brands.

- To optimize absorption, take a supplement with or after a meal.

and regular daily activity. I repeat, just as the wrong foods can be powerfully bad for your health, the right foods can be powerfully protective.

B Vitamins

In contrast to the antioxidant vitamins, the B-complex vitamins (folate, B-6, and B-12) seem to have a protective role against heart disease because they can lower the levels of homocysteine in the blood. High levels of homocysteine are associated with a higher risk of heart disease. Food folate (or folic acid, if found in supplements) lowers blood levels of homocysteine, more so when combined with B-6 and B-12, and this is associated with lower risk of heart disease (Fairfield and Fletcher 2002).

Folic acid is found primarily in foods that are scanty in many people's diets—dried beans, colorful vegetables, and certain fruits—as well as in enriched foods, such as breakfast cereals, breads, energy bars, and even many sports drinks. Because so many popular sports foods are enriched with B-6, B-12, and folic acid, you may be getting plenty. By reading the food labels on cereals, breads, energy bars, and pastas, you can see how you're doing with your consumption of these nutrients through food. See table 2.3 for a comparison of sources of folate or folic acid.

TABLE 2.3

Sources of Folate or Folic Acid

Folate is the natural form of this vitamin found in food. Folic acid is the synthetic form found in supplements or enriched foods. The recommended intake is 400 micrograms of folic acid per day.

Food	Amount	Folate or folic acid (micrograms)
Spinach	1 cup cooked	260
Lentils	1/2 cup cooked	180
Asparagus	6 spears	130
Avocado	1/2 medium	80
Broccoli	1 cup cooked	80
Romaine lettuce	1 cup shredded	80
Chickpeas	1/2 cup canned	80
Kidney beans	1/2 cup canned	65
Orange	1 medium	50
Peas, green	1/2 cup	50
Peanut butter	2 tablespoons	30
Egg	1 large	20
Enriched foods:		
PowerBar	1	400
Cheerios	1 cup	200
Oatmeal, instant	1 packet	80
Flour, enriched	1/2 cup	80
Bread, whole wheat	2 slices	60

Information from J. Pennington, 1998, *Bowes & Church's Food Values of Portions Commonly Used*, 17th ed. (Philadelphia: Lippincott) and food labels.

Diet and Cancer

In the United States, cancer follows heart disease as the most frequent cause of death. Cancer isn't one disease, it is many. Each has its own high-risk groups, its own attack and cure rates, and its own causes. Diet and obesity are factors in an estimated 35 percent of cancer cases, and a healthier diet and weight may cut your risk more than you may think.

Despite the gloomy news that two out of every five of us will get cancer, the encouraging news is that dietary changes can prevent perhaps one-third of cancer deaths. For example, people who eat at least five servings a day of fruits and vegetables have a 40 percent lower risk for certain cancers (lung, colon, stomach, esophagus, and mouth) compared with people who eat two or fewer servings of fruits and vegetables. A fruit-filled, high-fiber, cancer-protective diet is also a top-performance sports diet. Indulge in good health and high energy!

Protective Nutrients

One key to the role of diet in preventing cancer may lie in an anti-oxidative capacity—that is, the ability of a nutrient to deactivate harmful chemicals in the body known as free radicals. Free radicals form daily through normal body processes. Environmental pollutants such as cigarette smoke, automobile exhaust, radiation, and herbicides also generate free radical precursors. These unstable compounds can attack, infiltrate, and injure vital cell structures. Fortunately, our bodies have natural control systems that deactivate and minimize free-radical reactions within the cells. These natural control systems involve many vitamins and minerals, including the following:

- **Carotenoids.** These precursors of vitamin A are found in plants and then converted into vitamin A in the body. Beta-carotene, as well as the more than 40 other carotenoids found in orange and green fruits and vegetables, helps prevent the formation of free radicals. Some of the best sources include carrots, spinach, sweet potatoes, kale, apricots, and cantaloupe. (If you eat too many carotene-rich vegetables and fruits, your skin might turn yellow. If it does, cut back!)

- **Vitamin C.** This vitamin guards against harmful reactions within the cells. The best sources include kiwi, citrus fruits, broccoli, green and red peppers, and strawberries. Eating the recommended five daily servings of fruits and vegetables easily provides 200 milligrams a day of vitamin C, an amount that saturates body tissues.

- **Vitamin E.** Vitamin E protects the cell walls from free-radical damage. The best sources are plant oils (and foods made with them, such as salad dressings), almonds, peanuts, sunflower and sesame seeds, wheat germ, and whole grains (see table 2.4).

TABLE 2.4

Vitamin E in Foods

The best sources of vitamin E are in plant oils. You need to carefully consume E-rich foods because they are calorie-dense. Be sure to include some of these healthier high-fat foods when balancing your daily calorie budget. The Recommended Dietary Allowance for vitamin E is 15 milligrams.

Food	Portion	Vitamin E (mg)
Almonds	1/4 cup	14
Peanuts	1/4 cup	4
Sunflower seeds	1/4 cup	28
Oil, olive	1 tbsp	2
Oil, canola	1 tbsp	3
Oil, safflower	1 tbsp	6
Spinach, cooked	1 cup	2
Wheat germ	1/4 cup	5

Data from J. Pennington, 1998, *Bowes & Church's Food Values of Portions Commonly Used*, 17th ed. (Philadelphia: Lippincott).

- **Selenium.** Selenium protects the cell walls from free-radical damage and enhances the response of the immune system with increased resistance to cancer growth. The best sources of selenium include seafood such as tuna fish, meats, eggs, milk, whole grains, and garlic. Supplements are not recommended because of the danger of toxicity with long-term supplementation over 200 micrograms.

Other cancer protectors include foods rich in fiber. Although population studies suggest that people who eat a lot of fiber from grains, fruits, and vegetables have a lower risk of cancer, scientists are not sure if the fiber is the protective nutrient. In addition to the known vitamins and minerals in grains, fresh fruits, and vegetables, these fiber-rich foods contain hundreds, perhaps thousands, of lesser-known substances called phytochemicals that may protect our health (see table 2.5). That's why you want to put your energy into eating a varied diet rather than wondering which supplement to choose.

Although researchers at one time hoped that high intakes of antioxidants from pills would reduce the incidence of some types of cancer, the current evidence is disappointing. Apart from the possibility that vitamin E and selenium might reduce the risk of prostate cancer

TABLE 2.5

Nutrition and Cancer Prevention

Why should you push yourself to eat at least 5 servings a day of fruits and vegetables? The answer is plant foods contain active compounds called phytochemicals (*phyto* is the Greek word for *plant*) that provide protection not only against cancer but also against heart disease, hypertension, arthritis, and other degenerative diseases of aging. The following list contains some foods rich in phytochemicals.

Food	Phytochemical	Action
Soy milk, tofu	Genistein	Inhibits formation of blood vessels that assist growth of tumors
Spinach, collard greens	Lutein	Reduces blindness in the elderly
Carrots, squash, apricots, peaches	Beta-carotene	Protects the immune system
Fish oil	Omega-3 fatty acids	May decrease risk of heart disease
Rosemary	Quinones	Interfere with the action of cancer-causing substances
Chili peppers	Capsaicin	Prevents toxic molecules from damaging cells, discouraging the growth of cancerous cells
Beans, peas, peanuts	Isoflavones	Interfere with harmful estrogen action and may reduce the risk of breast and ovarian cancer
Cabbage, broccoli, cauliflower, kale	Isothiocyanates, indoles	Block carcinogens from damaging cells, interfere with the action of the harmful precancerous form of estrogen
Citrus fruits	Terpenes	Stimulate enzymes that block tumor growth
Strawberries, pineapple	Chlorogenic acid	Blocks the production of cancer-causing nitrosamines
Garlic, onions	Allylic sulfide	Intercepts and detoxifies carcinogens
Flaxseed	Lignans	Interfere with estrogen action and may reduce breast and ovarian cancer
All fruits and vegetables	Flavinoids	Prevent carcinogenic hormones from attaching to cells

and eye problems such as macular degeneration, several large studies have shown that supplemental antioxidants offer few health benefits. The studies that drove the hope that antioxidants would be cancer protective came from people who ate lots of fruits and vegetables (and had higher blood levels of antioxidants). Hence, most health professionals today emphasize the importance of obtaining these nutrients from food, not from supplements. Scientists have yet to pinpoint which of the thousands of substances in fruits and vegetables are protective. If you choose to take an antioxidant supplement, be sure to do so in addition to eating well—including lots of broccoli, carrots, sweet potatoes, and other colorful vegetables. No amount of supplementation will compensate for a fast-food diet low in fruits and vegetables and a stress-filled, health-eroding lifestyle.

Cancer and Fat

Eating a low-fat diet may be a second dietary key to reducing cancer risk. Population studies suggest that people who eat low-fat diets have a lower incidence of cancer. The National Research Council

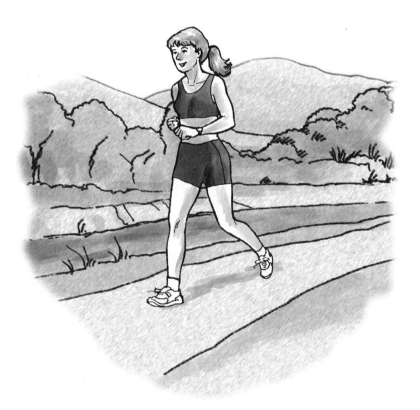

recommends that we eat less than 30 percent of our total calories as fat, eat more fruits and vegetables rich in beta-carotene and vitamin C (review the nutrients in fruits and vegetables in table 1.1 on page 10 and table 1.2 on page 12), and eat more whole grains. Voila—a high-carbohydrate sports diet that is conducive to fighting cancer and maintaining a healthy weight! Fatty fish can also be included among cancer-protective foods. The omega-3 fatty acids may slow tumor growth.

Besides your diet, your lifestyle can also affect cancer and other health problems. Relaxation, peace of mind, a positive outlook on life, a contented spirit, absence of envy, love of mankind, and faith are powerful, health-promoting factors which can help you achieve optimal health. This holistic approach to cancer prevention and health protection includes nourishing yourself with pleasant, well-balanced, low-fat meals; enjoying exercise as part of your daily routine; and taking time to smell the roses.

Diet and High Blood Pressure

High blood pressure, or hypertension, is a major risk factor for heart disease and the chief risk factor for stroke. Hypertension affects approximately 25 to 30 percent of Americans. By having your blood pressure measured, you can determine if it is in a healthy range. The normal pressure is 120 over 80, and a measure that exceeds 140 over 90 is considered high.

What Causes Hypertension?

Risk factors that can predispose people to hypertension include obesity, smoking, high stress, poor kidney function, and poor diet. Most health-conscious exercisers are not obese, do not smoke, and eat a healthier-than-average diet, thus eliminating several risk factors. Most active people, in fact, have low blood pressure. But you cannot change additional predisposing factors such as your genetics, age, and race, which can sometimes cause high blood pressure in spite of all your good health habits.

If you have high blood pressure, you may believe that salt causes the problem and that reducing salt intake will lower your high blood pressure, but that's not always true. Only 10 percent of American cases of high blood pressure have a known cause. In the remaining 90 percent, no one cause can be identified. Hence, health professionals debate whether the broad recommendation for everyone to reduce sodium intake is necessary. After all, Japan has the highest life expectancy in the world yet one of the highest rates of sodium intake.

Athletes and Salt

Salt is a compound of 40 percent sodium and 60 percent chloride. The sodium helps maintain proper fluid balance between the water in and around your body's cells; thus, you do need some sodium—about 1,000 milligrams per day. Many Americans, however, routinely consume up to seven times that amount.

The suggested daily value is 2,400 milligrams, but that number seems low for healthy athletes with low blood pressure. Because you lose salt when you perspire heavily, a low-salt diet may be a needless restriction if you are very active and have normal or low blood pressure and no family history of hypertension. Yet if you choose to restrict your sodium intake, your body will adjust by conserving more sodium and secreting less.

Even sweaty athletes can get adequate sodium from the sodium that naturally occurs in foods. For the most part, your body adapts to the heat by conserving salt and sweating proportionately more water. If you are unacclimated to the heat, such as on that first warm spring day when you overexercise to clear out the winter cobwebs, you will notice that your sweat is far saltier than it is at the end of the summer when you've adapted to the heat. If you really need salt, you will crave it. If you will be exercising for more than four to six hours in the heat, you should purposefully consume salt. Many ultramarathoners and long-distance cyclists snack on salted crackers, chips, pretzels, and other salty foods to satisfy their salt needs.

How to Reduce Your Salt Intake

If you want a diet that contributes to low blood pressure, your best bet is to buy foods in their natural state, such as raw unsalted peanuts, fresh (not canned) vegetables, and so on. Plan to eat lots of fresh fruits, vegetables, low-fat dairy products, and lean proteins. If you are over-

Food type	Average sodium content	Comments
Cereal (cold)	250 mg/oz	Read food label; varies by brand
Baked goods	250 mg/serving	Once a day, if at all
Cheese (low-fat)	200 mg/oz	Moderate amounts; 1-2 oz/day
Breads	150 mg/slice	
Milk, yogurt (low-fat)	125 mg/8 oz	
Meat, fish, poultry	80 mg/4 oz	
Eggs	60 mg/egg	
Vegetables	10 mg per serving	Fresh and frozen; if canned, rinse well
Fruit, juice	5 mg/serving	
Butter, margarine	50 mg/pat	

weight, try to lose a little weight, which will lower blood pressure. Eating less of the following foods will also lower your sodium intake and may contribute to a greater reduction in blood pressure:

Commercially prepared foods such as frozen dinners, canned soups, and instant meals unless they are labeled "low sodium."

Table salt. Remove the saltshaker from the table. Omit or reduce salt from cooking and baking. You can often leave it out without affecting the outcome.

Obviously salty foods such as salted crackers, chips, pretzels, popcorn, salted nuts, olives, and pickles. Buy low-sodium versions, if they're available.

Smoked and cured meats and fish such as ham, bacon, sausage, corned beef, hot dogs, bologna, salami, pepperoni, lox, and pickled herring. Choose low-sodium versions if you like these foods.

Cheeses, in particular processed and low-fat cheeses, some of which may be higher in sodium than the regular form.

Seasonings and condiments such as catsup, mustard, relish, Worcestershire sauce, soy sauce, steak sauce, MSG, and garlic salt.

Baking soda, seltzers, and antacids. Also, some laxatives may be high in sodium.

To add flavor to your foods, experiment with herbs and spices. When you try a new seasoning, cautiously add a small amount. Some tried-and-true combinations include the following:

- Beef—dry mustard, pepper, marjoram, red wine or sherry
- Chicken—parsley, thyme, sage, tarragon, curry, white wine or vermouth
- Fish—bay leaf, cayenne pepper, dill, curry, onions, garlic
- Eggs—oregano, curry, chives, pepper, tomatoes, pinch of sugar

The DASH Diet

To clarify the connection between blood pressure and diet, the National Institutes of Health funded a large study of Dietary Approaches to Stop Hypertension (DASH). The DASH diet requires twice the average daily servings of fruits, vegetables, and dairy foods; one-third the usual intake of beef, pork, and ham; one-half the typical use of fats, oils, and salad dressings; and one-quarter the ordinary number of snacks and sweets (Blackburn 2001). When more than 400 people followed the DASH diet for three months, their blood pressure dropped. The researchers concluded that a diet rich in calcium, potassium, magnesium, and fiber contributes to lower blood pressure. When people simultaneously reduce sodium intake, their blood pressure drops even more. Those consuming 1,500 milligrams of sodium a day experience a greater drop in blood pressure than those who eat 3,300 milligrams (the typical American intake). Fast-food eaters commonly consume more than 5,000 milligrams of sodium per day. (For more details about the DASH diet, go to www.nhlbi.nih.gov.)

The DASH study points out that blood pressure is affected by more than just sodium intake. The same fruits, vegetables, whole grains, and low-fat dairy products and meats that optimize your sports diet can also optimize your health. Eating a potassium-rich diet seems to guard against hypertension. Potassium helps make arteries stronger and better able to withstand the blood-vessel damage that can occur with aging. Calcium may offset the effect of too much sodium in the diet. See tables 1.1 and 1.2 for the potassium content of some popular fruits and vegetables and table 1.4 for a list of calcium-rich foods.

Increasing Your Potassium Intake

A high potassium diet is thought to be protective against high blood pressure. Potassium is found in most wholesome foods: fruits, vegetables, whole-grain breads and cereals, lentils, beans, nuts, and protein foods. Refined or highly processed foods, sweets, and oily foods (salad dressing, butter, and so on) are poor sources of potassium. You can increase your potassium intake by eating the following kinds of foods:

- Whole-wheat, oatmeal, and dark breads instead of white bread and flour products.
- More salads and raw or steamed veggies cooked in only a small amount of water, because the potassium leaches into the water. Steaming removes only 3 to 6 percent of the potassium, as compared with 10 to 15 percent with boiling. Microwaving is best for optimal potassium retention.
- Potatoes more often than rice, noodles, or pasta.
- Natural fruit juices instead of fruit-flavored beverages or soft drinks.

The suggested daily intake for potassium is 3,500 milligrams for the average person and 6,000 milligrams for the athlete not acclimated to the heat. The typical American diet contains 4,000 to 7,000 milligrams of potassium. One pound of sweat loss may contain 85 to 105 milligrams. For more information on salt and potassium for athletes, see chapter 6.

Diet and Diabetes

People with diabetes have an impaired ability to transport glucose from the blood into the muscles so that it can be used for energy. The resulting high levels of blood glucose increase the risk of heart attacks, strokes, kidney disease, blindness, and loss of limbs. The best cure for diabetes is prevention. Although one type of diabetes, insulin-dependent (type 1) diabetes, is the result of the body's inability to produce adequate insulin to carry the blood sugar into the cells, a second and more common type of diabetes, type 2 diabetes, commonly occurs in people who are overweight and underfit. With the current epidemic of obesity in America, a concurrent epidemic of diabetes is tagging alongside, particularly among children who have grown accustomed to eating supersized fast foods and spending too much time in front of TV and computer screens instead of being outside playing and moving their bodies.

Many people think eating lots of sugar causes diabetes. Wrong. Being overweight and underfit are the bigger culprits. The solution is to lose weight and exercise regularly. In a study of 3,200 people who were overweight, had an average age in the 50s, and had elevated blood glucose both when fasting and after eating meals (a risk factor for diabetes), some of the subjects were given medication to lower their blood glucose (metformin). Others were taught to exercise at least 150 minutes per week (five times a week for 30 minutes) and to lose weight (about 7 percent of their body weight, equivalent to about 11 pounds for a 160-pound person or 5 kilograms for a 73-kilogram person). And some, the control group, made no changes. The subjects who became more active and lost a little bit of weight dramatically reduced their risk of getting diabetes: 58 percent reduced incidence of getting diabetes during the almost three-year study versus 31 percent in the group that got medicine. The conclusion is that food and exercise are better than medicine. By becoming active and staying active throughout your life, you'll greatly reduce your risk of developing adult-onset diabetes, as well as other diseases of aging (Knowler et al. 2002).

Diet and Bone Health

Osteoporosis, or thinning of the bones with aging, results in hunched backs and brittle bones that break easily. Particularly among older postmenopausal women, osteoporosis is a serious health problem. In a survey of over 200,000 healthy women 50 years or older, 40 percent had osteopenia (reduced bone mass; the early stage of osteoporosis) and 7 percent had osteoporosis—and they didn't even know it. The women diagnosed with osteoporosis were four times more likely to fracture a bone within the next 12 months; those with osteopenia were almost two times more likely (Siris, Miller, Barrett-Connor, et al. 2001). Osteoporosis is also a major concern for men older than 70. Hence, men who plan to live a full life also need to take care of their bones in their earlier years.

Younger female athletes who have stopped having regular menstrual periods are also at risk for developing osteoporosis. Both amenorrheic and postmenopausal women lack adequate estrogen, a hormone that contributes to menstruation and helps to maintain bone density. The low bone density of a 29-year-old woman, a former amenorrheic runner, has left her living in pain from osteoporosis and doubting if her bones will be able to withstand the weight of a pregnancy.

The good news is that osteoporosis is a preventable condition. It is not an inevitable result of old age. You can reduce your risk of developing osteoporosis with these good-health habits:

- **Calcium-rich diet.** A lifelong calcium-rich diet, particularly in the three years surrounding puberty and up to about age 30, will help you build strong bones as well as maintain bone density by reducing the rate of calcium loss thereafter. (High calcium intake is associated with other health benefits, such as reduced risk of colon cancer and lower blood pressure.)

  In chapter 1 I talked about how to include in your daily diet the calcium necessary for lifelong fitness. Unfortunately, the typical 25- to 40-year-old woman consumes only 600 milligrams of calcium daily, almost half the recommended intake of 1,000 milligrams. This may be one reason why about 25 percent of women over 65 years are afflicted by osteoporosis (of whom 12 percent may die from medical complications). These women might have reduced their risk by consuming more calcium-rich foods throughout their lifetimes.

- **Regular exercise.** Participate in a regular exercise program that includes weight-bearing aerobic and muscle-building exercises. Accompany these bone-strengthening exercises with adequate calcium intake.

- **Normal hormones.** Women with estrogen deficiency have lower bone-mineral density despite high calcium intake and participation in a weight-bearing exercise program. (That's why amenorrheic female athletes are at high risk for stress fractures.) To compensate for lack of bone-protective hormones, athletes with amenorrhea commonly take the birth-control pill. But the latest research suggests that this may be ineffective and even potentially harmful (Weaver et al. 2001). The better bet for athletes with amenorrhea is to eat adequately to support regular menses (see chapter 12).

- **Low sodium intake.** Because too much salt interferes with the retention of calcium (Sellmeyer, Schloetter, and Sebastian 2002), your best bet is to moderate your salt intake, especially if you have a genetic predisposition to osteoporosis.

Unfortunately, too many women follow too few of these guidelines. I once counseled a very thin 24-year-old amenorrheic aerobics instructor who had the bones of a 60-year-old. She rarely drank milk (believing it to be a fattening fluid), ate a restrictive diet low in calories and protein, and was always trying to be thinner despite her obvious leanness. Little did she know that diet was contributing to the amenorrhea and that she was putting herself at risk of developing stress fractures, an early sign of poor bone health and premature osteoporosis. She thought that exercise would keep her bones strong because she'd heard that exercise helps maintain bone density. Exercise does help, but calcium and estrogen are simultaneously essential.

Her doctor advised her to regain her menstrual period to protect her bone health. Because lack of menstruation is associated with inadequate nutrition, I recommended that she boost her calorie and protein intake by consuming more calcium-rich low-fat milk and yogurt. Within two months she regained her menstrual period and started promoting her lifelong health. See chapter 12 for more information about how to resolve amenorrhea. For more information about osteoporosis, see the National Osteoporosis Foundation Web site, www.nof.org.

Fiber for Good Health

Fiber is the part of plant cells that humans can't digest. Having heard claims that fiber promotes regular bowel movements, lowers blood cholesterol, improves blood sugar control, and protects against colon cancer, sports-active Americans are seeking out high-fiber, carbohydrate-rich foods—the fruits, vegetables, beans, legumes, and whole grains that easily fit into a sports diet.

Types of Fiber

You should try to eat a variety of fiber-rich foods on a daily basis because different foods offer different types of fiber with different health benefits. The two main types of fiber are:

- **Insoluble fiber.** This type of fiber gives plants their structure. It does not dissolve in water. Common sources are wheat bran, vegetables, and whole grains. Insoluble fiber absorbs water, increases fecal bulk, and makes the bowels easier to pass.
- **Soluble fiber.** This type of fiber forms a gel in water. It is in oatmeal, barley, and kidney beans (as well as in pectin and guar gums, two fibers often added to foods and listed among the

ingredients). Soluble fiber lowers blood cholesterol, particularly in people with elevated cholesterol. Soluble fiber can also help stabilize blood glucose levels, making fiber-rich snacks a wise preexercise choice (assuming they settle comfortably). Some sustaining preexercise snacks include oatmeal—and oatmeal breads, cookies, muffins—as well as beans and legumes, such as lentil soup, refried beans, hummus, chili, and chickpeas. The information in table 2.6 can help you choose the foods richest in fiber.

The soluble fiber in beans, legumes, oat bran, psyllium, and pectin and guar gums (two fibers often added to foods and listed among the ingredients) lowers blood cholesterol, particularly if you start with elevated cholesterol. The soluble fibers transport bile acids (needed to make cholesterol) out of the body, which results in lower blood

TABLE 2.6

Fiber in Foods

Fiber is lost through food processing, such as milling whole wheat into white flour, peeling skins, pureeing vegetables, and juicing fruits. To reach the target intake of at least 25 grams of fiber per day, you should try to eat foods that have not been processed. You should also try to eat a variety of fiber-rich foods, because different types of fiber have different positive health effects.

Cereal	Fiber (g)	Grain	Fiber (g)
Fiber One	14	Bulgur, 1 cup	8
All-Bran with Extra Fiber, 1/2 cup	13	Brown rice, 1 cup	4
All-Bran, 1/2 cup	10	Triscuits, 7	4
Fruit & Fibre, 1 cup	6	Branola bread, 1 slice	3
Bran flakes, Complete, 3/4 cup	5	Popcorn, 3 cups	3
Cheerios, 1 cup	3	Spaghetti, 1 cup	2
Oatmeal, 1 packet instant	3	White rice, 1 cup	1
Vegetables	**Fiber (g)**	**Fruits**	**Fiber (g)**
Brussels sprouts, 1 cup	6	Pear, 1 medium	4
Spinach, 1 cup	5	Apple, medium	4
Potato, 1 large with skin	5	Prunes, 5 dried	3
Peas, 1/2 cup	4	Orange, 1 medium	3
Carrot, 1 medium	2	Banana, 1 medium	3
Corn, 1/2 cup	2	Kiwi, 1 medium	3
Lettuce, 1 cup	1	Raisins, 1/4 cup	2
Legumes	**Fiber (g)**		
Lentils, boiled, 1/2 cup	8		
Chickpeas, canned, 1/2 cup	5		
Kidney beans, canned, 1/2 cup	5		
Peanut butter, 2 tbsp	2		

Data from food labels and J. Pennington, 1998, *Bowes & Church's Food Values of Portions Commonly Used*, 17th ed. (Philadelphia: Lippincott).

cholesterol. Eating more oat bran, oatmeal, and oatmeal breads, cookies, and muffins will help, as will more beans and legumes. Corn bran, barley, and rice bran are other rich sources that are becoming more readily available.

A Fiber Myth

Despite popular belief, fiber does not hasten the time it takes for food to pass through your system. Fiber may increase fecal weight and the number of trips to the bathroom, but it usually does not increase transit time. Transit time varies for each person, but it normally averages two to four days and varies according to stress, exercise, and diet. Your best bet as an active person is to determine the right combination of fiber-rich foods that promotes regular bowel movements for your body. You may need to restrict your fiber intake if exercise itself becomes a powerful bowel stimulant.

To Your Good Health

By combining the best food choices from the Food Guide Pyramid with a regular exercise program, you can invest in your future well-being. Although genetics does play a strong role in heart disease, cancer, hypertension, and osteoporosis, you can help put the odds in your favor by eating wisely. As Hippocrates said, "Let food be thy medicine."

Nutrition for the Pregnant Athlete

Each woman experiences a unique pregnancy. Some feel fine, eat well, exercise regularly, and breeze through the nine months of pregnancy. Others suffer from fatigue, nausea, low-back pain, and other discomforts. Some gain more weight than expected. Others gain according to the standard guidelines shown in the following chart.

Regardless of your personal experience, your job during pregnancy is to eat as healthfully as you can and focus on foods rich in calcium, protein, iron, and folic acid. Eat according to your appetite and trust that regularly scheduled meals and snacks will contribute to the weight gain appropriate for your body, the enjoyment of a comfortable exercise program, and the building of a blue-ribbon baby.

Your best bet for nutrition during pregnancy is to follow the good nutrition guidelines offered in the first two chapters of this book, as well as read some of the books about pregnancy suggested in the reading list. Your diet should focus primarily on calcium-rich foods, dark green or colorful vegetables, fresh

(continued)

(continued)

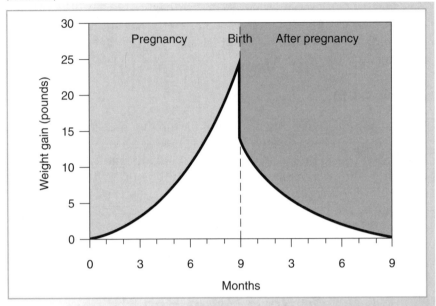

fruits such as orange and other citrus fruits, whole grains, and protein-rich foods.

You want to eat a healthful prepregnancy diet to be sure you start the pregnancy well nourished. Your body may experience strange cravings and morning sickness that limit your food intake during the pregnancy. For about two-thirds of women, tastes change during pregnancy. You may develop strong aversions to meat, vegetables, or coffee. If you can hold down nothing but a few crackers, rest assured that your baby will still manage to grow on the nutrients you've stored up from your prepregnancy diet. If your intake is very limited because of nausea that lasts for more than three months, you might want to consult with a registered dietitian who can suggest ways to balance your diet.

If you experience unusual cravings, such as for salt, fat, or red meat, it's possible that nature is telling you that those foods have nutrients you need. Food cravings tend to be harmless and probably won't lead to a nutrient deficiency, so listen to your body and respond appropriately.

Try to resolve your cravings for sweets with the most healthful choices, such as frozen yogurt instead of ice cream or raisins and dried fruits instead of candy. The reality may be that only one food will do the trick—the food you crave!

Better Diets Begin With Breakfast

Just as your car works better when it has gas in its tank, your body works better when you give it adequate morning fuel. Yet many people push their bodies through a busy day with an empty gas tank. The result is low energy, cravings for sweet foods, high intake of cookies and treats, and often undesired weight gain. Breakfast is the most important meal of the day. Eat up!

Don't Skip Breakfast

Of all the nutritional mistakes that you might make, skipping breakfast is the biggest. Marsha, a group exerciser at the Y, learned this the hard way: She fainted from low blood sugar after one of her morning workouts. Marsha managed to struggle through the hour-long step-aerobics class but felt lightheaded and dizzy. She ended up in a heap on the floor, surrounded by the other frightened exercisers. She had blacked out because she had no fuel to feed her brain.

Marsha's story is a dramatic example of how skipping breakfast can hinder your workouts and leave you drained for the rest of the day. In comparison, a high-energy breakfast sets the stage for a high-energy day. Nevertheless, many active people come up with familiar excuses for skipping the morning meal: I don't have time . . . I'm not hungry in the morning . . . I don't like breakfast foods . . . I'm on a diet . . . If I eat breakfast, I feel hungrier all day.

Excuses, excuses. If you skip breakfast, you're likely to concentrate less effectively in the late morning, work or study less efficiently, feel irritable and short tempered, or fall short of energy for your afternoon workout. For every flimsy excuse to skip breakfast, there's an even better reason to eat it. Keep reading!

You Do Have Time for Breakfast

"I just don't have time to eat breakfast. I get up at 5:30, go to the rink, skate for an hour, then dash to school by 7:45." Obviously, this ice-hockey player's morning schedule didn't allow him to relax and enjoy a leisurely meal. But Nick still needed the energy to tackle his high school classes.

I reminded Nick that breakfast doesn't have to be a sit-down, cooked meal. It can be a substantial snack after hockey practice while riding to school. I advised him to plan and prepare a breakfast-to-go the night before. If he could make time to train for hockey, he could make time to eat right for training.

Nick discovered that his duffle-bag breakfast was worth the effort. Two peanut butter and banana sandwiches and two juice boxes satisfied

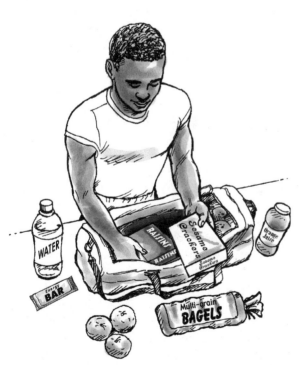

his ravenous appetite and improved his ability to concentrate at school. No longer did he sit in class counting the minutes until lunch and listening to his stomach grumble. Rather, he was able to concentrate on his classes and even improve his grades.

Jane, a nurse who was training for her first marathon, had the same excuse of no time for breakfast. She'd rise at 6:00 and be at the hospital by 6:45, and she didn't want to eat breakfast at that early hour. But by 10:00 she'd be devouring the jellybeans at the nurses' station!

I recommended that Jane eat some nutritious food between 8:00 and 9:00 to prevent the overwhelming hunger that contributed to her overeating and subsequent weight gain. Jane made the effort to do one of the following every day:

- Take a sandwich to work to eat within four hours of waking.
- Buy a bagel, yogurt, and orange juice at the coffee shop.
- Take an early break and enjoy a hot breakfast at the cafeteria.
- Keep emergency food in her desk drawer: granola bars, crackers, peanuts, and dried fruits.

She soon became a breakfast advocate, feeling much better when well fueled rather than half starved.

If you lack creative quick-fix breakfast ideas, these suggestions can help you make a fast break to becoming a regular breakfast eater.

- **Yogurt.** Keep your refrigerator well stocked; add cereal for crunch.
- **Banana.** Eat an extra-large one, chased by a large glass of milk.
- **Blender drink.** Whip together juice, fruit, and yogurt or dried milk powder. (See the smoothie recipe on page 357).
- **Raisins and peanuts.** Prepacked in small plastic bags, these are easy to tuck in your pocket.
- **Bran muffin.** Add raspberry jam for a tiny bit more fiber.
- **Bagel.** Spread it with peanut butter and then wash it down with a half pint of low-fat milk.
- **Graham crackers.** Refresh yourself with this childhood favorite—graham crackers and low-fat milk.
- **Pita bread.** Stuff it with low-fat cheese, cottage cheese, hummus, sliced turkey, or other handy fillings.

No Morning Appetite?

If you are not hungry for breakfast, you probably ate too many calories the night before. I often counsel people who routinely devour a bag of chips while watching TV or eat a pint of ice cream at 2 A.M. These snacks can curb a morning appetite, contribute to weight gain, and even result in an inadequate diet if too many munchies replace wholesome meals.

Mark, a 35-year-old computer programmer and runner, wasn't hungry for breakfast for another reason: His morning workout killed his appetite. But by 10:00 his appetite came to life again. He'd try to hold off until lunchtime, but he raided the candy machine three out of five workdays. I recommended that Mark take a bagel, yogurt, or banana to work. These portable foods are much more nutritious than candy, especially for breakfast.

For morning exercisers like Mark, a wholesome breakfast of cereal, fruit, and whole-grain toast, bagels, or muffins promptly replaces the depleted glycogen stores and helps refuel the muscles for the next training session. Exercised muscles are hungriest for carbohydrates within the first two hours after a hard workout. For more information on recovery foods, see chapter 6.

A recovery breakfast is particularly important if you do two workouts per day. For example, I often talk with triathletes who say they're not hungry for breakfast after the first workout, let's say a morning run. They then skimp at lunchtime, afraid that a substantial meal might interfere with the afternoon swim. They end up dragging themselves through a poor workout.

In this situation I recommend having brunch or a substantial snack around 10:00 or 11:00. The food will be adequately digested in time to fuel the muscles that afternoon. Refreshing liquids, such as juices and smoothies, also can help refuel you as well as quench your thirst. You'll discover that you have more energy for the second workout.

Breakfast for Dieters

Everyone knows diets start at breakfast, right? Wrong! Skipping breakfast to save calories is an unsuccessful approach to weight loss. If you are tempted to save calories by skimping on breakfast, remember that you don't gain weight eating this meal. You do gain weight if you skip breakfast, get too hungry, and then overindulge at night. If you are going to skip any meal, skip dinner but not breakfast. Your goal should be to fuel by day and eat a little less at night.

A survey of almost 3,000 dieters who have lost more than 30 pounds (14 kilograms) and have kept it off for at least a year suggests that 78 percent of the dieters ate breakfast every day and 88 percent ate breakfast five or more days a week. Only 4 percent reported never eating breakfast. The breakfast eaters reported being slightly more active during the day. This study suggests breakfast is indeed an important part of a successful weight-loss program (Wyatt et al. 2002). Another study of breakfast and weight control suggests the dieters who ate breakfast did less impulsive snacking later in the day and ate a lower fat diet overall (Schlundt et al. 1992). You can't go wrong with eating breakfast.

I repeatedly advise dieters to fuel during the day and eat less (diet) at night, and they always look at me with fear in their eyes. As Pat, an at-home mom who wanted to lose a few pounds, explained, "If I eat breakfast, I get hungrier and seem to eat more the whole day." Her breakfast was only half of a dry bagel, enough to get the digestive juices flowing but not enough to satisfy her appetite. When she ate a substantial 500-calorie breakfast, she felt fine and didn't blow it later in the afternoon. Although she initially couldn't believe that the following 500-calorie breakfasts (appropriate for a 1,500–1,800-calorie diet) would help her lose weight, she discovered that they did.

Breakfast on the run

Bagel, medium large	300
Vanilla yogurt	200
Total:	500

Nontraditional breakfast

2 slices of cheese pizza	500
Total:	500

Desk-drawer breakfast

Instant oatmeal, 2 packets	250
Raisins, 1 small box (1.5 oz)	130
Powdered milk, 1/2 cup	120
Total:	500

Kristen, a 28-year-old mother who worked out at the health club three days per week, also insisted that eating breakfast triggered her to overeat the whole day. She complained, "When I eat breakfast, I keep eating the rest of the day. I find it's easier to not start eating than it is to stop." I invited her to experiment for just three days to determine whether a heartier 500-calorie breakfast really did make her hungrier and fatter.

Kristen quickly discovered that she no longer craved hard candies all day and that she snacked less in the afternoon, had a better afternoon workout, and was able to enjoy a relaxed dinner rather than wolf down whatever food was in sight, without even waiting to sit down at the dinner table. She felt less hungry and snacked less throughout the night. By trading 600 to 800 snack calories in the evening for 500 breakfast calories, she discovered that breakfast, for her, would become the most important meal of the day.

If you are watching your weight and for some reason overeat at breakfast, don't continue to overeat for the rest of the day. Simply acknowledge that you ate part or all of your lunch calories early. You will then naturally eat less at lunch because you won't be hungry! Listen to your body, which is likely feeling content. Disregard the wayward mental voices that encourage last-chance eating: "Keep eating because this is your last chance before the diet starts again."

Number-One Breakfast for Champions

My clients commonly ask what I recommend for breakfast. In general my answer is any combination of wholesome choices from three food groups. Specifically, my answer is cereal because it's a simple way to get those three types of foods—grains, milk, and fruit—plus a host of other benefits.

What's So Great About Cereal?

I'm big on cereals because they are all these positive things:

Quick and easy. People of all ages and cooking abilities can easily pour a bowl with no cooking or messy cleanup.

Convenient. By simply stocking the cupboard or desk drawer, breakfast will be ready for the morning rush. A baggie of dry cereal is better than nothing. Keep some in your gym bag!

Carbohydrate rich. Your muscles need carbohydrates for energy. Cereal, a banana, and juice constitute a superior carbohydrate-rich meal.

Fiber rich. When you select bran cereals, you reduce your risk of becoming constipated, an inconvenience that can certainly interfere with enjoyment of exercise, and you also consume a health-protective, anticancer food.

Iron rich. By selecting fortified or enriched brands, you can easily boost your iron intake and reduce your risk of becoming anemic. Drink orange juice or another source of vitamin C with the cereal to enhance the iron absorption from the cereal.

Calcium rich. Cereal is rich in calcium when eaten with low-fat milk or yogurt or calcium-fortified soy milk. Women and children, in particular, but also men benefit from this calcium booster that helps maintain strong bones and protects against osteoporosis.

Low in fat and cholesterol. Cereals are a heart-healthier choice than the standard breakfast alternatives of buttered toast, a bagel slathered with cream cheese, or bacon and eggs.

Versatile. Rather than always eating the same brand, try mixing cereals to concoct endless flavors. I typically have 10 to 18 varieties in my cupboard. My friends laugh when they discover this impressive stockpile. I further vary the flavors by adding different mix-ins, such as banana, raisins, applesauce, cinnamon, maple syrup, or vanilla extract.

The Scoop on Cereal

Cereal, in general, is a breakfast for champions, but some brands offer far more nutritional value than others do. Here are five tips to help you make wise choices.

1. **Choose iron-enriched cereals.** An iron-rich diet is particularly important for active people, because iron is the part of the red blood cell that carries oxygen from your lungs to your muscles. If you are anemic (have iron-poor blood), you will feel tired and fatigue easily during exercise. Iron-rich breakfast cereal is a handy way to boost your iron intake, particularly if you eat little or no red meat (the best source of dietary iron).

    You can tell which cereals have iron added to them by looking for the words fortified or enriched on the label, or by checking the nutrition facts panel. You should choose a brand that supplies at least 25 percent of the daily value. Table 3.1 provides information that can help you select the brands enriched with iron to supplement the small amount naturally occurring in grains.

    If you prefer all-natural cereals with no additives, remember that "no additives" means that no iron is added, as is often the case with granola, shredded wheat, puffed rice, and other all natural brands. If you like, you can mix all-natural cereals with iron-enriched varieties (for example, granola with Cheerios, Shredded Wheat with Wheat Chex), or you can choose iron-rich foods at other meals or take an iron supplement (for more information on iron, see chapter 8).

    Because the iron in cereal is often poorly absorbed, you can enhance iron bioavailability, your body's ability to absorb iron, by drinking some orange juice or eating fruit rich in vitamin C along with the cereal (try oranges, grapefruit, cantaloupe, and strawberries).

2. **Choose cereal fortified with folic acid.** The B vitamin folic acid is found in small amounts in grains but in higher amounts (100 to 400 micrograms, 25 to 100 percent of the Daily Value) in fortified foods such as breakfast cereals. Folic acid is associated with a lower risk of not only certain types of birth defects but also heart disease. People with heart disease often have high blood

TABLE 3.1

Nutritional Value of Some Commonly Eaten Cereals

Cereal	Amount	Cal	Sugar (g)	Fat (g)	Fiber (g)	Sodium	Iron (% DV)
All-Bran Extra Fiber	1/2 cup	50	0	1	13	120	25
Complete Bran Flakes	3/4 cup	90	5	Trace	5	210	100
Cap'n Crunch	3/4 cup	110	12	1.5	1	200	25
Cheerios	1 cup	110	1	2	3	280	45
Corn bran	3/4 cup	90	6	1	5	230	45
Corn Flakes, Kellogg	1 cup	100	2	Trace	1	200	45
Cracklin' Oat Bran	3/4 cup	200	15	7	5	140	10
Crispix	1 cup	110	3*	—	<1	210	45
Fiber One	1/2 cup	60	0	1	14	130	25
Frosted Flakes	3/4 cup	120	12	—	1	150	25
Froot Loops	1 cup	120	15	1	1	150	25
Grape-Nuts	1/2 cup	210	5	1	5	340	90
Great Grains	1/2 cup	200	26*	5	4	135	50
Honey Nut Cheerios	1 cup	120	11	1.5	2	270	25
Kashi Go Lean	3/4 cup	120	7	1	10	35	8
Life	3/4 cup	120	6	1.5	2	160	45
Quaker Oat Squares	1 cup	210	10	2.5	5	250	90
Nutri-Grain Wheat	3/4 cup	100	24	Trace	4	220	6
Product 19	1 cup	100	4	—	1	210	100
Puffed Wheat, Quaker	1 cup	50	0	Trace	1	1	2

Cereal	Amount	Cal	Sugar (g)	Fat (g)	Fiber (g)	Sodium	Iron (% DV)
Quaker 100% Natural	1/2 cup	220	13	9	4	25	6
Lowfat Granola, Kellogg's	1/2 cup	190	14	3	3	—	10
Raisin Bran, Kellogg's	1 cup	190	19	1.5	7	350	25
Rice Krispies	1 1/4 cup	120	3	—	0	320	10
Shredded Wheat, Post	2 biscuits	160	0	1	6	—	6
Smart Start	1 cup	180	15	0.5	2	280	100
Special K	1 cup	110	4	—	4	20	45
Total	3/4 cup	110	5	1	3	190	100
Wheat Chex	1 cup	180	5	1	5	—	80
Wheaties	1 cup	110	4	1	3	220	45

*Includes raisins

Compiled from information provided on cereal boxes, 2003.

levels of homocysteine; folic-acid supplementation can reduce the levels. Hence, a hefty bowl of breakfast cereal can potentially contribute to optimal health (Malinow, Duell, Hess, et al. 1998) (see chapter 2).

3. **Choose high-fiber bran cereals.** Cereal with at least four grams of fiber per ounce is the best breakfast choice. Fiber is beneficial for people with constipation. Research suggests that fiber also has protective qualities that may reduce your risk of colon cancer and heart disease, as well as curb your appetite and assist with weight loss (see chapters 2 and 11).

   Bran cereals can provide far more fiber than most fruits and vegetables. High-fiber cereals include All-Bran, corn bran, raisin bran, oat bran, bran flakes, Fruit & Fibre, and any of the many cereals with bran or fiber in the name (see table 3.1). You can also boost the fiber content of any cereal by simply sprinkling raw bran on it.

4. **Choose wholesome cereals.** By wholesome cereals, I mean those with sugar not listed among the first ingredients. (Ingredients

What to Look for In a Cereal

If your favorite cereal doesn't meet these criteria, combine it with others to achieve a healthy mix.

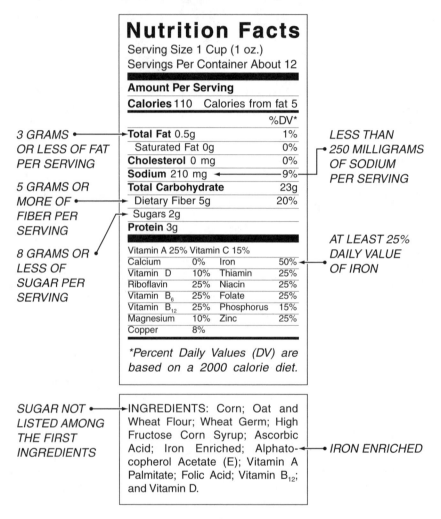

3 GRAMS OR LESS OF FAT PER SERVING

5 GRAMS OR MORE OF FIBER PER SERVING

8 GRAMS OR LESS OF SUGAR PER SERVING

LESS THAN 250 MILLIGRAMS OF SODIUM PER SERVING

AT LEAST 25% DAILY VALUE OF IRON

SUGAR NOT LISTED AMONG THE FIRST INGREDIENTS

IRON ENRICHED

Nutrition Facts

Serving Size 1 Cup (1 oz.)
Servings Per Container About 12

Amount Per Serving

Calories 110   Calories from fat 5

%DV*

Total Fat 0.5g		1%
Saturated Fat 0g		0%
Cholesterol 0 mg		0%
Sodium 210 mg		9%
Total Carbohydrate		23g
Dietary Fiber 5g		20%
Sugars 2g		
Protein 3g		

Vitamin A 25%		Vitamin C 15%	
Calcium	0%	Iron	50%
Vitamin D	10%	Thiamin	25%
Riboflavin	25%	Niacin	25%
Vitamin B$_6$	25%	Folate	25%
Vitamin B$_{12}$	25%	Phosphorus	15%
Magnesium	10%	Zinc	25%
Copper	8%		

Percent Daily Values (DV) are based on a 2000 calorie diet.

INGREDIENTS: Corn; Oat and Wheat Flour; Wheat Germ; High Fructose Corn Syrup; Ascorbic Acid; Iron Enriched; Alphato-copherol Acetate (E); Vitamin A Palmitate; Folic Acid; Vitamin B$_{12}$; and Vitamin D.

are listed by order of weight, from most to least.) By reading the nutrition facts on box labels, you can learn the amount of sugar in a cereal. Simply multiply grams of sugar (listed under total carbohydrate) by four calories per gram to determine the calories of sugar per serving. Quaker Toasted Oatmeal Squares, for example, has sugar listed as the third ingredient. A one-cup serving contains 9 grams of sugar (9 grams of sugar × 4 calories per gram = 36 calories) in 210 calories, so about 15 percent of the calories are from added sugar.

Some kids' cereals are 45 percent sugar, more like dessert than breakfast. Although sugar fuels the muscles and is not the poison it is reputed to be, sugary cereals tend to pamper your sweet tooth rather than promote your health.

Hannah, a flight attendant and avid exerciser, avoided all cereals with sugar listed among the ingredients, even the lightly sweetened ones like Total, Wheaties, and bran flakes. She restricted herself to the sugar-free puffed wheat and corn flakes, cheating herself of variety and flavor. She failed to recognize that sugar is a carbohydrate that fuels, not poisons, the muscles.

The small amount of sugar in cereal is relatively insignificant in comparison to the sugar Hannah ate in frozen yogurt, licorice, and gummy bears. The overall healthfulness of the cereal breakfast far outweighed those few nutritionally empty sugar calories. I told her that 10 percent of daily calories could appropriately come from sugar; the 16 calories (four grams) of sugar in a cereal could certainly fit into her day's 240-calorie sugar budget. Given this perspective, she decided to relax her sugar rules to include more variety, especially brands with health-protective fiber and iron.

5. **Choose low-fat cereals.** Rather than fretting about sugar content in a cereal, you should focus more on its fat calories. Fat is the bigger health threat because it's linked with weight gain, heart disease, and cancer. If you like the higher-fat cereals, such as granola or Cracklin' Oat Bran, use them for a topping sprinkled on a foundation of a lower-fat cereal.

Cereal Alternatives

Cereal may be one breakfast of champions, but it's not the only one. For you noncereal eaters, rest assured that other breakfasts can fuel you for a high-energy day. See the recipes in part III for some wholesome, high-carbohydrate breakfast breads you might want to enjoy with a glass of low-fat milk and some fruit or juice.

Whatever your choice, always remember that any breakfast is better than no breakfast, and a wholesome, carbohydrate-based breakfast that includes three different types of foods is best for your health and performance.

Quick Service Breakfasts

If you are destined to buy breakfast on the run, be sure to make wise food choices.

- Instead of egg, bacon, sausage, croissant, or biscuit combinations, choose pancakes, hot or cold cereal, juice, unbuttered bagels, english muffins, or other (low-fat) muffins. Spread whole-wheat toast with jelly or jam for extra carbohydrates, if desired, but go easy on the butter.
- Because fresh fruits can be hard to find on the menu, remember to tuck an apple or orange into your pocket. Or, take a big swig of juice before you leave home.
- Treat yourself to a latte (with low-fat milk), instead of coffee with cream, for more protein and calcium.
- Find a deli with fresh bagels, fruit, juice, and yogurt.
- Skip the breakfast temptations (cinnamon rolls, doughnuts, croissants, and so on) and bring a box of cereal to the office. On your way to work, pick up some milk and a banana, along with your coffee, if desired. If you are traveling and staying at a hotel, you can save yourself time, money, and temptation by taking your own cereal and dried fruit (and spoon). Take powdered milk or buy a half pint of low-fat or skim milk at the corner store. A water glass or milk carton can double as a cereal bowl.

Nontraditional Breakfasts

If you skip breakfast because you don't like breakfast foods, just eat something else. Who said you have to eat cereal or toast? Any food you eat at other times of the day you can eat for breakfast. I happen to love leftover pizza or Chinese food for a morning change of pace.

You might even want to eat most of your treats at breakfast. One of my clients found that by enjoying a chocolate croissant in the morning, she killed her desire for sweets for the rest of the day. Instead of craving cookies in the afternoon, she enjoyed the bowl of cereal that seemed humdrum at 8:00 A.M.

A good goal is to eat about one-third of your daily calories in the morning. Some acceptable choices include dinner leftovers, a baked potato with cottage cheese, a peanut butter and honey sandwich, a yogurt sundae with sliced fruit and sunflower seeds, tomato soup with crackers, or even special holiday foods. Why not enjoy for breakfast those high-calorie treats like left-over birthday cake or Thanksgiving pie? You're better off eating them during the day and burning off their calories than holding off until evening, when you may succumb to overconsumption in a moment of weakness.

Coffee: The Morning Eye-Opener

Coffee is a universally loved beverage. Every culture the world around enjoys some type of caffeinated beverage, be it tea in England and China, espresso in Italy, or coffee in America. Questions abound about the role of coffee in a healthy diet. Here are some answers to commonly asked questions. For more information about coffee as it relates to exercise, see chapter 5.

Q: Is coffee bad for me? That is, will it hurt my health?

A: Because coffee is so widely consumed, it has been extensively researched. To date, there is no obvious connection between caffeine and heart disease, cancer, or blood pressure. Hence, the general answer, according to leading medical and scientific experts, is that normal coffee consumption produces no adverse health effects. (The average American consumes 200 milligrams of caffeine per day, the equivalent of about 10 to 12 ounces—a large mug—of coffee.) For the 10 percent of Americans who ingest more than 1,000 milligrams of caffeine per day and sustain themselves on the cream and sugar in coffee plus a few cigarettes alongside, heart disease is indeed more common—and linked to the poor diet and unhealthful lifestyle.

Besides smokers, those who should abstain from caffeine include ulcer patients and others prone to stomach distress (caffeine stimulates gastric secretions and may cause "coffee stomach") and athletes with anemia. Substances in coffee and tea can interfere with the absorption of iron. If you suffer from anemia and routinely drink coffee or tea with meals or up to one hour after a meal, you might be cheating yourself nutritionally. A cup of coffee consumed with a hamburger can reduce by about 40 percent the absorption of the iron in the hamburger. Drinking caffeinated beverages up to an hour before eating, however, seems to have no negative effect on iron absorption.

The biggest health worries about coffee have to do with the following habits surrounding that beverage:

Adding cream or coffee whiteners containing coconut oil. These add saturated fat that contributes to heart disease. At least switch to milk or powdered milk for whitening your coffee.

Drinking coffee instead of eating a wholesome breakfast. A large coffee with two creamers and two sugars contains 70 nutritionally empty calories. Multiply that by three mugs, and you could have had a nourishing bowl of cereal for the same number of calories. Many people who say they live on coffee could easily drink much less if they would eat a satisfying breakfast and lunch. Food is better fuel than caffeine. See table 3.2 for a comparison of calorie and fat contents in popular coffee drinks.

Drinking coffee to stay alert. A good night's sleep might be a better investment. You could also try drinking a tall glass of ice water to perk yourself up. Sometimes dehydration contributes to fatigue, and you'd be better off drinking water than pumping caffeine.

These bad habits are more likely to harm your health than the caffeine itself. If you are concerned about caffeine and health, you might want to switch to tea. Tea drinkers tend to have a lower risk of heart disease, perhaps because tea is a rich source of flavonoids that protect against heart disease, or because tea drinkers, in general, tend to be more health conscious, smoke less, and eat more fruits and vegetables (Geleijnse et al. 2002).

TABLE 3.2 GULP!

It's a Calorie Cafe!

Beware of the fat and calories in the popular beverages that are readily available at coffeehouses. A large coffee Coolatta can accommodate half the day's recommended fat allowance (for a person eating 2,000 calories, a low-fat diet offers 55 to 65 grams of fat). Replacing whole milk or cream with low-fat or skim milk can save considerable calories. In general, be cautious with sugary beverages. They do not always register as food and can lead to weight gain.

Beverage	Calories	Fat (g)
Dunkin' Donuts		
Iced coffee with cream and sugar, 16 oz	110	6
Coffee Coolatta with skim milk, 16 oz	230	0
Coffee Coolatta with 2% milk, 16 oz	240	1.5
Coffee Coolatta with cream, 16 oz	370	16
Coffee Coolatta with cream, 32 oz	740	32
Strawberry Fruit Coolatta, 16 oz	270	0
Vanilla chai, 10 oz	220	8
Starbucks		
Latte with whole milk, 12 oz	210	11
Latte with skim milk, 12 oz	120	0.5
Coffee Frappuccino, 12 oz	200	2
Coffee Frappuccino, 24 oz	405	5

Nutrition information from Starbucks (800-23-LATTE) and www.dunkindonuts.com, July 2002.

Q: What does coffee do to my body?

A: The caffeine in coffee is a mild stimulant that increases the activity of the central nervous system. Hence, caffeine helps you stay alert and enhances mental focus. The stimulant effect peaks in about one hour and then declines as the liver breaks down the caffeine. If you are an occasional coffee drinker, you'll tend to be more sensitive to the stimulant effects of caffeine as compared with the daily coffee consumer who has developed a tolerance to caffeine.

Q: Do people get addicted to coffee?

A: Although coffee has been a popular beverage for centuries, its sustained popularity fails to classify it as addictive. Coffee is not associated with the behaviors found with hard drugs (such as a need for more and more coffee, antisocial behavior, severe difficulty stopping consumption). If you are a regular coffee drinker who decides to cut coffee out of your diet, you may develop headaches, fatigue, or drowsiness. The solution is to decrease your caffeine intake gradually rather than eliminate coffee cold turkey. And be aware that if you should get a headache because of caffeine withdrawal, caffeine-containing medicines such as Anacin or Excedrin will foil your efforts to reduce your caffeine intake.

If you drink too much coffee, sleep poorly, and are chronically nervous, jittery, and irritable, then you should slowly cut back. Switching to tea reduces caffeine intake (and also increases your intake of a beverage that has potential benefits in terms of reducing heart disease and cancer). Other ways to reduce your caffeine include drinking more of the following caffeine-free alternatives: decaffeinated coffee, decaffeinated tea, herbal tea, hot water with a lemon wedge, Postum, Pero, and other cereal-based coffee alternatives, broth, bouillon (low-sodium or regular), hot chocolate, Ovaltine, other hot milk-based drinks, mulled cider, hot cranberry juice, or apple juice.

Q: How much caffeine is in espresso?

A: Ounce for ounce, espresso is about twice as strong as coffee (35 versus 18 milligrams of caffeine per ounce of Starbucks). But because the espresso serving is so small, you end up with less caffeine: 35 milligrams from one shot (one ounce) of espresso versus 140 milligrams from an eight-ounce Starbucks coffee.

Q: How much caffeine do Coke and Pepsi have compared with coffee?

A: The typical 12-ounce mug of coffee averages 200 milligrams of caffeine, about four times more than the 35 to 50 milligrams in a can of cola. The real kick from soft drinks comes from sugar, not caffeine.

Q: What about coffee and women?

A: Pregnant women should prudently limit their caffeine to less than 300 milligrams per day (less than 18 ounces of coffee). Caffeine readily crosses the placenta and, in excess, may be associated with premature birth. Women who are breastfeeding should also limit their intake. Caffeine crosses into breast milk and can make babies agitated and poor sleepers. Women who are trying to become pregnant might want to reduce caffeine intake even more, but more research is needed to clarify the controversy over the effects of caffeine on fertility. Women who are worried about getting osteoporosis may have heard that caffeine is linked to low bone density. The solution is to consume at least eight ounces of milk per day. Simply put more milk in your coffee or enjoy some lattes.

Q: If I drink too much alcohol, will coffee help me sober up?

A: No. Coffee will just make you a wide-awake drunk. Coffee does not speed the time needed for the liver to detoxify alcohol. But coffee does get some water into your body, and that can have a positive effect.

Q: Does coffee count toward my daily fluid needs?

A: Yes. All fluids count—plain water, juice, soup, watermelon—and even coffee. The rumor that coffee dehydrates people lacks scientific support (Armstrong 2002). Even during exercise in the heat, athletes can consume coffee and not be concerned about dehydration.

Q: What's a good alternative to drinking coffee?

A: Without doubt, the best caffeine-free alternative to an eye-opening cup of coffee is exercise. A quick walk and some fresh air may be far more effective than a cup of brew. For more information about caffeine and performance, see chapter 5.

Meals to Fight Stress and Fatigue

Relaxing lunches and dinners—nicely prepared, attractively served, and shared with family and friends—are a rare occurrence for many active people and sports families. Lunch tends to be catch it if you can—especially if you have no interest in making a bag lunch in the morning or have little time to enjoy lunch at noon. You might end up with a salad bar at best, an energy bar as a handy alternative, or a huge cookie at worst.

Dinner presents a similar dilemma. If you are responsible for preparing your own food, you likely arrive home tired from work and your workout with little desire to cook. The easy options become a take-out meal, a frozen dinner, or frozen yogurt. If you are trying to plan dinner for a sports family with kids who have practices scheduled at mealtime, drive-through dinners are a tempting choice.

Whatever the scenario, my clients commonly express dissatisfaction with their mealtime eating. Yet, when life is full, stress is high, and schedules are crazy, eating well-balanced, healthful meals can provide the energy you need to manage stress and prevent fatigue. The purpose of this chapter is to provide meal management tips so that you can care for your health while balancing work, workouts, family, and stress.

Lunch Bunch

For active people who should be in the continuous cycle of fueling up for workouts and refueling afterward, lunch is the second most important meal of the day. Breakfast remains number one. Lunch refuels morning or noontime exercisers and offers fuel to those preparing for an afternoon session. Given that active people tend to get hungry every four hours (if not sooner), if you eat breakfast at 7:00 or 8:00 A.M., you are certainly ready for lunch at 11:00 or 12:00. But if you eat too little breakfast (as commonly happens), you'll be hungry for lunch by 10:00 A.M.—and that throws off the rest of the day's eating schedule.

The solution to the "I cannot wait until noon to eat lunch" dilemma is simple: You could either eat a bigger breakfast that sustains you until noon, eat a midmorning snack (more correctly, the second half of your too-small breakfast), or eat the first of two lunches, one at 10:00 and the other at 2:00.

For a nation of lunch skippers, eating two lunches may seem a wacky idea. But why not? Ideally, you should eat according to hunger, not by the clock. After all, hunger is simply your body's request for more fuel. If you've eaten only a light breakfast or have exercised hard in the morning, you can easily be ready for lunch #1 at 10:00 A.M. and for lunch #2 at 2:00. That's what I do—and have found that this system keeps me evenly fueled and helps me arrive home agreeably ready for dinner, but not starving.

In general, when you plan your intake for the day, you should try to divide your calories evenly. Given the tendency to become hungry every 4 hours, active people can appropriately eat 25 percent of their calories at each of four meals (breakfast, lunch #1, lunch #2, and dinner); this covers a 16-hour time span. By experimenting with this concept of evenly sized and spaced meals, you'll eradicate your afternoon sweet cravings or after-dinner dietary disasters. A hearty lunch (or two) truly invests in a higher-energy day.

Lunchtime Logistics

Despite the importance of lunch, logistics tend to be a hassle. If you pack your own lunch, what do you pack? If you buy lunch, what's a healthful bargain? If you're on a diet, what's best to eat? Here are some helpful tips to improve your lunch intake.

Brown Bagging It

If you pack your lunch, the what-to-pack dilemma quickly becomes tiring. Hence, most people tend to pack more or less the same food every day and end up with yet another turkey sandwich, salad, or bagel. As long as you're content with what you choose, fine. But if you're tired of the same stuff, consider these suggestions:

- Strive for at least 500 calories (even if you are on a reducing diet) from three types of food at lunch. This means bagel, yogurt, and banana, or salad, turkey, and pita. Just a bagel or just a salad is likely too little fuel.

- Remember peanut butter. Peanut butter is an outstanding sports food—even for dieters—because it's satisfying and helps you stay fueled for the whole afternoon. Yes, it has 200 more calories than a standard turkey sandwich, but a satisfying peanut butter sandwich allows you to nix the afternoon cookies and snacks that would otherwise sneak into your intake for the day. In addition, the fat in peanut butter is health protective and can lower your risk of heart disease. Refresh your memory of this childhood staple! See page 34 for more information on peanut butter.

- Pack planned leftovers from dinner and heat them in the microwave oven. They're preferable to the cup of noodles or frozen lunches that cost more than they're worth.

If you're lucky enough to have a cafeteria at work or to participate in a business lunch, take advantage of the opportunity to enjoy a hot meal. Eating a dinner at lunch

1. fuels you for a high-energy after-work exercise session,

2. simplifies the "what's to eat for dinner" routine because you'll feel less hungry and may be content to enjoy a bowl of cereal or a sandwich, and

3. reduces the hungry horrors that you might otherwise fight if you were to skip lunch or hold off until dinner. Why hold off? You are going to eat the calories eventually, so you might as well honor your hunger and eat now!

Lunch for Dieters

Because most Americans regard meals as fattening, dieters tend to skip or skimp on lunch. As one overweight walker confided, "I have only a very light lunch. Because I'm fat and should be dieting, I don't give myself permission to eat lunch." That sad statement is common in our society. I urged her to take care of herself better and at least eat enough "diet foods" to keep her metabolism going and fuel her muscles for her walking program. Once she started to have a turkey sandwich, yogurt, and orange for lunch, she discovered the benefits of eating this meal. She was more effective at work, less hungry in the afternoon, less likely to raid the refrigerator the minute she arrived home, and better able to lose weight. She learned that lunch works.

Super Salads

Salads are a popular lunch and a super way to boost your intake of vegetables. In just one big bowlful you can get your five daily vegetable servings—if not more! Yet lunchtime salads can be either good news or bad news, depending on the salad.

If you are a dieter who deems salads an appropriate lunch, take heed. A meager salad offers too few calories. You'll likely end up visiting the vending machine that afternoon. I suggest that dieters have a salad for dinner but eat a substantial meal at lunch. If you take full advantage of a brimming salad bar, take heed. A typical salad-bar meal can easily contain 1,000 calories, with 45 percent of those from fat. This is not a diet meal.

To create a high-energy sports salad that is the mainstay of your lunch or dinner, include enough carbohydrate-rich foods to make it substantial but limit the fats to control the calories. Here are five tips to help you get the most in your salad bowl.

Tip #1. Boost the carbohydrate content of the salad by adding

- carbohydrate-dense veggies such as corn, corn relish, peas, beets, and carrots;
- beans and legumes such as chickpeas, kidney beans, and three-bean salad;
- cooked rice, pasta, or potato chunks;
- orange sections, diced apple, raisins, banana slices, and berries;
- toasted croutons (limit your intake of buttered croutons that leave you with greasy fingers); and
- thick slices of whole-grain bread and a glass of low-fat milk for accompaniments.

Tip #2. Choose a variety of dark, colorful veggies such as red tomatoes, green peppers, orange carrots, and dark lettuces. Colorful vegetables nutritionally surpass paler lettuces, cucumbers, onions, celery, and mushrooms. For example, a salad made with spinach has seven times the vitamin C as one made with iceberg lettuce; one made with dark romaine has twice the vitamin C. See table 4.1 for ranking salad fixings. In addition, colorful vegetables are brimming with the antioxidant nutrients and phytochemicals that protect your health. Exceptions include beets and corn; although colorful and carbohydrate-rich, they have fewer vitamins than their deeply colored peers do. Cauliflower, although colorless, is a good source of vitamin C (70 milligrams per cup, raw) and the cancer-protective nutrients found in the cruciferous vegetable family to which it belongs.

TABLE 4.1

Ranking Vegetables

The Center for Science in the Public Interest (CSPI) has developed a system for ranking vegetables in order of their nutritional value and fiber content. The higher the score, the better and more nutrient dense the vegetable. In general, notice how the vegetables with more color also have more nutrients. Here's how some popular salad ingredients compare:

Ingredients	Score based on six nutrients and fiber
Spinach, 1 cup raw	287
Red pepper, 1/2 medium raw	261
Carrot, 1 medium raw	204
Romaine lettuce, 1 cup shredded	174
Broccoli, 1/2 cup raw florettes	160
Cabbage, 1/2 cup raw	135
Boston or Bibb lettuce, 1 cup	134
Green pepper, 1/2 raw	109
Green peas, frozen, 1/2 cup	104
Avocado, 1/2 Haas raw	82
Tomato, 1/2 raw	78
Corn, 1/2 cup	67
Green beans, 1/2 cup cooked	65
Cauliflower, 1/2 cup raw	62
Iceberg lettuce, 1 cup	45
Beets, 1/2 cup canned	33
Mushrooms, 1/2 cup cooked	33
Cucumber, 1/2 cup raw	14
Alfalfa sprouts, 1/2 cup raw	7

Copyright 2002, CSPI. Adapted from *Nutrition Action Healthletter* (1875 Connecticut Ave., N.W., Suite 300, Washington, D.C. 20009-5728.

Tip #3. Pile on the potassium-rich veggies. This mineral, which gets lost in sweat, protects against high blood pressure. You should try to get at least 3,500 milligrams of potassium per day—an easy task for salad lovers (see table 1.2 on page 12). Some of the veggies richest in potassium include

- romaine, four large leaves (400 milligrams),
- broccoli, one cup chopped, raw (380 milligrams),
- tomato, one medium (370 milligrams), and
- carrot, one large (340 milligrams).

Tip #4. Include adequate protein by adding low-fat cottage cheese, flaked tuna, canned salmon, sliced turkey, chicken, or other lean meats.

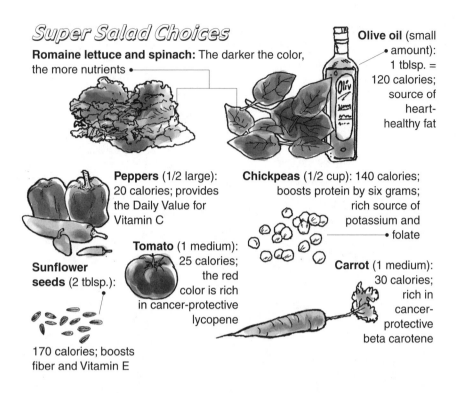

Super Salad Choices

Romaine lettuce and spinach: The darker the color, the more nutrients

Olive oil (small amount): 1 tblsp. = 120 calories; source of heart-healthy fat

Peppers (1/2 large): 20 calories; provides the Daily Value for Vitamin C

Chickpeas (1/2 cup): 140 calories; boosts protein by six grams; rich source of potassium and folate

Sunflower seeds (2 tblsp.):

Tomato (1 medium): 25 calories; the red color is rich in cancer-protective lycopene

Carrot (1 medium): 30 calories; rich in cancer-protective beta carotene

170 calories; boosts fiber and Vitamin E

For vegetarian proteins, toss in diced tofu, chickpeas, three-bean salad, walnuts, sunflower seeds, almonds, and peanuts. Too often vegetarians eat just the greens and neglect the protein. They often end up anemic, injured, and chronically sick with colds or the flu.

Tip #5. Remember the calcium. For calcium (and protein), add grated part-skim mozzarella cheese; cubes of tofu; dressing made from plain yogurt seasoned with oregano, basil, and other Italian herbs; or a scoop of low-fat cottage cheese (a better source of protein than calcium). Drink low-fat milk or skim milk along with the salad, or have a cup of yogurt for dessert. Don't try to live on lettuce alone!

A Word About Salad Dressings

On a large salad, dressing can easily add 800 to 1,000 calories. On even a small side salad, a few ladles of dressing can drown the healthfulness of the salad in 400 calories of fat. These fat calories appease the appetite, add to your waistline, and fail to fuel the muscles with carbohydrates. I often advise my clients to educate themselves about salad dressing calories by measuring out the amount of dressing they normally use on a salad—they tend to be shocked.

Dressing Well

A few innocent ladles of salad dressing can transform a potentially healthful salad into a high-fat, nutritional nightmare. Even lite dressings have calories. Use them sparingly! A large salad can easily accommodate six tablespoons of dressing—an extra 60 to 650 calories that still count, whether it's fat free or not.

Dressing, 2 tbsp	Calories	Fat (g)
Plain olive oil	240	26
Plain vinegar	5	0
Herbs, sprinkling	5	0
Blue cheese, Wishbone	170	17
Blue cheese, Wishbone fat-free	35	0
Ranch, Kraft regular	110	11
Ranch, Kraft Light Done Right	70	4
Ranch, Kraft fat-free	50	0
Italian, Wishbone regular	80	8
Italian, Wishbone Just 2 Good	35	2
Italian, Wishbone fat-free	20	0

Nutrition information from food labels, July 2002.

To reduce the fat and calories from salad dressing, choose low-fat dressings or simply dilute a regular dressing with extra vinegar, lemon juice, water, or milk in creamy dressings. By using only small amounts of this diluted version, you'll get lots of flavor and moistness with fewer calories. At restaurants, always request that the dressing be served on the side so that you can control the amount you consume. Add the dressing sparingly or dip a forkful of salad into the dressing before each bite. And be aware that even fat-free dressings have calories in them, so use them sparingly.

At home you might want to create your own creamy low-calorie dressing by adding a little blue cheese or Italian seasonings to plain low-fat yogurt. Or adventure into the world of exotic vinegars. Balsamic is one of my favorites.

Replacing these fat calories with more carbohydrates—an extra dinner roll or a baked potato—can improve the capacity of your body for exercise. This idea also holds true for athletes who want to maintain or gain weight. Athletes who are eating generous amounts of olive oil (a heart-healthy fat) to boost their calorie intake should also remember they need a foundation of carbohydrates to fuel their muscles.

Dinners: Home and Away

In America, dinners are commonly the biggest meal of the day—the reward for having survived yet another busy, stress-filled day. I invite you to start putting dinner on the bottom of the meal-priority list and place more focus on breakfast and lunch (or lunches). This way you'll have more energy to cope with daytime stresses, enjoy a good workout, and feel less in need of high calorie rewards at night. Yes, you can and should enjoy a pleasant meal, but you won't need a humongous meal followed by endless snacks.

Dinner at Home

When dinner is home based, you need a game plan to pull together a team of nutritious foods. The following tips can help you plan for and prepare wholesome dinners without much time or effort—with little or no cooking. The recipes in part III offer additional tried-and-true menu suggestions.

Tip #1. Don't arrive home too hungry. One prerequisite for successful nighttime dining is to eat a hearty lunch plus a second lunch or afternoon snack. Jen, a busy stockbroker, experimented with my suggestion to eat a heartier lunch plus a preexercise snack before her 5:30 P.M. kick-boxing class. In one day, she discovered that this food enhanced her energy for exercise and transformed her 7:00 bowl of ice cream for dinner into a bowl of salad.

This approach prevents you from attacking the refrigerator the minute you walk in the house in the evening. A substantial lunch supports greater energy in the afternoon, higher quality afternoon workouts, the physical and mental energy you need to prepare a nourishing supper, and better ability to cope with the stress of the day.

Tip #2. Plan time to food shop. Good nutrition starts in the grocery store. By stocking your kitchen shelves and freezer with a variety of wholesome foods that are ready and waiting, you will be more likely to eat a better dinner. Kirsten, a 24-year-old dental assistant, used to spend most of her food budget in restaurants on the way home from work because at home she faced bare cupboards and an empty refrigerator. Although she liked to cook, she rarely did so because she simply didn't plan the time to grocery shop. In addition, she became discouraged by meats and vegetables that often spoiled before she got around to cooking them.

I advised Kirsten to write into her schedule book a time to food shop. She kept that appointment and was then able to stock her freezer with individually wrapped chicken breasts, lean hamburger patties, turkey burgers, and frozen vegetables, particularly vitamin-rich broccoli, spinach, and winter squash. Freezing does not destroy the nutritional value of food, so frozen foods provide quick nutrition with less fuss and waste than fresh items do. The frozen broccoli provides far more nutrients than the wilted, five-day-old stalks that Kirsten occasionally dragged from her refrigerator. Once she had stocked her kitchen with frozen foods and other staples, Kirsten discovered that she enjoyed coming home for dinner.

I always stock basic foods that won't spoil quickly. On days when I arrive home to an empty refrigerator, I can either pull together a no-cook meal or quickly prepare a hot dinner. Some of my standard menus include these items:

- English muffin pizzas
- Stoned-wheat crackers, peanut butter, and milk
- Lentil soup with extra broccoli, leftover pasta, and a sprinkling of parmesan
- Refried beans and cheese rolled in a tortilla and heated in the microwave
- Tuna sandwich with tomato soup
- Bran cereal with banana and raisins

My standard ingredients include the following:

Cupboard		Refrigerator	Freezer
Spaghetti	Salsa	Low-fat cheese	English muffins
Rice	Minced clams	Grated parmesan	Pita bread
Potatoes, white	Tuna	Low-fat cottage cheese	Multigrain bread
Potatoes, sweet	Spaghetti sauce	Low-fat yogurt	Bagels
Wheat crackers	Canned salmon	Low-fat milk	Broccoli
RyKrisp crackers	Kidney beans	Eggs (omega)	Winter squash
Pretzels	Refried beans	Oranges	Spinach
Bran flakes	Soups (lentil, tomato)	Carrots	Peas
Oat bran	Peanut butter	V-8 juice	Chicken breasts
Muesli	Raisins	Orange juice	Ground turkey
Bananas	Dried apricots	Tortillas	Extralean hamburger

When creating a meal from these staples, I choose items from three of the five food groups, using carbohydrates as the foundation for each meal. The following are samples of well-balanced meals that contain about 650 calories, 60 percent carbohydrates, and require no cooking.

Food group	Menu 1: crackers with tuna	Menu 2: peanut butter and raisin sandwich
1. Grain	8 stoned-wheat crackers	2 slices multigrain bread
2. Protein	1/2 can tuna with 1 tbsp lite mayo	2 tbsp peanut butter
3. Fruit		1/4 cup raisins
4. Vegetable	12 oz can V-8 juice	1 raw carrot
5. Dairy	1 cup fruit yogurt	1 cup low-fat milk

Food group	Menu 3: pizza	Menu 4: burrito
1. Grain	2 English muffins	2 tortillas
2. Protein	(cheese)	1 cup vegetarian refried beans
3. Fruit	1 cup orange juice	Apple
4. Vegetable	3/4 cup spaghetti sauce	Chopped tomatoes, lettuce
5. Dairy	2 oz mozzarella cheese, low-fat	1 cup low-fat cottage cheese

The portions are appropriate for an active woman who needs about 1,800 to 2,000 calories per day. A hungry man may want more.

Tip #3. Eat more than just plain pasta at a meal. Pasta in any shape—spaghetti, ziti, twists, whatever—is without question a popular and easy-to-cook meal among active people. Although carbohydrate-rich pasta does provide muscle fuel (gas for your body's engine), pasta is a marginal source of vitamins and minerals (the spark plugs needed for top performance). Pasta is made from refined white flour with a few vitamins added to replace those lost during processing. Whole-wheat pastas offer little nutritional superiority, because wheat and other grains, in general, are better respected for their carbohydrate value than their vitamin density. Even spinach and tomato pastas are over-rated; they contain little of the vegetables.

Remember the Food Guide Pyramid (chapter 1) and the value of eating at least three out of five food groups with each meal. Pasta becomes a nutritional powerhouse when topped with any combination of vegetables and protein-rich foods, such as:

- tomato sauce (fresh or from a jar),
- spinach and garlic sauce,
- fresh or frozen broccoli, spinach, or green peppers from the freezer, or
- canned beans, cottage cheese, tofu, nuts, or tuna for cook-free protein.

Tip #4. Plan cook-a-thons. Lauren, a 53-year-old high school teacher, enjoyed cooking on the weekends when she had the time. She always created a big batch of something on Sunday so that it would be waiting for her when she arrived home tired and hungry after work and work-outs. She preferred convenience to variety and thrived on beans and rice for a week; then spinach lasagna the next week; split-pea soup the third, and so on. When Lauren couldn't face another repetitious dinner, she cooked something else and put the leftovers in the freezer.

Dinner Out

Some people eat in restaurants because the cupboards are empty or because they prefer not to cook. Others enjoy dining in restaurants with their friends. And some end up in restaurants because of business meetings. Whatever the situation, every active person who relies on restaurants for a balanced sports diet faces the challenge of finding healthful meals among all the rich temptations. Unfortunately, many people select whatever is fast and happens to tempt their taste buds at the moment, particularly when they are tired, hungry, stressed, anxious, or lonely.

Selecting the Right Restaurant

Here are a few suggestions for successfully selecting healthful restaurant meals. The most important first step is to patronize restaurants that offer carbohydrate-rich sports foods. Don't go to a steak house if you're looking for muscle fuel! Study the menu before you sit down to see if the restaurant offers pasta, baked potatoes, bread, juices, and other carbohydrate-based foods. Try to avoid places that have only fried items. Also check to see if they allow special requests. If the menu clearly states "no substitutions," you might be in the wrong place.

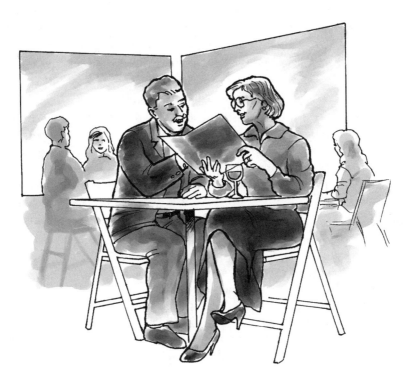

When you're in an appropriate restaurant, choose your foods wisely. In general, you should request foods that are baked, broiled, roasted, or steamed—anything but fried. Low-fat poultry and fish items tend to be better choices than items naturally high in fat, such as prime rib, cheese, sausage, and duck.

Low-Fat and Healthful Restaurant Choices

Keep the following foods in mind as you peruse a menu.

- **Appetizers.** Tomato juice, fruit juice, shrimp cocktail, fruit cocktail, melon, and crackers make great starters for your meal.

- **Breads.** Unbuttered rolls and breads are great—particularly if they are whole grain; ask for extras! If the standard fare is buttered (as in garlic bread) request some plain bread as well and enjoy the buttery bread in moderation.

- **Soups.** Broth-based soups (such as vegetable, chicken and rice, and Chinese soups) and hearty minestrone, split-pea, navy bean, and lentil soups can be good sources of carbohydrates and are more healthful than creamy chowders and bisques. They are also a source of fluids.

- **Salads.** Enjoy the veggies but limit the chunks of cheese, bacon bits, grated cheese, olives, and other high-fat toppings. Be extra generous with chickpeas and toasted croutons.

- **Salad dressings.** Always request that the dressing be served on the side so that you can control how much you use. You want to fill up on carbohydrates, not oily dressings.

- **Seafood and poultry.** Request chicken or fish that's baked, roasted, steamed, stir-fried, or broiled. Because many chefs add a lot of butter when broiling foods such as fish, you might want to request that your entree be broiled dry, that is, cooked without the extra fat. If the entree is sautéed, request that the chef sauté it with very little butter or oil and add no extra fat before serving.

- **Beef.** Many restaurants pride themselves on serving huge slabs of beef or 12-ounce steaks. If you order beef, plan to cut this double portion in half and take the rest home for tomorrow's dinner, share it with a companion (who has ordered accordingly), or simply leave it. Trim all the visible fat and request that any gravy or sauce be served on the side so that you can use it sparingly, if at all. Your goal is to eat meat as the accompaniment to the meal, not as the focus. Your muscles will perform better if two-thirds of your plate is covered with carbohydrate-based potatoes, vegetables, and bread.

- **Potatoes.** Order extra to make potatoes the mainstay of your dinner. Baked potatoes are a great source of carbohydrates, unless the chef loads them up with butter or sour cream. Request that these toppings be served on the side so that you can control how much you eat. Better yet, trade those fat calories for more carbohydrates. Add moistness by mashing the potato with some milk (special request). This may sound a bit messy, but it's a delicious, low-fat way to enjoy what might otherwise be a dry potato.

- **Pasta.** Enjoy a pile! Pick pasta served with tomato sauces (carbohydrates) rather than the high-fat cheese, oil, or cream sauces.

Also be cautious of cheese-filled lasagna, tortellini, and manicotti, which can be high-fat choices.

- **Rice.** In a Chinese restaurant you'll be better off filling up on an extra bowl of plain rice, another good source of carbohydrates, rather than on egg rolls or other fried appetizers. Choose brown rice, if available.

- **Vegetables.** Request plain, unbuttered veggies with any special sauces (hollandaise, lemon butter) served on the side.

- **Chinese food.** Plain rice with stir-fry combinations such as chicken with veggies or beef with broccoli are the best choices. You can request that the food be cooked with very little oil.

- **Dessert.** Sherbet, low-fat frozen yogurt, angel cake, and fruit cups or berries are among the best choices for your sports diet. Fresh fruit is often available, even if it isn't listed on the menu. If you can't resist a decadent dessert, just be sure that you enjoy it after you eat a wholesome dinner. That is, don't have a carbohydrate-poor meal to save room for a high-fat dessert.

When you are faced with a meal that's all wrong for you, try to make the best of a tough situation. For example, you can scoop the sour cream off the potato, drain the dressing from the salad, scrape off the gravy, or remove the fried batter from the chicken. You can also top off a carbohydrate-poor meal with your own high-carbohydrate after-dinner snacks, such as fig bars, a bagel, pretzels, animal crackers, a banana, graham crackers, dried pineapple, raisins, and juice boxes. Pack these emergency foods to take with you. But also try to make special requests. Remember, you are the boss when it comes to restaurant eating. The job of the restaurant is to serve you the low-fat foods that enhance your health and your sports diet. Bon appetit!

Fast Foods That Fuel

Eating at a quick-service restaurant is like visiting Fat City. You have an easy opportunity to select a dietary disaster and choose items that are high in saturated fat and calories but low in carbohydrates, fiber, fruits, and vegetables. Although an occasional meal of a burger and fries is of little health concern, you need to balance fast foods that are a common part of your diet with wholesome, lower-fat choices. Fortunately for our health, most quick-service food centers offer healthful, low-fat options.

Travelers, in particular, need to learn how to fuel themselves wisely, even if on a budget. If you are a 140-pound (65-kilogram) athlete who needs 2,700 to 3,000 calories a day, the cheapest way to stave off hunger is to fill up on fatty foods—like tempting value meals. Bad idea. These high-fat meals not only clog the arteries and bulk up the waistline but also fail to fuel the muscles adequately. Table 4.2 provides some examples of healthful meals appropriate for a carbohydrate-rich sports diet. An even better bet is to carry carbs with you. Some easy-to-tote choices include bagels, crackers, fig bars, breakfast cereals, dried fruits, and trail mix.

The following menu ideas can help you healthfully navigate the world of fast foods without emptying your food budget.

- Any way you look at them, burgers and french fries have high fat content. You'll be better off going to an eatery that offers more than just burgers. Find a menu that offers grilled chicken or roast-beef sandwiches accompanied by soups (brothy or beany ones). Other options include roast or grilled chicken meals with mashed potatoes, rice, vegetables, and salad bars complete with kidney beans, chickpeas, and bread.

- If you order a burger, request a second roll or extra bread. Squish the grease into the first roll, then replace it with the fat-free roll. Boost carbohydrates with beverages such as juice, smoothies, or low-fat shakes. Pack supplemental carbohydrates, such as pretzels or fig bars.

- Shy away from value meals. You'll be better off having a burger and milk than having your money go "to waist" by choosing the meal deal.

- Beware of chicken sandwiches topped with a special mayonnaise-based sauce, which can make the sandwich as fatty as a fried-chicken sandwich. Request that the server hold the sauce or wipe off the mayo yourself.

- Meals with chicken that is roasted or grilled are generally preferable to fried-chicken meals. If you order fried chicken, get the larger pieces, remove all the skin, and eat just the meat. Order extra rolls, cornbread with honey or jam, corn on the cob, and other vegetables for more carbohydrates.

  Even though roasted chicken is preferable to fried, be aware that the roasted skin is still fatty. For example, by removing the skin and wing from a KFC Rotisserie Gold quarter breast, you remove 13 grams of fat and 115 calories.

  Although many of the accompaniments to chicken meals are laden with butter, any vegetable tends to be better than no vegetable. Ask if unbuttered, steamed veggies are an option.

TABLE 4.2

Sample Carbohydrate-Rich Restaurant Menus

The optimal sports diet gets most of its calories from carbohydrates. At quick-service restaurants, you can easily consume a suboptimal sports diet because fatty foods are readily available, inexpensive, and often tempting. Hence, you have to plan, bring wholesome snacks with you, and make special requests when possible.

The following menus are sample sports meals that offer at least 60 percent carbohydrates. Some of the food items (such as soft drinks) are not generally recommended as a part of an optimal daily diet, but you can incorporate them into a meal on the road from time to time.

The purpose of these sample meals is simply to give you an idea of what a carbohydrate-based sports diet looks like, so that you can use it to guide your food choices. The menus are appropriate for active women and men who need 2,000 to 2,600 or more calories per day. For extra carbohydrates, eat more of the foods listed in italics.

Meal	Item	Calories
Breakfast		
McDonald's	*Orange juice*, 6 oz	85
	Pancakes with *syrup*	420
	English muffin with *jelly*	155
	Total: 660 calories, 85% carbohydrates	
Dunkin' Donuts	*Bran muffin*, large	480
	Hot chocolate	210
	Total: 690 calories, 65% carbohydrates	
Family restaurant	*Apple juice*, large (10 oz)	145
	Raisin bran, 2 small boxes	220
	1% milk, 8 oz	110
	Sliced banana, medium-large	135
	Total: 610 calories, 90% carbohydrates	
Lunch		
Sub shop	Turkey sub, no mayo	590
	Cranapple juice (8 oz)	160
	Total: 750 calories, 60% carbohydrates	
Wendy's	*Baked potato*, plain	310
	Chili, large (12 oz)	300
	Frosty dairy dessert, small	340
	Total: 950 calories, 70% carbohydrates	

(continued)

TABLE 4.2 *(continued)*

Meal	Item	Calories
Lunch (continued)		
Salad bar	Lettuce, 1 cup	15
	Green pepper, 1/2	10
	Broccoli, 1/2 cup	20
	Carrots, 1/2 cup	20
	Tomato, large	50
	Chickpeas, 1/2 cup	160
	Feta cheese, 1 oz	75
	Italian dressing, 2 tbsp	100
	Bread, 1 slice	200
	Total: 650 calories, 60% carbohydrates	
Dinner		
Pizza	Cheese pan pizza, 2 slices	500
	Cola, 12 oz (no ice)	150
	Total: 650 calories, 60% carbohydrates	
Italian restaurant	*Minestrone soup*, 1 cup	90
	Spaghetti, 2 cups	400
	Tomato sauce, 2/3 cup	120
	Parmesan cheese, 1 tbsp	30
	Rolls, 2 large	280
	Total: 920 calories, 75% carbohydrates	
Family restaurant	Turkey, 5 oz white meat	250
	Stuffing, 1 cup	200
	Mashed potato, 1/2 cup	100
	Peas, 2/3 cup	70
	Cranberry sauce, 1/4 cup	100
	Orange juice, 8 oz	110
	Sherbet, 1 scoop	120
	Total: 950 calories, 65% carbohydrates	

- At a salad bar, be generous with the colorful vegetables and hearty breads but be careful to choose lite dressings. Also note that a caesar salad is not a dieter's delight. For example, Boston Market's Chicken Caesar Salad with dressing totals more than 800 calories. You'd have been better off eating a chicken breast (remove the skin and wing), corn bread, steamed vegetables, and whole kernel corn for 225 fewer calories and 46 grams less fat.
- Resist the temptation to choose baked potatoes smothered with high-fat toppings. Your best bet is to order an extra plain potato and split the broccoli and cheese topping (14 grams of fat) be-

tween the two. That way, you end up with a hearty 800-calorie, high-carbohydrate meal, with only 15 percent of the calories from fat. For additional protein, drink a glass of low-fat milk.

- Order thick-crust pizza that has extra crust rather than extra cheese. More dough means more carbohydrates. For example, a slice of Pizza Hut's pan pizza has 10 grams more carbohydrates than a slice of their thin crust pizza does. Pile on veggies (green peppers, mushrooms, onions) but shy away from the pepperoni, sausage, and hamburger. Don't be shy about using a napkin to blot the fat that cooks out of the cheese.

- Seek out the deli that offers wholesome breads. Request a sandwich that emphasizes the bread rather than the filling. A large submarine roll (preferably whole wheat) provides far more carbohydrates than half a small pita. Hold the mayo and add moistness with lite salad dressings (if available), mustard, or ketchup. The lowest fat fillings are turkey, ham, and lean roast beef.

- Hearty bean soups accompanied by crackers, bread, or corn bread provide a satisfying, carbohydrate-rich, low-fat meal. Chili, if not glistening with a layer of grease, can be a good choice. For example, a Wendy's large chili with eight saltines provides a satisfying 400 calories, and only 20 percent are from fat (nine grams).

Yes, you can eat a high-carbohydrate sports diet, even if you are eating fast foods. You simply need to balance the fats with the carbohydrates. Table 4.3 provides some appropriate choices (as well as some choices that are best avoided!).

Some Last Words About Supper

As I mentioned earlier, active people commonly eat a huge dinner as a result of having eaten too little during the day. If this sounds familiar, experiment with reorganizing your good-nutrition game plan so that you put more emphasis on breakfast and lunch as a means of fueling up and remaining fueled throughout the busy day. Use the evening meal as a time to refuel, but whenever possible keep it relatively equal in size to breakfast and lunch or lunches. As Gretchen, a kindergarten teacher said, "I used to stuff myself at night as a reward for having survived a hectic day. I'd arrive home stressed and tired, then overeat and feel lousy. Now I eat breakfast like a king, lunch like a prince, and dinner like a pauper. I've found that by eating this way, I have lots more energy for my students during the day and family in the evening. By eating a lighter dinner, I sleep much better and feel better overall."

TABLE 4.3

Fast-Food Calories

Although fast foods are often loaded with fat, they are certainly convenient and popular. If you routinely eat fast foods, you should make the lower fat choices—or at least balance the rest of your intake that day with low-fat fruits, vegetables, and fiber-rich breads and cereals. Bran cereal for breakfast and pasta with tomato sauce for dinner can balance a burger and fries for lunch. Remember, most sports-active women can target 600 to 700 calories per meal; sports-active men can consume 800 to 1,000 calories per meal.

McDonald's (www.mcdonalds.com)

	Cal.	Fat		Cal.	Fat
Hamburger	280	100	McDonaldland cookies	230	8
Quarter-Pounder	430	21	Fruit 'n Yogurt Parfait with granola	380	5
Quarter-Pounder with cheese	530	30	Egg McMuffin	290	12
Big Mac	590	34	Apple bran muffin, low-fat	300	3
Chicken McGrill	450	18	Bagel with ham, egg, cheese	480	31
without mayo	340	7	Biscuit	240	11
Chicken McNuggets (6)	290	17	Biscuit with bacon, egg, cheese	480	31
Sauce, sweet-n-sour	50	0	Hash browns	130	8
Filet-o-Fish	470	26	Hotcakes with 2 margarine, syrup	600	17
Grilled chicken caesar salad, plain	100	2	Hotcakes, plain	340	8
Fat-free vinaigrette	35	0	Breakfast burrito	290	16
Caesar dressing (1 package)	170	13	Orange juice, 6 oz	80	0
Garden salad, no dressing	100	6	Milk, 1%	100	2
French fries, small	210	10	Cola, large	310	0
French fries, medium	450	22	Shake, small chocolate or vanilla	360	9
French fries, supersize	610	29	McFlurry, M&M	630	23

Burger King (www.burgerking.com)

	Cal.	Fat		Cal.	Fat
Whopper	680	39	Chicken sandwich	660	39
Whopper without mayo	530	22	Chicken tenders (6 pieces)	250	14
Whopper, double with cheese, mayo	1,020	65	Fries, medium	360	18
BK Broiler Chicken	550	25	Onion rings, medium	320	16
BK Broiler Chicken without mayo	390	8	Croissanwich with sausage, egg, cheese	500	36

Domino's Pizza (www.dominos.com)

	Cal.	Fat		Cal.	Fat
Classic cheese, 1/4 of 14 in. large	515	15	Deep dish, 1/4 of 14 in. large	675	30
Thin-crust cheese, 1/4 of 14 in. large	380	16	Buffalo wings, hot (6)	270	14
Handtossed Deluxe Feast, 1/4 of			Handtossed Pepperoni Feast, 1/4 of		
14 in. large	625	24	14 in. large	730	34

Pizza Hut

	Cal.	Fat		Cal.	Fat
Pepperoni personal pan pizza	640	28	Supreme personal pan pizza	720	34

Kentucky Fried Chicken (www.kfc.com)

	Cal.	Fat		Cal.	Fat
Original recipe, breast 5.5 oz	400	24	Tender roast sandwich	270	5
Extra crispy, breast 6 oz	470	28	Corn on the cob	150	2
Crispy strips	400	24	Macaroni and cheese	130	6

Boston Market (www.bostonmarket.com)

	Cal.	Fat		Cal.	Fat
Chicken, 1/4, breast	170	4	Chicken sandwich, no cheese or sauce	390	5
Chicken, 1/4 with skin and wing	280	12	Chicken sandwich, with sauce, cheese	630	28
Chicken pot pie	750	46	Cornbread, 1 piece	200	6
Mashed potato, 3/4 cup	210	9	Butternut squash	150	6

Taco Bell (www.tacobell.com)

	Cal.	Fat		Cal.	Fat
Taco	210	12	Mexican pizza	550	31
Taco Supreme	260	16	Bean burrito	370	12
Soft taco, grilled chicken	190	7	Taco salad	850	52
Gordita, chicken baja	320	15	Nachos supreme	450	26
Gordita, beef	360	21	Pintos 'n Cheese	180	7

Au Bon Pain (www.aubonpain.com)

	Cal.	Fat		Cal.	Fat
Soup			*Sandwiches*		
Garden vegetable, medium	45	0	Thai chicken	420	6
Tomato Florentine, medium	90	2	Fields and feta	560	17
Vegetarian chili, medium	220	4	*Croissant*		
Salad without dressing			Plain	220	10
Garden, 1 container	160	1	Chocolate	400	24
Chicken caesar, 1 container	360	11	Sweet cheese	420	23
Oriental chicken	230	5	Spinach and cheese	290	16
Sandwich fillings			Ham and cheese	370	20
Smoked turkey, 3.75 oz	120	1	Turkey and cheddar	410	22
Roast beef	150	7	*Cookies*		
Tuna salad	310	24	Chocolate chip	280	15
Grilled chicken	130	4	Oatmeal raisin	250	10
Provolone cheese, 3 oz	300	22	Peanut butter	290	15
Rolls			*Muffin, Bagel, Danish*		
Petit pain	200	1	Bagel, plain	350	1
Hearth	220	2	Bagel, raisin	390	1
Sandwich rolls			Bran muffin	390	11
French	240	1	Low-fat triple berry muffin	270	3
Multigrain	260	2	Blueberry muffin	430	18
Croissant	300	14	Pecan roll	800	45

Dunkin' Donuts (www.dunkindonuts.com)

	Cal.	Fat		Cal.	Fat
Glazed, raised type	180	8	Chocolate-chip muffin	590	24
Jelly filled	210	8	Bagel, plain	340	2
Powdered sugar, cake type	270	15	Bagel, sesame	380	4
Glazed chocolate, cake type	310	17	Bagel sandwich (egg, cheese, bacon)	490	14
Munchkin, cake, cinnamon, 1	60	3	Croissant	290	18
Munchkin, glazed yeast, 1	40	2	Coffee with cream, sugar, 10 oz	90	6
Blueberry muffin (large)	490	17	Coffee Coolatta, 16 oz with cream	410	22
Blueberry muffin, reduced fat	450	12	Coffee Coolatta, 16 oz with skim milk	230	0
Bran muffin	490	16	Chocolate-chunk cookie	200	10

(continued)

TABLE 4.3 *(continued)*

Cinnabon				Cal.	Fat
	Cal.	Fat		Cal.	Fat
Cinnabon roll	670	34	Caramel pecan	890	41

Finagel a Bagel					
	Cal.	Fat		Cal.	Fat
Plain	360	0	Honey wheat	390	0

Mrs. Field's					
	Cal.	Fat		Cal.	Fat
Chocolate-chip cookie	250	13	Double fudge brownie	420	25
White chunk macadamia cookie	270	16			

Starbucks (1-800-23-LATTE)					
	Cal.	Fat		Cal.	Fat
Blueberry scone, cholesterol free	420	15	Cinnamon scone	530	26

Nutrition information from *Bowes & Church's Food Values of Portions Commonly Used*, 17th ed. (Philadelphia: Lippincott), food labels, Web sites, and corporate communications, July 2002.

5

Snacks for Cravings and Preexercise Energy

Once upon a time people ate three square meals a day. They rarely snacked. Today, people are forever seeking a quick energy fix, and snacks commonly make up 20 to 50 percent of total calories. If you are a big-time snacker, I encourage you to redefine snacks as meals so that you end up choosing wholesome food instead of cookies, chips, soft drinks, and other traditional energy boosters. In fact, I generally eliminate the word *snack* from my vocabulary. I teach my clients to think *two lunches* instead of *lunch* and *afternoon snack*. That way, they end up choosing wholesome foods (like vegetable soup) and not typical snacks (like sweets) in the afternoon.

Wise Snacking

Many of my clients believe that snacking is bad, because they snack on glazed doughnuts, snack cakes, candy bars, cookies, colas, and other

89

lackluster choices that fail to offer the nutrients needed for optimal performance. If this sounds like you, remember: Just as a car needs gasoline and spark plugs to function, your body needs calories (gas) and the vitamins, minerals, and proteins (spark plugs) found in wholesome foods to function well. If you want to have quality workouts, high energy, and good health, you need to fuel your body with quality calories. You can do this by thinking *second lunch* instead of *sweet snack.*

Some people try not to snack because they believe that eating between meals is sinful and fattening. The truth is that snacking is important. Active people tend to get hungry at least every four hours, so even if you have breakfast at 8:00 and lunch at noon, your body will still want a snack by 4:00 P.M., if not sooner. If you will be exercising in the afternoon, you need added fuel to energize your workout. Snacking is good for you and your workouts, and you should plan it as part of your sports diet.

Fast Snacks

When you are eating on the run and grabbing snacks instead of real meals, be sure to choose wholesome foods for these minimeals. You can make wise choices from among many nutritious and conveniently available items. Some popular suggestions include

- whole-grain bagel with peanut butter and a yogurt;
- thick-crust pizza with green peppers;
- peanut butter, crackers, and V-8 juice;
- trail mix with nuts and dried fruit;
- granola with low-fat milk and banana;
- Chinese takeout—stir-fry chicken with vegetables and steamed rice; and
- instant oatmeal made with low-fat milk.

Note that each of these minimeals includes foods from at least two food groups. The following list provides additional ideas for snacks and grazing at home and on the road. Ideally, you'll choose foods from different groups to help balance your diet. That way, even people who graze throughout the day can get a variety of nutrients needed for good health and top performance.

- **Dry cereal.** Mix your favorite cereal with raisins, dried fruits, cinnamon, or nothing!
- **Instant oatmeal.** Microwave the oatmeal in milk instead of water to boost its nutritional power. Sprinkle with raisins and chopped nuts.
- **Popcorn.** Eat plain or sprinkled with spices such as chili powder, garlic powder, onion powder, or soy sauce. If you like, spray with low-calorie butter-flavor sprays so that the spices stick.

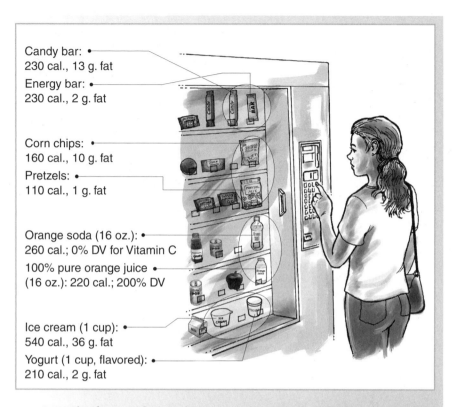

Candy bar:
230 cal., 13 g. fat
Energy bar:
230 cal., 2 g. fat

Corn chips:
160 cal., 10 g. fat
Pretzels:
110 cal., 1 g. fat

Orange soda (16 oz.):
260 cal.; 0% DV for Vitamin C
100% pure orange juice
(16 oz.): 220 cal.; 200% DV

Ice cream (1 cup):
540 cal., 36 g. fat
Yogurt (1 cup, flavored):
210 cal., 2 g. fat

- **Pretzels.** If you wish to reduce your salt intake, knock off the salt or buy salt-free pretzels.

- **Crackers.** Stoned wheat, sesame, bran, and other reduced-fat or fat-free brands are good choices.

- **Muffins.** Homemade with canola oil are best. If store bought, choose low-fat muffins; wholesome bran or corn muffins are better than those made with white flour (see the recipes in part III).

- **Bagels.** Whole-grain varieties provide more vitamins and minerals than do bagels made with white flour.

- **Fruits.** Choose oranges, bananas, apples, or any fresh fruit. When traveling, pack along dried fruit for concentrated carbohydrates. See the table at the end of this list for some of the best fruits.

- **Smoothies.** Whip together milk or juice, fresh or frozen fruit, and wheat germ or flax meal (see recipes beginning on page 355).

- **Frozen fruit bars.** You can slowly savor these pleasant treats in good health.

- **Yogurt.** Buy plain low-fat yogurt and flavor it with vanilla, honey, cinnamon, instant decaffeinated coffee, applesauce, fruit cocktail, or berries.

(continued)

(continued)

- **Energy bars, breakfast bars, low-fat granola bars.** Prewrapped and portable, these travel well in pockets and gym bags and can be very handy.
- **Nuts, seeds.** Peanuts, pistachios, almonds, sunflower seeds, pumpkin seeds, and other nuts and seeds are excellent for protein, B vitamins, vitamin E, and healthful fat.
- **Sandwiches.** Sandwiches don't have to be just for lunch; they are great for snacks. Use peanut butter, turkey, hummus, lean roast beef, or tuna with lite mayo.
- **Baked potatoes.** Microwave ovens make these a handy snack. They're tasty warm or cold, and because of their high glycemic effect, they are excellent for refueling your muscles after a hard workout. Try sweet potatoes with a dash of nutmeg—mmm!

Fruitful Snacks

Vitamin-packed and health-protective, fruit is a top-notch sports snack. To help you make the best choices, use this list, which orders fruits according to their content of nine vitamins and fiber. The higher the score, the more nutrient-dense the fruit.

Fruit	Nutrition score
Watermelon, 2 cups	310
Grapefruit, 1/2 pink or red	263
Papaya, 1/2	223
Cantaloupe, 1/4	200
Orange, 1 average	186
Strawberries, 1 cup	173
Kiwi, 1	115
Raspberries, 1 cup	106
Tangerine, 1 average	105
Mango, 1/2	94
Honeydew, 1/8 melon	85
Apricots, 2 fresh	78
Banana, 1	54
Peach, 1 large	47
Pear, 1 average	44
Apple, with skin, 1	43
Raisins, 1/4 cup packed	24
Pears, canned, 2 halves	20
Apple juice, unsweetened, 1/2 cup	14

Copyright 1995, CSPI. Adapted from *Nutrition Action Healthletter* (1875 Connecticut Ave., N.W., Suite 300, Washington, D.C. 20009-5728. $24.00 for 10 issues).

Energy Bars: Costly but Convenient

PowerBars, PRBars, Zone Bars, Balance Bars—a plethora of energy bars await you at every convenience store, each boasting its ability to enhance your performance. You can spend a fortune on these prewrapped bundles of energy, thinking they offer magic ingredients (not true). Here is some information to help you decide how much of your food budget to dedicate to these popular snacks.

- **Energy bars are convenient.** In today's eat-and-run society, when meals are a rare occurrence in a busy schedule, an energy bar suits the need for many hungry people who seek a hassle-free, somewhat nutritious snack.

- **Energy bars are portable.** You can easily tuck these compact and lightweight vitamin-enriched bars into a pocket for "emergency food." Energy bars are handy for runners and bikers who want to carry a durable snack on a long run or ride, or for hikers who want a light backpack.

- **Energy bars promote preexercise eating.** Snacking before exercising is a great way to boost stamina and endurance. The energy bar industry has done an excellent job of educating us that preexercise eating is important in optimizing performance. The associated energy boost likely does not result from magic ingredients (chromium, amino acids) but from eating 200 to 300 calories. These calories (which usually include some form of sugar) clearly fuel you better than the zero calories in no snack. Note that calories from tried-and-true fig bars, graham crackers, bananas, and granola bars are also effective preexercise energizers.

- **Energy bars promote eating during endurance exercise.** Energy bars are also a great way to boost stamina and endurance. Instead of relying on what you eat before you exercise, you can consume about 0.5 grams of carbohydrate per pound of body weight per hour during endurance exercise. This comes to 200 to 300 calories for most active people—exactly what an energy bar offers.

- **Most energy bars claim to be highly digestible.** One could debate whether energy bars are easier to digest than standard food, because digestibility varies greatly from athlete to athlete. I've heard some people comment about how a PowerBar settles heavily in the stomach, whereas others swear it is the only food they can tolerate during exercise. As with all sports snacks, you have to learn through trial and error during training what foods work for your system and what foods don't. Do not try this pricey treat for the first time before a special event, such as a marathon, bike race, or rugby game only to discover it causes discomfort. One key to tolerating energy bars is to drink plenty of water along with the bar. Otherwise, the product will settle poorly. Energy bars have a very low water content to make them more compact than fresh fruit, for example, which has high water content.

- **Some energy bars are touted as fat free or very low in fat.** The claim is that they digest quickly and empty from the stomach without causing problems.

- **Some energy bars boast about a higher fat content.** A higher fat content supposedly promotes greater fat burning to help you lose body fat and exercise longer before you hit the wall. To date, I know of no professional research that suggests that preexercise fat enhances weight loss (see chapter 11 for more information about fat burning and weight control).

  One possible advantage to including a little fat in the pre-exercise snack may be to provide sustained energy. A little fat can provide longer lasting energy for people who will be exercising for more than 90 minutes, such as long-distance bikers, runners, or cross-country skiers. The value of the preexercise fat will vary according to individual tolerance.

- **Energy bars are expensive.** You'll have to fork over at least one dollar, if not two, to buy most sports bars. The better value is to buy low-fat granola bars or breakfast bars from the supermarket at a much lower price. A handful of raisins can also do a great job at a low price (see table 5.1).

TABLE 5.1

Energy Bars Versus Standard Foods

Although energy bars are a convenient and popular energy source for sports snacks, standard foods can be just as effective at a much lower price.

Sports snack	Cal/oz	Carbs/oz	Cost /100 cal
Banana	20	5	$0.20
Raisins	90	22	$0.18
NutriGrain Cereal Bar	105	20	$0.26
Nature Valley Granola Bar	120	19	$0.24
PowerBar	100	19	$0.55
Luna Bar	107	15	$0.88
Balance bar	112	12	$0.75

Nutrition information from food labels and J. Pennington, 1998, *Bowes & Church's Food Values of Portions Commonly Used*, 17th ed. (Philadelphia: Lippincott).

Prices based in Boston, August 2002.

Snack Attacks

I always plan for an afternoon snack (rather, a second lunch) to boost my energy. This approach helps me concentrate better by maintaining my blood sugar level, taking the edge off my appetite, and fueling me for my after-work bike commute. I pack the snack along with lunch and take the time to eat it. I've learned that if I don't enjoy a few crackers with peanut butter at the office, I can easily devour too many crackers the minute I get home from work. Not snacking is a bad practice; I get too hungry and later overeat.

Snacks prevent not only hunger sensations but also cravings for sweets. Many of my clients complain about their constant cravings for sweets. They believe they are hopelessly, and helplessly, addicted to sugary snacks. I believe they are not addicted and that they can change their behavior. I've helped many clients resolve their problematic sweets cravings easily and painlessly. The solution is simple: Eat before you get too hungry. When you are ravenous, you tend to crave sweets and overeat.

If you frequently experience uncontrollable snack attacks, examine the following case studies and solutions to learn how to tame the cookie monster within you. Remember, snack attacks, not snacks per se, are the problem.

Case #1: Predinner Snack Attack

"I have the worst sweet tooth. I manage to fight sweet cravings until I get home and then I inevitably attack the chocolate-chip cookies. I feel as though I'm powerless and have no control over sweets. I hope you can put me on the straight and narrow."

—*David, 47-year-old marathon runner, accountant, and father*

Stories like David's are typical among my clients. He came to me feeling guilty about his lack of control over sweets. He required about 3,000 calories per day but ate zero calories at breakfast and barely ate lunch, only a 200-calorie yogurt, because he claimed he had no time. No wonder he was uncontrollably ravenous by the time he got home; he had accumulated a 2,800-calorie deficit! Nature took control by encouraging him to eat more than enough so that he would get adequate energy into his system.

I suggested that David eat his 1,600 cookie calories in the form of wholesome meals during the day. He started eating 800 calories for breakfast (cereal, milk, banana, juice, and bagel) and 1,000 calories of easy-to-eat snack-type foods for lunch and throughout the afternoon (two yogurts, two large bananas, two juices). Within one day he discovered that he wasn't a cookie monster after all. He could come home in a better mood, feel untempted by cookies, and have the energy to enjoy his family rather than be focused on eating cookies. This switch reduced his intake of fat, improved the quality of his overall diet, helped him flatten the spare tire that had been inflating around his middle, and lowered his cholesterol.

Case #2: Premenstrual Snack Attack

"Once a month I feel driven to devour a bag of chocolate kisses. I can easily tell the time of the month by my eating habits. Premenstrual chocolate cravings do me in."

—Charlene, 20-year-old active college student

Charlene, like many women, recognized that her eating patterns change with the stages of the menstrual cycle. In the week before her period, she has overwhelming sweet cravings; the week afterward, she tends to crave more protein foods or have very little appetite. Researchers have verified these eating patterns and report that a complex interplay of hormonal changes seems to influence women's food choices. High levels of estrogen may be linked with the premenstrual carbohydrate cravings.

Women also may crave carbohydrates because they are hungrier. Before menstruation, a woman's metabolic rate may increase by 100 to 500 calories (Barr, Janelle, and Prior 1995). That addition can be the equivalent of another meal. But when Charlene felt bloated and fat because of premenstrual water weight gain, she, like most women, would put herself on a reducing diet. The result was double deprivation. She had a physiological need for extra calories just when she put herself on the calorie-deficient reducing diet. No wonder she experienced overwhelming hunger and craved sweets.

I told Charlene not to diet but instead, when she felt hungry in the week before her period, to give herself permission to eat up to 500 additional wholesome calories. She started adding a slice of toast and jam to her standard breakfast, a hot cocoa at lunch, and an afternoon snack of some raisins. She successfully curbed the nagging hunger that had previously plagued her, and she was less irritable. Even her friends and family noticed a difference in her moods. She also lost interest in chocolate and was thrilled to survive a menstrual cycle without gaining weight from chocolate gluttony. By reading the nutrition information on the candy bag label, she was able to limit herself to 500 calories of chocolate kisses—no more!

Case #3: Chocolate Snack Attack

"Chocolate is my favorite food. I fight the urge to feed myself chocolate bars for lunch, brownies for snacks, and chocolate ice cream for dinner!"
—*Jocelyn, 17-year-old high school basketball player*

Some folks simply love sweets. They need no excuse to indulge in sugary goo. They eat sweets daily, three times if not more, starting with chocolate doughnuts for breakfast, cookies for lunch, sweet-and-sour pork for dinner, and then ice cream for dessert. Naturally, this high consumption of sweets results in a poor diet because sugar lacks vitamins and minerals.

Being a healthy, active teen, Jocelyn had space in her diet to fit in some sweets without jeopardizing health. For people eating an overall wholesome diet, about 6 to 10 percent of the calories can appropriately come from refined sugar, if desired (Institute of Medicine 2002). Because Jocelyn required 2,800-plus calories per day, she could certainly fit in 280 calories of sugar, a reasonable amount.

Sweets abusers are more at risk for nutritional problems than those who enjoy an occasional treat. Eating a little chocolate as a fun food for dessert after a nourishing meal is far different from eating a box of chocolates to replace that meal.

Chocoholics commonly skip breakfast because they're not hungry in the morning after eating a whole bag of chocolate-chip cookies the night before. They would nourish themselves better by eating one or two cookies for dessert and then waking up hungry for a wholesome breakfast the next morning.

In Jocelyn's case the chocolate problem stemmed from having no time for breakfast, disliking school lunch, and having easy access to the vending machine. I encouraged her to eat breakfast on her way to school, which helped her consume less chocolate during the day.

Snack Attacks: Bottom Line

Here are the key points you should remember about snacking and snack attacks:

- Snacks can be an important part of your training diet; they help prevent your becoming overwhelmingly hungry. Remember that when you get too hungry you may not care about what you eat, and you may blow your good intentions on fat and goo.

- A sugary treat can fit into a well-balanced diet. Eating a cookie for dessert after lunch is fine. The nutrition problems arise when you have cookies *for* lunch.

- If you find yourself craving sweets, determine whether you've eaten adequate calories to support your activities. Chances are you've let yourself get too hungry. Sweet cravings are commonly a sign that you are physiologically ravenous.
- Prevent sweet cravings by eating more calories at breakfast and lunch (and plan an afternoon snack or second lunch if you will be eating a late dinner) so that you curb the cookie monster that tends to arise in the late afternoon and evening.

Energizing Your Exercise

Snacking before you exercise will help energize your workout. A pre-exercise snack has four main functions:

1. To help prevent hypoglycemia (low blood sugar) with its symptoms of lightheadedness, needless fatigue, blurred vision, and indecisiveness—all of which can interfere with top performance
2. To help settle your stomach, absorb some of the gastric juices, and abate hunger
3. To fuel your muscles, both with food eaten in advance that is stored as glycogen, and with food eaten within an hour of exercise
4. To pacify your mind with the knowledge that your body is well fueled

Yet many people purposefully exercise on empty because they believe that exercising without having eaten beforehand enhances fat burning. True, but they assume that by burning more body fat, they will lose more body fat. False. To lose body fat, you need to create a calorie deficit by the end of the day. Whether you burn carbs or fats has less to do with losing body fat than it does with your calorie balance at the end of the day. The truth is you'll be able to exercise harder and burn more calories if you eat a preexercise snack. The harder exercise might contribute to the desired calorie deficit. See chapter 11 for more information on appropriate methods to lose weight.

Many people are also afraid that preexercise food will result in an upset stomach, diarrhea, and sluggish performance. Of course, too much of the wrong kinds of foods can cause intestinal problems, but lack of fuel is more often the cause of sluggish performance. Morning exercisers, in particular, need to be sure they have fueled themselves adequately, even if they work out before breakfast.

Snacks Before Morning Workouts

Skipping breakfast is a common practice among people who exercise in the morning. If you roll out of bed and eat nothing before you jump into the swimming pool, participate in a spinning class, or go for a run, you may be running on fumes. You will probably perform better if you eat something before you exercise. During the night, you can deplete your liver glycogen, the source of carbohydrates that maintains normal blood sugar levels. When you start a workout with low blood sugar, you fatigue earlier than you would have if you had eaten something.

How much one should eat varies from person to person, ranging from a few crackers to a slice of bread, a glass of juice, a bowl of cereal, or a whole breakfast. If you've had a large snack the night before, you'll be less needy of early morning food. But if you've eaten nothing since a 6:00 P.M. dinner the night before, your blood sugar will definitely need a boost. Most people feel good results with 0.5 grams of carbohydrate (2 calories) per pound (1 gram per kilogram) of body weight one hour before moderately hard exercise, and 2 grams of carbohydrates (8 calories) per pound (4 grams per kilogram) of body weight four hours beforehand. For a 150-pound (68-kilogram) person this is 75 to 300 grams (300 to 1,200 calories) of carbohydrate—the equivalent of a small bowl of cereal with a banana to a big stack of pancakes (ACSM et al. 2000).

Defining the best amount of preexercise food is difficult because tolerances vary greatly from person to person. Some athletes get up an hour early just to eat and then go back to bed and allow time for the food to settle. Others have a few bites of a bagel, a banana, or some other easy-to-digest food as they dash out the door. Then there are those who habitually run on empty. If that's you, an abstainer, here is a noteworthy study that might convince you to experiment with eating a morning snack before you work out.

Researchers asked a group of athletes to bike moderately hard for as long as they could. When they ate breakfast (400 calories of carbohydrates) 3 hours before the exercise test, they biked for 136 minutes, as compared with 109 minutes with only water (Schabort et al. 1999). Clearly, these athletes were able to train better with some gas in their tank. Preexercise morning fuel will likely work for you, too!

Four hundred calories is the equivalent of an average bowl of cereal with some milk and banana; it's not a pile of pancakes. You need not eat tons of food to notice a benefit; some food is helpful but more food may not be better. Eat what's comfortable for you and learn what is the right amount to fuel your workouts but still settle well.

Snacks Before Afternoon Workouts

Joe, an afternoon runner, wondered if eating a bagel at 3:00 would provide energy for his 4:00 workout or simply sit in his stomach. I explained that, despite popular belief, the food one eats before a workout is digested and used for fuel during exercise. The body can indeed digest food during exercise, as long as you are exercising at a pace you can maintain for more than 30 minutes. Cyclists who ate 300 calories before exercise absorbed all 300 calories during the hour of moderate to somewhat hard exercise (Sherman, Pedan, and Wright 1991).

If Joe were to do extremely intense sprint activity such as a track workout or time trial, the food would be more apt to sit in his stomach and talk back to him. During intense exercise the stomach shuts down so that more blood can flow to the muscles. Therefore, you need to plan your schedule and eat a hearty lunch at noon if you will be doing a hard workout at 4:00 (with no preexercise snack because of the intensity of the workout).

Here is a second study that demonstrates the importance of eating before you exercise. In this study cyclists ate either nothing or 1,200 calories of carbohydrates (two grams of carbohydrates per pound of body weight) four hours before an exercise test to exhaustion. When they ate the 1,200-calorie meal they were able to bike 15 percent harder during the last 45 minutes, as compared with when they ate nothing. Given that road races and many competitive events are won or lost by fractions of a second, to be 15 percent stronger offers a huge advantage (Sherman et al. 1989). The carbohydrates the cyclists ate before they exercised supplied extra fuel for the end of the workout, when their glycogen stores were low.

Although these studies looked at cyclists, who tend to report fewer gastrointestinal complaints than do athletes in running sports that jostle the stomach, the benefits are worth noting. If you've always exercised on an empty stomach, you may discover that you can exercise harder and longer with an energy booster. Experiment during training with eating some carbohydrate-based snacks within a few minutes to four hours before you exercise. If you swim at 6 A.M., munch on a bagel on the way to the pool. If you work out at lunch, be sure to eat carbs such as cereal for breakfast and a banana for a 10 A.M. snack. If you exercise after work, have a substantial lunch and then a yogurt and energy bar for a second lunch later that afternoon.

What's the Best Time to Eat?

The trick to completing your workout with energy to spare is to fuel up at the right time before the event. Here are some suggestions for different types of events at different times of the day.

Time: 8 A.M. event, such as a road race or swim meet

Meals: Eat a high-carbohydrate dinner and drink extra water the day before. On the morning of the event, about 6:00 or 6:30, have a light 200- to 400-calorie meal (depending on your tolerance), such as yogurt and a banana or one or two energy bars, tea or coffee if you like, and extra water. Eat familiar foods. If you want a larger meal, consider getting up to eat by 5:00 or 6:00.

Time: 10 A.M. event, such as a bike race or soccer game

Meals: Eat a high-carbohydrate dinner and drink extra water the day before. On the morning of the event, eat a familiar breakfast by 7:00 to allow three hours for the food to digest. This meal will prevent the fatigue that results from low blood sugar. If your body cannot handle any breakfast, eat a late snack before going to bed the night before. The snack will help boost liver glycogen stores and prevent low blood sugar the next morning.

Time: 2 P.M. event, such as a football or lacrosse game

Meals: An afternoon game allows time for you to have either a big, high-carbohydrate breakfast and a light lunch or a substantial brunch by 10:00, allowing four hours for digestion time. As always, eat a high-carbohydrate dinner the night before and drink extra fluids the day before and up to noon.

Time: 8 P.M. event, such as a basketball game

Meals: You can thoroughly digest a hefty, high-carbohydrate breakfast and lunch by evening. Plan for dinner, as tolerated, by 5:00 or have a lighter meal between 6:00 and 7:00. Drink extra fluids all day.

Time: All-day event, such as a hike, 100-mile bike ride, or triathlon training

Meals: Two days before the event, cut back on your exercise. Take a rest day the day before to allow your muscles the chance to replace depleted glycogen stores. Eat carbohydrate-rich meals at breakfast, lunch, and dinner (see chapter 7 for information about carbo loading). Drink extra fluids. On the day of the event, eat a tried and true breakfast depending on your tolerance.

While exercising, at least every 1 1/2 to 2 hours plan to eat carbohydrate-based foods (energy bars, dried fruit, sports drinks) to maintain normal blood sugar. If you stop at lunchtime, eat a comfortable meal, but in general try to distribute your calories evenly throughout the day. Drink fluids before you get thirsty; you should need to urinate at least three times throughout the day.

Preexercise Caffeine: A Stimulating Topic

Caffeinated beverages are popular with some athletes who believe caffeine enhances exercise performance by making the effort seem easier and allowing them to exercise longer. But for others, preexercise coffee puts them over the edge. When they are already jittery before a competitive event, a caffeine jag is the last thing they need.

Because caffeine stimulates the release of fats into the blood, researchers originally thought that the working muscles would burn more of these fats for energy and spare the limited muscle glycogen stores. Recent research does not support this hypothesis (Hawley 2002), particularly among competitive athletes who are already wired on adrenaline with similar fat-releasing effects.

Caffeine's energy-enhancing effect is more likely related to its ability to make exercise seem easier. Through its stimulant effect upon the brain, caffeine may reduce the fatigue associated with long bouts of exercise. If you are chronically tired from the rigors of your training program, you may be particularly attracted to caffeine for this reduction in perceived exertion.

If you do not commonly drink coffee or consume caffeinated beverages, you may receive greater energy-enhancing effects for preexercise caffeine than if you are a regular coffee drinker. A study comparing nonusers to regular caffeine users reports that the nonusers exercised for 8 1/2 minutes longer on an exercise test (biking very hard to exhaustion) compared with when they had no preexercise caffeine. The regular users exercised for only 4 minutes longer when they had the caffeine (Bell 2002). You might think that the results of this study would put caffeine high on my recommended list. It's not. The jitters and other adverse effects of coffee may negate those reported benefits. If you are already hyper with precompetition adrenaline, you are unlikely to need the additional stimulation of caffeine.

Caffeine taken before exercise has been reputed to have a diuretic effect. The newest research, however, negates that belief. According to Dr. Larry Armstrong, an exercise physiologist at the University of Connecticut, caffeine does not contribute to water loss and is OK for athletes even in hot weather (Armstrong 2002).

Although a cup or two of coffee before exercise may be a helpful energizer, more may be of little value. A 1995 study (Pasman et al. 1995) showed that well-trained cyclists performed equally well with about 350 milligrams of caffeine as they did with 850 milligrams. So if you're tempted to jazz yourself up with a second mugful, think again. You may find that the second mug will do you in with the caffeine jitters. In addition, too much caffeine is illegal according to the International Olympic Committee. Caffeine is 1 of more than 50 drugs banned by the International Olympic Committee. The irony is that small doses of caffeine (such as taken socially) may enhance performance, whereas high doses (such as amounts that are banned) are counterproductive to performance. Table 5.2 lists the caffeine amounts in some common perk-me-ups.

TABLE 5.2

Caffeine Sources

Source of caffeine	Average caffeine content (mg)
Coffee, 12 oz.	
Brewed, drip method	200
Instant	115
Decaffeinated	6
Tea, 12 oz brewed	25-110
Iced tea, 12 oz	40-75
Hot cocoa, 12 oz	8
Soft drink, 12 oz*	
Coca Cola, regular or diet	45
Pepsi	40
Diet Pepsi	35
Pepsi One	55
Sunkist Orange Soda	40
Barq's Root Beer	20
Mello Yello, regular or diet	50
Mountain Dew, regular and diet	55
Snapple, Decaffeinated Lemon Tea	5
Snapple, Lemon Tea	30
Snapple, Peach Tea	30
Drug	
Anacin, 1 tablet	32
Excedrin, 1 tablet	65
Dexatrim, 1 tablet	80
No Doz, Maximum strength, 1 tablet	200

*Small children who drink a can of cola can receive the equivalent in caffeine to the adult who drinks a cup of coffee.

Caffeine data from International Food Information Council, 1998 (www.ific.org); the National Soft Drink Association (www.nsda.org/whatsin/caffeinecontent.html); food labels; and J. Pennington, 1998, *Bowes & Church's Food Values of Portions Commonly Used*, 17th ed. (Philadelphia: Lippincott).

Many folks drink a warm mug of coffee not for an energy boost but because a warm liquid promotes regular bowel movements and helps empty them out before they exercise. This may be the most justifiable reason for some people to include this brew in their preexercise diet. After all, if you are so tired that you seek coffee for its stimulant effect, you should probably be resting and not dragging yourself through a workout. Be sure no trouble is brewing in your desire for caffeine!

Quick Fixes

If you have failed to eat enough breakfast, first lunch and second lunch, or lunch and afternoon snack, you can easily start hankering for some candy. As I mentioned earlier in this chapter this craving is a sign you have become too hungry. You can prevent sweet cravings and the need for a quick energy fix by eating a bigger breakfast and lunch. But questions arise about preexercise sugar. Is it detrimental to performance?

Eating a high-sugar food during the period 15 to 45 minutes before you exercise might have a negative effect if you are sensitive to swings in blood sugar. Sugary soft drinks and even fruit juices offer a short-term energy boost that later may hinder performance by contributing to hypoglycemia (low blood sugar) shortly after you start to exercise.

A concentrated dose of sugar (either natural sugar in fruit juice or refined sugar in soft drinks and jelly beans) rapidly boosts your blood sugar but simultaneously triggers the pancreas to secrete an abnormally large amount of insulin. Insulin transports excess sugar out of the blood and into the muscles. Exercise, like insulin, similarly enhances this transport. Thus, your blood sugar can drop to an abnormally low level once you start to exercise. Some athletes are more susceptible than others to negative effects caused by this rebound hypoglycemia.

Such was the case with Jackson, a teacher who liked to take a spin class after work, at about 4:00 in the afternoon. Because he was trying hard to lose weight, he ate only small portions at breakfast and lunch. By the time he left work for the 4:00 spin class, he was drained and searched for a quick energy boost—a can of soda pop. Within 10 to 15 minutes after beginning the spin class, he felt lightheaded, shaky, uncoordinated, and unmotivated to continue. On some days he even had to stop for a rest. The rapid drop in blood sugar interfered with his ability to exercise. I suggested that he trade his quick-fix calories for more calories at lunch. That change did the trick. He ate an extra half sandwich at lunch (150 calories) instead of an afternoon can of cola (150 calories), and he enjoyed his higher energy level.

Despite popular belief, most athletes can tolerate a preexercise sugar fix without physical problems (Horowitz and Coyle 1993). Even a candy bar eaten five minutes beforehand is unlikely to hurt performance. But a better solution than consuming preexercise sweets is to maintain a high energy level throughout the day by eating adequate calories at breakfast and lunch. Research shows that people who eat a good meal four hours before they exercise perform better than those who eat no snack, and that a meal plus a snack just five minutes before exercise helps them work best.

Without doubt, breakfast and lunch are the best energy boosters. But if for whatever reason you have skipped breakfast or lunch and are hungry and craving sweets before your afternoon workout, eat the sweets within 10 minutes of exercise if you are concerned about experiencing a sugar low. This plan will minimize the risk of a possible hypoglycemic reaction, because the insulin will not have greatly increased in that short period.

Going by Your Gut

Although a preexercise meal or snack can improve your workout, it can also hinder your workout if it results in gastric distress. Each person has unique food preferences and aversions, so no one food or magic meal will ensure top performance for everyone.

- Frank, a competitive runner, avoids any food within four hours of training or competing. Otherwise, he has horrible stomach cramps.
- Kristin, a loyal exerciser at a health club, thrives best on a plain bagel an hour before her morning routine. "It absorbs the stomach juices and settles my stomach."
- Sarah, a gymnast and eighth-grade student, snacks on a banana before practice sessions but on nothing before a competition. She gets so nervous that she can't keep anything down. "I make sure I eat extra the day before a competition."

Choices of what to eat before exercising vary from person to person and from sport to sport, with no single right or wrong choice. My experience has shown that each athlete has to learn though trial and error during training and competitions what works best for his or her body and what doesn't work. Some people can eat almost anything, others want special foods, and then there are the abstainers who have absolutely no desire to eat anything.

Athletes in running sports, in which the body moves up and down, tend to experience more digestive problems than those in sports in which the stomach is relatively stable. Jostling seems to be a risk factor for abdominal distress; food eaten too close to exercise time can often talk back. For that reason, Walter, a 21-year-old triathlete and college student, eats according to his sport of the day. "When I bike, I enjoy a reasonable meal before the ride and munch on goodies during the workout, or even stop for a frozen yogurt. When I run, I have to abstain from food for three hours before a workout, or I get diarrhea. That's one reason why I prefer biking to running."

To Eat or Not to Eat

Certainly, preexercise foods that settle comfortably can enhance stamina, endurance, strength, and enjoyment. But with the possibility that preexercise food can create intestinal chaos, the threat of diarrhea can turn the thought of pancakes into panic. Adverse reactions occur in 30 to 50 percent of endurance athletes. Complaints include stomach and upper gastrointestinal (GI) problems (heartburn, vomiting, bloating, heaviness of food, and stomach pain) and intestinal and lower GI problems (gas, intestinal cramping, urge to defecate, loose stools, and diarrhea).

You should know about some of the predisposing factors for GI problems:

- **Type of sport.** Cyclists, swimmers, cross-country skiers, and others who exercise in a relatively stable position report fewer GI problems than do athletes in sports that jostle the intestines.

- **Training status.** Untrained people who are starting an exercise program report more GI problems than do well-trained athletes who have built up tolerance to exercise. If you are a novice who is experiencing GI distress, gradually increase your training volume and intensity so that your body can adjust to the changes.

- **Age.** GI problems occur more frequently in younger athletes than in veterans, because the younger athlete may be less trained and possibly have less nutrition knowledge and experience with precompetition eating. Veterans, on the other hand, have had the opportunity to learn from years of nutritional mistakes.

- **Gender.** Women, as compared with men, report more GI problems, particularly at the time of the menstrual period. The hormonal shifts that occur during menstruation can contribute to looser bowel movements.

- **Emotional and mental stress.** Athletes who are tense are more likely to report that food in the stomach lingers longer and settles like a lead balloon.

- **Exercise intensity.** During easy and even moderately hard exercise, the body can both digest food and comfortably exercise. But during intense exercise, the shift of blood flow from the stomach to the working muscles may be responsible for GI complaints.

- **Precompetition food intake.** Eating too much high-protein and high-fat food (such as bacon and eggs or greasy burgers) shortly before exercise can cause GI problems. Tried-and-true low-fat, carbohydrate-rich favorites (such as oatmeal or bananas) that are part of your day-to-day training diet are a safer bet.

- **Fiber.** High-fiber diets intensify GI complaints. If you are eating large amounts of bran cereal or high-fiber energy bars, try cutting back for a week to see if you feel better.

- **Caffeine.** Some athletes seek enhanced performance from drinking a larger-than-usual mug of coffee but end up with an upset stomach, diarrhea, and substandard performance.

- **Gels and concentrated sugar solutions.** Highly concentrated sugar solutions consumed during exercise may cause stomach distress. Don't confuse the high-carb recovery drinks (about 200 calories per eight ounces, or per one-quarter liter) with low-carb fluid replacers.

- **Level of hydration.** Dehydration enhances the risk of intestinal problems. During training, be sure to practice drinking different fluids on a regular schedule (eight ounces every 15 to 20 minutes of strenuous exercise) to learn how your body reacts to water, sports drinks, diluted juice, and any fluids that you will be drinking during competition.

- **Hormonal changes that occur during exercise.** The digestive process is under hormonal control, and exercise stimulates changes in these hormones. For example, the postmarathon levels of GI hormones in marathon runners tend to be two to five times higher than resting levels. These hormonal changes can result in food traveling faster through the digestive system and explain why some people experience GI problems regardless of what they eat.

Preexercise Snack Guidelines

To determine the right pretraining or precompetition snack or meal for your body, experiment with the following guidelines. You may find your food preferences vary with the type of exercise, level of intensity, and time of day. For example, cyclists and skiers often eat differently than do high-intensity runners and basketball players.

- On a daily basis eat adequate high-carbohydrate meals to fuel and refuel your muscles so that they'll be ready for action. Snacks eaten within an hour before exercise primarily keep you from feeling hungry and maintain your blood sugar; they don't significantly replenish muscle glycogen stores. The best refueling starts within an hour after exercise. (See chapter 6.)

- If you will be exercising for more than 60 to 90 minutes and will be unable to consume calories during that time, choose slowly digested carbohydrates with a moderate to low glycemic effect (see table 7.1 on page 142 and table 7.2 on page 148). Yogurt, bananas, oatmeal, bean soup, lentils, and apples are just a few choices. When eaten an hour before exercise, the foods will be digested enough to be burned for fuel and then will continue to provide sustained energy during the long workout. Chapter 7 contains detailed information about carbohydrate loading for endurance events.

- If you will be exercising for less than an hour, simply snack on any tried-and-true foods that digest easily and settle comfortably. Bread, english muffins, bagels, crackers, and pasta are a few of the most popular high-carb, low-fat preexercise choices.

- Limit high-fat proteins like cheese omelets, hamburgers, and fried chicken because they take longer to empty from the stomach. This occurs because fat delays gastric emptying. Cheeseburgers with french fries, large ice cream cones, and pancakes glistening with butter have been known to contribute to sluggishness, if not to nausea. Note that small servings of lean protein-rich foods (turkey, eggs, low-fat milk), however, can settle well and keep you from feeling hungry.

- Be cautious with sugary foods (such as soft drinks, jelly beans, gels, and even lots of maple syrup or sports drinks) or foods with a high glycemic effect (a large plain potato, honey, corn flakes, or a bowl of plain white rice). Although most athletes perform well after a preexercise sugar fix, some athletes who eat these types of carbohydrates within 15 to 120 minutes before hard exercise experience a drop in blood sugar that leaves them feeling tired, lightheaded, and needlessly fatigued. By experimenting with eating sugary or high-glycemic foods before training sessions, you can learn how your body responds.

- Allow adequate time for food to digest. Remember that high-calorie meals take longer to leave the stomach than hearty, lighter snacks. The general rule is to allow at least three to four hours for a large meal to digest, two to three hours for a smaller meal, one to two hours for a blended or liquid meal, and less than an hour for a small snack, according to your own tolerance.

If you are going to participate in a road race at 10:00, you might want to eat only a light 400-calorie breakfast such as a bowl of cereal between 7:00 and 8:00 a.m. A hefty 1,000- to 1,200-calorie pancake breakfast might weigh you down. For a noon event, you could adequately digest a pancake breakfast that you ate at 8:00 a.m.

- Allow more digestion time before intense exercise than before low-level activity. Your muscles require more blood during intense exercise than they do at rest, so your stomach may get only 20 percent of its normal blood flow during a hard workout. This shortfall slows the digestive process. Any food in the stomach jostles along for the ride and may feel uncomfortable or be regurgitated.

  During exercise of moderate intensity, blood flow to the stomach is 60 to 70 percent of normal and you can still digest food. The snacks that recreational skiers, cyclists, and even ultrarunners eat before and during exercise do get digested and contribute to lasting energy during long-term, moderate-intensity events.

- If you have a finicky stomach, experiment with liquid meal replacers to see whether they offer you any advantage. Liquid foods tend to leave the stomach faster than solid foods do. In one research study, a 450-calorie meal of steak, peas, and buttered bread remained in the stomach for six hours. A liquefied version of the same meal emptied from the stomach two hours earlier (Brouns, Saris, and Rehrer 1987). Before converting to a liquid pre-event meal, be it a homemade blenderized meal or a can of a commercial meal replacement, experiment during training to determine if this new food offers you any advantage.

- If you know that you'll be jittery and unable to tolerate any food before an event, make a special effort to eat well the day before. Have an extralarge bedtime snack in lieu of breakfast. Some athletes can comfortably eat before they exercise, but others prefer to abstain. Both sorts perform well, and both have simply learned how to fuel their bodies in the best way.

- If you have a "magic food," be sure to pack it along with you when traveling to an event. Even if it's a standard item such as bananas, pack it so that you will be certain to have it on hand. Even if you have no favorite foods, you still might want to pack a tried-and-true favorite in case of an emergency. If you should encounter delays, such as being stuck in traffic or stranded at an airport, you'll still be able to eat adequately. Emergency foods might include durable carbohydrates that don't easily crumble, such as fig bars, dried fruits, granola bars, or bagels.

- Always eat familiar foods before a competition. Don't try anything new! New foods always carry the risk of settling poorly; causing intestinal discomfort, acid stomach, heartburn, or cramps; or necessitating pit stops. Schedule a few workouts of intensity similar to and at the same time of day as an upcoming competition and experiment with different foods to determine which (and how much) will be best on race day. Never try anything new before a competition, unless you want to risk impairing your perfor- mance.

- Drink plenty of fluids. You are unlikely to starve to death dur- ing an event, but you might dehydrate. I suggest you drink an extra four to eight glasses of fluid the day before, so that you overhydrate. Drink about two or three glasses of fluid up to two hours before the event and drink another one to two glasses 5 to 10 minutes before the start.

Sports Supplements for Quick Fixes

When athletes get tired and experience poor workouts, they often start to think about sports supplements that might offer more energy. Substances like ginseng, ephedra, Echinacea, and ma huang start to become a source of curiosity. Perhaps you feel that one or two of these will help you feel better.

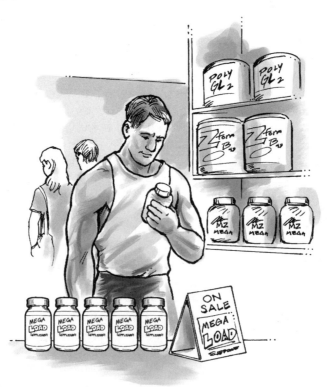

Many people do not know that the Food and Drug Administration poorly regulates dietary supplements for quality and purity. What you take may not be what's on the label. You have to ask yourself: Do I really want to take a questionable product? It's not uncommon for a collegiate athlete to be disqualified from his or her sport because of positive drug testing related to the consumption of questionable sports supplements.

Rather than look for a quick fix, the best bet is to be responsible and fuel your body on a regular schedule. Breakfast, lunch, and a preexercise snack are the best and safest quick fixes around. If you have questions about sports supplements, the National Agricultural Library's Food and Nutrition Information Center offers abundant Internet information on supplements as well as links to other sources of credible information. Log on to www.nal.usda.gov/fnic and click on Dietary Supplements.

Snacking Is Important

Most active people need and should eat snacks to keep them fueled throughout the day. The snack also prevents extreme hunger that commonly leads to extreme cravings for sweets and other such treats. By snacking on grains, fruits, vegetables, and low-fat dairy foods from the base of the food pyramid, you'll be able to curb hunger and be content to enjoy carrots rather than carrot cake, and apples rather than apple pie.

When and if you choose to snack on sweets and treats, be sure to eat only a small amount from the tip of the pyramid, after you have climbed to the top by first eating basic foods. Otherwise, your diet will end up the shape of an upside-down pyramid that topples your health and sports performance.

Appropriate preexercise snacks benefit optimal performance by preventing dehydration and maintaining normal blood sugar. You should consume adequate preexercise fluids and carbohydrates, as tolerated by your body. In general, most active people can enhance their performance with 200 to 300 calories of carbohydrates within an hour or two before the workout.

6

Fueling During and After Exercise

Just as what you eat *before* you exercise greatly affects your energy levels, so does what you eat *during* extensive exercise. Hence, students who practice after-school sports from 3:30 to 5:30, businesspeople who work out at the health club from 5:30 to 7:00 P.M., marathoners who train for one to two hours, and others who exercise for more than 60 to 90 minutes need to think about fueling during exercise. Unfortunately, many of these folks are in such a rush to start their workouts that they fail to bring with them the foods and fluids that will enhance their exercise efforts.

If you have concerns about how to prevent fatigue during your workouts, this chapter will help you enjoy high energy and enhanced stamina during exercise sessions that last longer than an hour. Standard healthy eating practices should take care of shorter sessions. That is, if you are doing fitness exercise for 30 to 45 minutes, a simple preexercise snack and plenty of water should fuel you well. But when you're pushing the limits, you'll want to pay proper attention to what you eat and drink during and after your hard workouts.

Eating During Extensive Exercise

Ideally, during extensive exercise that lasts for more than 60 to 90 minutes, you should try to balance your water and energy output with enough fluid to match your sweat losses and enough carbohydrates to provide energy and maintain normal blood sugar level. You can significantly increase your stamina by consuming about 100 to 250 calories (30 to 60 grams) of carbohydrates per hour while performing endurance exercise, after the first hour (ACSM et al. 2000). This might be four eight-ounce glasses (about one liter) of a sports drink (50 calories per eight ounces), two cups (500 milliliters) of a sports drink and a banana, or an energy bar (plus extra water).

During a moderate to hard endurance workout, carbohydrates supply about 50 percent of the energy. As you deplete carbohydrates from muscle glycogen stores, you increasingly rely on blood sugar for energy. By consuming carbohydrates during exercise, such as the sugar in sports drinks, your muscles have an added source of fuel. Sports drinks also help maintain normal blood sugar level. Because much of performance depends on mental stamina, you should maintain normal blood sugar level to keep your brain fed and help you think clearly, concentrate well, and remain focused.

Your body doesn't care if you ingest solid or liquid carbohydrates; both are equally effective (Mason, McConell, and Hargreaves 1993). You just have to learn which foods and fluids settle best in your body. Despite popular belief, even sugar can be a positive snack during exercise and is unlikely to cause rebound hypoglycemia, because sugar feedings during exercise result in only small increases in both insulin and blood glucose. For snacks during exercise, some people prefer the natural sugars from fruits and juices, some choose gels or energy bars, and others prefer sports drinks or hard candy. You need to experiment to determine what foods or fluids work best for you and how much is appropriate.

Also keep in mind that too much sugar or food taken at once can slow down the rate at which fluids leave the stomach and become available to replace sweat losses. Be more conservative with your sugar fixes during intense exercise in hot weather, when rapid fluid replacement is perhaps more important than carbohydrate replacement. In cold weather, however, when the risk of becoming dehydrated is lower, sugar fixes can provide much-needed energy.

Because consuming 100 to 250 calories or more per hour (after the first hour) may be far more than you are used to consuming during exercise, you need to practice eating during training to figure out what foods and fluids do or do not work. Alex, a novice marathoner, tucked hard candies, gummy bears, and chocolate mints in a waist pack that he wore on his long runs. He also hid a cooler with a granola bar, a banana, and bottles filled with sports drink on his running loop. Between the snacks and the sports drink, he was able to maintain adequate energy during his three-hour training runs and simultaneously learn what he liked to eat during exercise. On marathon day, he assigned friends to specific checkpoints along the route. Their jobs were to keep him well supplied with a variety of these carbohydrates. He never hit the wall, and he was pleased with his time.

Whatever the situation, endurance athletes such as marathon runners, ultradistance cyclists, and Ironman triathletes need to make a nutrition plan far in advance of the event and experiment during training to learn if they prefer grape or lemon sports drinks, solid foods or liquids, energy bars or bananas. By developing a list of several tried-and-true foods that taste good even when you are hot and tired, you need not worry about what to eat (and what not to eat) on race day.

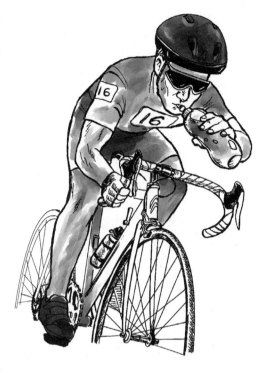

Ideally, you should have a defined feeding plan for the event and know

- your fluid targets, as determined by weighing yourself naked before and after a workout in different temperatures to determine sweat loss per hour, and

- your calorie targets. By working with a sports nutritionist or exercise physiologist and the information in tables 11.1 and 11.2 on pages 221 and 223, you can calculate your calorie needs per hour.

You should also figure out how to have these foods and fluids available for you, by using methods such as hiding a bottle of sports drink behind a bush on your training loop, tucking a small bag of raisins into a pocket, putting snacks in a waist pack, or using a support crew that meets you at designated spots along the route.

During the event, you should try to replace the majority of those calories as tolerated, or target about 250 calories of carbohydrates per hour. If you have a support crew, instruct them to feed you on a defined schedule so that you can prevent hypoglycemia and dehydration. How much you are able to consume will likely depend on the sport. That is, runners and swimmers have a harder time with eating and drinking during exercise than do cyclists and hikers.

Fluids During Extensive Exercise

Some people sweat a lot. For example, James had to put a towel under the exercycle to mop the sweat that dripped from his body. Although this was a source of embarrassment, I reminded James that sweating is good. It's the body's way of dissipating heat and maintaining a constant internal temperature (98.6 degrees F, or 37.0 degrees C).

During hard exercise, your muscles can generate 20 times more heat than they do when you are at rest. You dissipate this heat by sweating. As the sweat evaporates, it cools the skin. This in turn cools the blood, which cools the inner body. If you did not sweat, you could cook yourself to death. A body temperature higher than 106.0 degrees F (41.1 degrees C) damages the cells. At 107.6 degrees F (42.0 degrees C), cell protein coagulates (like egg whites do when they cook), and the cell dies. For this reason you shouldn't push yourself beyond your limits in extremely hot weather.

James, like many men, produced more sweat than he needed to cool himself. He'd sweat large drops of water, which dripped off his skin instead of evaporating, resulting in less cooling effect. In comparison, women tend to sweat more efficiently than men do. But both men and women need to be diligent in replacing sweat losses.

James wondered how much he needed to drink to replace this loss. I suggested that he learn his sweat rate by weighing himself before and after an hour of exercise. For every pound (16 ounces) he lost, he needed to learn how to drink about 80 to 100 percent of that loss (13 to 16 ounces) while exercising. To do this, he would have to train his gut to handle the volume. I also suggested that he figure out how many gulps of water equated to 16 ounces. By knowing his sweat rate (two pounds, or 32 ounces, an hour), he was able to practice programmed drinking during exercise to minimize sweat losses. James started to drink 8 ounces (eight gulps) every 15 minutes, regardless of thirst. Doing this required having the right quantity of enjoyable fluids (chilled, palatable) readily available and even setting an alarm wristwatch to remind him to drink on schedule.

Thirst, as defined by a conscious awareness of the desire for water and other fluids, usually controls water intake. An abnormally high concentration of body fluids triggers the sensation of thirst. When you sweat, you lose significant amounts of water from your blood. The remaining blood becomes more concentrated and has, for example, an abnormally high sodium level. This triggers the thirst mechanism and increases your desire to drink. To quench your thirst, you have to replace the water losses and bring the blood back to its normal concentration.

Unfortunately for athletes, this thirst mechanism can be an unreliable signal to drink. Hence, you should plan to drink before you are thirsty. By the time your brain signals thirst, you may have lost 1 percent of your body weight, which is the equivalent of 1 1/2 pounds (three cups, or 24 ounces) of sweat for a 150-pound person. This 1 percent loss corresponds with the need for your heart to beat an additional three to five times per minute (Casa et al. 2000). A 3 percent loss (4 1/2 pounds) can significantly hurt your performance (Coyle and Montain 1992). Exercise can blunt thirst, and the mind can override it. You may voluntarily replace less than half of sweat losses. To be safe, always drink enough to quench your thirst, plus a little more.

Young children, in particular, have poorly developed thirst mechanisms. At the end of a hot day, children often become very irritable, which may be partially because of dehydration. If you are going to spend the day with children at a place where fluids are not readily available, such as at the beach or a baseball game, take a cooler stocked with lemonade, juice, and ice water, and schedule frequent fluid breaks to increase everyone's enjoyment of the whole day.

Senior citizens also tend to be less sensitive to thirst sensations than younger adults are. Research with active, healthy men aged 67 to 75 years shows that they were less thirsty and voluntarily drank less water after having been water deprived for 24 hours than were similarly deprived younger men aged 20 to 31 years (Phillips et al. 1984). Older hikers (average age of 56 years) became progressively dehydrated during 10 days of strenuous hill walking. The younger hikers (average age of 24 years) remained adequately hydrated (Ainslie et al. 2002). Athletic seniors who participate in any sports should monitor their fluid intake.

How Much Fluid Is Enough?

On a daily basis, the simplest way to tell if you are adequately replacing sweat loss is to check the color and quantity of your urine. If your urine is dark and scanty, it is concentrated with metabolic wastes and you need to drink more fluids. When your urine is pale yellow, your body has returned to its normal water balance. Your urine may be dark if you are taking vitamin supplements; in that case, volume is a better indicator than color is.

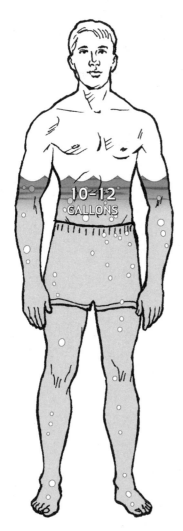

150-lb. man

Water and You

Water...

◊ in blood transports glucose, oxygen, and fats to working muscles and carries away metabolic by-products such as carbon dioxide and lactic acid.

◊ in urine eliminates metabolic waste products. The darker the urine, the more concentrated the wastes.

◊ in sweat dissipates heat through the skin. During exercise water absorbs heat from your muscles, dissipates it through sweat, and regulates body temperature.

◊ in saliva and gastric secretions helps digest food.

◊ throughout the body lubricates joints and cushions organs and tissues.

Besides monitoring urine and weight loss, you should also pay attention to how you feel. If you feel chronically fatigued, headachy, or lethargic, you may be chronically dehydrated. This condition is most likely to happen during long hot spells in the summertime. Dehydration is cumulative.

When the weather is hot and you (or your exercise partner) are losing your cool, be aware of the signs and symptoms of heat illness. Be sure to consume appropriate fluids to prevent the problem. If you fail to drink enough, don't tough it out to finish your workout. Watch for these signs:

- Muscle cramps
- Nausea, vomiting
- Headache, dizziness
- Confusion, disorientation
- Weakness, reduced performance
- Inability to concentrate
- Irrational behavior

Can You Drink Too Much Water?

For the most part, people who drink too much water are simply inconvenienced by frequent trips to the bathroom. But in some cases, drinking too much water can be lethal if it dilutes body fluids and creates a sodium imbalance.

Athletes affected by hyperhydration tend to be those who habitually limit their daily dietary sodium intake and exercise for more than four hours in the heat. They are commonly slow marathoners, triathletes, ultrarunners, and unfit weekend warriors who have higher sweat losses of sodium than do their fitter counterparts. They may diligently consume high amounts of preexercise water and consistently drink water during their events. They accumulate too much water by consuming water faster than their bodies can make urine. They end up with a relative excess of water compared with sodium (in part because of large losses of sodium through sweat and urine). The plain water dilutes their electrolyte balance.

The symptoms of hyperhydration include fatigue, nausea, and headache. If an athlete's blood sodium levels drop (a condition known as hyponatremia), he'll be confused and uncoordinated and may have a seizure. In the 2000 Houston Marathon, 21 of 5,082 finishers developed hyponatremia. Of these runners, 14 required hospitalization (Reuters 2001).

To prevent hyponatremia, people who will be exercising for more than four hours in the heat should

- eat salty foods (or lightly salt their food) the week before the endurance event,
- stop drinking water during exercise if the stomach is sloshing (as may happen if they drink more than a quart of water per hour for extended periods), and
- consume a sodium-containing sports drink or snacks (pretzels, baked chips, and stoned-wheat crackers are some common choices) during extended (more than four hours) exercise in the heat.

Cramping Your Style?

Muscle cramps are often associated with dehydration. If you have ever experienced the excruciating pain of a severe muscle cramp, you may fearfully wonder if it will strike again. Because no one totally understands what causes muscle cramps, these unpredictable spasms are somewhat mysterious. They most commonly occur among athletes who work their muscles to the point of exhaustion. They are likely related to overexertion, but fluid loss, inadequate conditioning, and electrolyte imbalance may also be predisposing factors. The solution often can be found with massage and stretching. Other times, nutrition may be involved. Although the following nutritional tips are not guaranteed to resolve this malady, I recommend that people who are predisposed to getting cramps rule out these possible contributing causes:

- **Lack of water.** Cramps commonly coincide with dehydration. To prevent dehydration-induced cramps, drink more than enough fluids before, during, and after you exercise. Always drink enough fluids daily so that your urine is clear, pale yellow, and copious. During a long exercise session, you should target eight ounces (250 milliliters) of fluid every 15 to 20 minutes.

- **Lack of calcium.** Calcium plays an essential role in muscle contractions. Some active people report that their problem with cramping disappears when they boost their calcium intake. For example, one ballet dancer found that once she reintroduced yogurt and skim milk into her diet, her cramping disappeared. A mountaineer resolved his muscle cramps by taking antacid tablets containing calcium when hiking. But some exercise scientists question the accuracy of these anecdotes. Calcium imbalance seems an unlikely cause of muscle cramps because the bones are a huge calcium reservoir. If a dietary deficiency should occur, calcium would be released from the bones to provide what is needed for proper muscle contraction.

  Nevertheless, to rule out any possible link between a calcium-poor diet and muscle cramps, athletes plagued by cramps should consume dairy products at least twice each day, such as low-fat milk on cereal and yogurt for a snack. This good nutritional practice certainly won't hurt them and possibly may help.

- **Lack of potassium.** Electrolyte imbalance, such as lack of potassium, may play a role in muscle cramps. You can rule this out by eating potassium-rich foods on a daily basis, focusing on fruits and vegetables. But a potassium deficiency is unlikely to occur as a result of sweat losses, because the body contains much more potassium than even a marathoner might lose during a hot, sweaty race. Nevertheless, a daily potassium-rich diet certainly won't hurt anyone, and in fact is a health-protective choice.

- **Lack of sodium.** Active people who restrict their sodium (salt) intake on a daily basis despite losing a significant amount of sodium through sweat may be putting themselves at risk of developing a sodium imbalance that could contribute to cramps. This circumstance is most likely to occur in athletes with habitual low-sodium diets who exercise hard for more than four hours in the heat, such as tennis players, triathletes, or ultrarunners. The risk increases if they consume only water during the event and have eaten no foods or beverages that contain sodium. Sports drinks and salted pretzels would be wise snack choices during exercise.

Although the suggestions for resolving muscle cramps are only suggestions and not proven solutions, you might want to experiment with these dietary improvements if you repeatedly suffer from muscle cramps. Adding extra fluids, low-fat dairy products, potassium-rich fruits and vegetables, and a sprinkling of salt certainly won't harm you, and it may resolve the worrisome problem. I also recommend that you consult with a physical therapist, athletic trainer, or coach regarding proper stretching and training techniques.

As I mentioned above, nutrition may play no role at all in your cramps. Given that cramps occur when muscles are fatigued, the problem may be related to a nerve malfunction that creates an imbalance between muscle excitation and inhibition, which prevents the muscle from relaxing. When that's the case, stretching the cramp is the best solution.

All-Day Fueling

If you are a competitive swimmer, wrestler, tennis buff, or soccer or basketball player, you may frequently face the nutrition challenge presented by back-to-back events and tournaments that require top performance for hours on end, sometimes for days in a row. If you pay careful attention to what you eat, you'll be able to win with good nutrition. But as one soccer mom commented, "Most players don't even think about what they will be eating during and between games. They just eat whatever is around—hot dogs, doughnuts, chips, or nothing." Athletes who give no thought to their nutrition game plan for a full day of activity can cheat themselves of the ability to perform well throughout the day.

When you will engage in extended periods of exercise, your goals are to maintain proper hydration and normal blood sugar level. You have to think constantly about fueling for the upcoming event and then refueling as soon as possible after the first event to prepare for the next session. Knowing your calorie and fluid goals can guide your calorie intake and menu planning. Having tried-and-true sports foods readily available in your gym bag or a cooler can also make this an easier task.

Making use of good nutrition can certainly give a team the winning edge. But persuading a team to dedicate themselves to eating a proper sports diet can be a challenge. One college coach felt frustrated by his team's ritual of pre-event high-fat pepperoni pizza and beer parties that filled the stomach but left the muscles unfueled and the players dehydrated. No wonder the team was having a bad season. The coach took a strong stance.

- He hired a sports nutritionist to educate the players about the importance of pre-event carbohydrates and fluids, and he gave the players lists of foods highest in carbohydrates (see chapter 7 and table 7.3 on page 156) and pregame meal suggestions.

- He instructed all coaches and athletic trainers to enforce appropriate between-game eating. With the financial support of the booster club, they started to provide bagels, bananas, juices, pretzels, and other high-carbohydrate sports snacks and drinks for tournament days.

- When traveling to a game, the coach preselected an appropriate restaurant that could handle the whole team, and he prearranged an economical buffet with minestrone soup, crackers, spaghetti with tomato sauce, meatballs on the side, green beans, fresh whole-grain rolls, low-fat milk, juice, and frozen yogurt.

- He instructed each player to pack his gym bag with personal favorite sports foods (such as sports drinks, oatmeal raisin cookies, trail mix, oranges, bagels) to eat before, during, and between practice sessions and games.

Each player noticed that proper fueling helped him perform better, and the team as a whole respected the value of this "win with nutrition" program. Sure enough, they did start to have greater stamina and strength. Although they didn't always win, they no longer got clobbered in the final minutes, and they felt better about their overall effort.

If you are among the many athletes who give no thought to a sports-nutrition game plan during daylong tournaments and repeated events, think again. The right sports diet can indeed enhance your performance. Athletes and teams who are doing well despite poor food choices can do better when they pay attention to their diets. Be responsible. Plan your day-long sports foods and enjoy your higher energy!

Pit Stops

Gastrointestinal (GI) problems such as constipation or diarrhea are common among athletes. If you've ever been plagued by one or the other during training or competition, you know how worrisome this is and how much it can interfere with top performance. That's why most athletes go to great extremes to promote regular bowel movements.

People who fear becoming constipated should faithfully eat fiber-rich foods and plenty of fresh fruits and vegetables (see chapter 2) to help prevent constipation, drink warm liquids in the morning to encourage regular bowel movements, and drink more than enough fluids.

If you struggle with "rapid transit," you should try to determine what triggers the diarrhea by carefully charting for weeks every food and fluid that you ingest, as well as the times you exercise and the times you have diarrhea. Be sure to include sugar-free gum and candies that contain sorbitol, a type of sugar that can cause gastrointestinal problems if taken in excess.

You should also try to eliminate suspected problem foods like milk, broccoli, onions, corn, kidney beans, sugar-free foods with sorbitol, and other possibly hard-to-digest foods for a week to see if the problem goes away. Then look for bowel changes when you reintroduce these foods into your diet.

Some people never do find a simple dietary solution to their intestinal problems. Sometimes they are simply training too much or too fast. Easy exercise of any type can at times stimulate bowel movements. Peter, a jogger, was plagued with diarrhea when he started to increase his training mileage. I recommended that he cut back to his baseline mileage for a week and then gradually add one mile per week rather than four to five. I also advised him to talk with a sports doctor to determine whether he had a medical problem. For Peter, the solution was to train less intensely. He was trying to run too much, too fast. Like many novice athletes whose bodies have not yet adapted to the stress of intense exercise, he ended up with diarrhea.

If you have persistent problems with diarrhea, intestinal distress, and GI cramping, you should consult your physician. He or she may prescribe some medication to control the problem. You should also consult a sports nutritionist, especially if you are making radical long-term dietary changes. For example, when Larry, a basketball player, recognized that milk contributed to GI problems, he needed help finding alternative, nondairy sources of calcium, riboflavin, and protein—some of the key nutrients in milk. A sports nutritionist who was a registered dietitian helped him find substitutes without sacrificing nutrition.

Digesting Sports Nutrition Advice

Advice about what to eat before and during exercise must be taken with a grain of salt, so to speak, because each person's digestive tract is metabolically unique. By experimenting with a variety of fluids, foods, and eating patterns before, during, and after practice, you'll gradually discover the best choices for your body. In contrast to the wrong foods, which can destroy your performance, the right foods in the right amounts can optimize your chances for success. Be wise; eat wisely!

Recovering From Extensive Exercise

When you've exercised hard and feel stiff, sore, and tired, you may wonder, *If I were to eat better, would I recover faster?* Without doubt, consuming the appropriate foods and fluids can affect your recovery (as can doing light exercise for 10 to 20 minutes while you are cooling down to assist with removal of lactic acid from the blood and muscles, and then stretching). Many of my clients have questions about their recovery diets:

- Football players want to know what they should eat after morning practice to prepare for the afternoon session.
- People who lift weights wonder if they should eat extra protein after workouts to repair muscles.
- Squash players seek foods that will prepare them for the next day's match.
- Swimmers search for the proper foods that will get them through a heavy season of training and competing without deterioration and chronic fatigue.

When you deal with the rigors of a tough training schedule, remember that what you eat after a hard workout or competition affects your recovery. For the serious athlete, foods eaten after exercise require the same careful selections as the meal before exercise. By wisely choosing your foods and fluids, you will recover more quickly for the next workout.

If you are a recreational exerciser who works out three or four times per week, you need not worry about your recovery diet because you have enough time to refuel your muscle glycogen stores before your next workout. But you should be concerned about your recovery diet if you are a competitive athlete who does two or more workouts per day, such as a soccer player at training camp who practices morning and afternoon, a competitive swimmer who competes in multiple events per meet, a triathlete who trains twice per day, an aerobics instructor who teaches several classes daily, or a basketball player who needs to endure an entire season of intense training and competing. To recover and refuel for the next bout, you should pay particular attention to what you eat after the first session.

Recovery Fluids

After you finish a hard workout, your top dietary priority should be to replace the fluids you lost by sweating so that your body can get back into water balance. Ideally, you should have minimized dehydration during the event by consuming at least 80 percent of sweat losses, but that can be hard to do during intense exercise. Hence, the best choices for replacing sweat losses include one or more of the following:

- Juices, which supply water, carbohydrates, vitamins, and potassium
- Watery foods such as watermelon, grapes, and soups that supply fluids, carbohydrates, vitamins, and potassium
- High-carbohydrate sports drinks or soft drinks, which supply fluids and carbohydrates (but minimal, if any, vitamins or minerals)
- Commercial fluid replacers, which supply fluids, some carbohydrates and sodium, and a few vitamins if fortified with them
- Water, which tends to be convenient, well tolerated, and least expensive

To determine how much fluid to replace, you need to know how much water you lose during a strenuous event. You can estimate this by weighing yourself before and after a hard training workout. Your goal is to lose no more than 2 percent of your body weight (for example, 3 pounds for a 150-pound person). By drinking on a schedule (eight ounces every 15 to 20 minutes of hard exercise), you can prevent or at least minimize dehydration.

One large, muscular man who spent two hours at the gym doing an hour of cardio and an hour of strength training was shocked to discover he'd lose about 8 pounds (3.5 kilograms) during the morning sessions—5 percent of his body weight and the equivalent of a gallon (4 liters) of sweat! (One pound of sweat loss represents 16 ounces of fluid.) He became aware of the importance of drinking more. He started bringing a gallon of water to the gym. He drank one quart every half hour and made sure that he finished the whole gallon. These steps to prevent dehydration helped him recover easily. Drinking large volumes of fluid during training will help you adapt to the fluid load and prevent stomach sloshing and discomfort during competitions.

If you become dehydrated during an unusually long and strenuous bout of exercise, you should drink frequently for the next day or two. Your body may need 24 to 48 hours to replace the sweat losses. You'll know that you are adequately rehydrated when your urine is clear or pale yellow and you have to urinate frequently. If you urinate only a small amount of dark colored urine, it is still concentrated with metabolic wastes. (If you take vitamin supplements, your urine may be a dark color, so you'll need to judge your hydration status by the volume of urine.)

Recovery Carbohydrates

To optimize muscle glycogen replenishment, you should consume carbohydrate-rich foods and beverages within 15 minutes after your workout. During that time the enzymes responsible for making glycogen are most active and will most rapidly replace the depleted glycogen stores. More precisely, your target intake is about 0.5 grams of carbohydrate per pound (about 1 gram per kilogram) of body weight every hour, taken at 30-minute intervals for four to five hours (Ivy 2001). Let's assume that you weigh 150 pounds:

$$150 \text{ lb} \times 0.5 \text{ g carbs} = 75 \text{ g carb} = 300 \text{ calories carb}$$

One gram of carbohydrate contains 4 calories, so 75 grams converts to 300 calories. This means that you'll need about 300 calories of carbohydrates within the first hour, some taken as soon as tolerable after exercise, let's say 15 minutes after the workout ended, and then again in 30 more minutes. After another 30 minutes, you should consume another 150 of the 300 calories of high-carbohydrate foods.

Your body will naturally want this amount, if not more. If you've been exercising so hard that you have concerns about replacing depleted glycogen stores, the chances are good that you are hungry for lots more calories. You can eat more than the calculated amount, but extra carbohydrates will not hasten the recovery process.

Liquids and solid foods will refuel your muscles equally well, and foods with a moderate to high glycemic effect will provide the quickest replenishment (see chapter 7). Some popular 300-calorie, carbohydrate-rich food suggestions are 8 ounces (250 milliliters) of orange juice and a medium bagel, 16 ounces (500 milliliters) of cranberry juice, one 12-ounce (375-milliliter) can of soft drink (not diet) and an 8-ounce fruit yogurt, or one bowl of corn flakes with milk and a banana.

Commercial high-carbohydrate sports drinks and carbohydrate powders can also refuel your muscles. But be aware that these carbo drinks lack most of the vitamins and minerals that accompany wholesome natural foods (unless the drinks are fortified). They also tend to be more expensive than standard foods.

Take note: You need not eat only carbs. As I talk about in the following section, some protein is also OK (Ivy 2001). Hence, there's little wrong with a lean roast-beef sandwich on a thick kaiser roll or minestrone soup with crackers. Think of the roast beef as being an accompaniment to the other carbohydrate-rich choices, and you'll still end up with a carbohydrate-rich diet recovery after all.

Recovery Protein

You don't need to avoid protein in your recovery diet. In fact, some protein might enhance glycogen replacement in the initial hours after hard exercise. Protein, like carbohydrate, stimulates the action of insulin, a hormone that transports glucose from the blood into the muscles. Some researchers contend a little protein eaten along with carbohydrates (such as milk with cereal, a slice or two of turkey on a bagel, a little lean meat in spaghetti sauce, and even an energy bar with at least six grams of protein) provides a winning combination (Ivy et al. 2002). Other researchers contend that consumption of adequate calories of carbs is the key to optimal recovery. At least five carefully controlled studies have shown that adding protein to recovery carbohydrates is no more effective for replacing muscle glycogen than consuming equal calories of carbohydrates alone (Zachweija 2002).

Despite the debate regarding how to optimize glycogen replacement, there is certainly no harm in eating some postexercise protein as an enjoyable part of the refueling process. In addition, the availability of amino acids (from protein) may enhance the process of building and repairing muscles (Ivy 2001).

Eating a little protein (as little as six grams, the amount in one egg) before exercise may also optimize recovery. This preexercise protein provides a readily available supply of the amino acids required for optimal muscular development at that moment (Zachweija 2002).

Recovery Electrolytes

When you sweat you lose not only water but also some minerals (electrolytes) such as potassium and sodium that help your body function normally. You can easily replace electrolyte losses with the foods and fluids you consume after the event (see tables 6.1 and 6.2). Based on the assumption that the harder you exercise, the hungrier you'll get and the more you'll eat, you'll consume more than enough electrolytes from standard postexercise foods. You won't need salt tablets or special potassium supplements. For example, the marathoner who guzzles a quart (liter) of orange juice after completing the 26.2-mile event replaces three times the potassium he might have lost. Munching on a bag of pretzels will more than replace sodium losses.

The concentration of sodium in your blood increases during exercise because you lose proportionately more water than sodium (unless you overhydrate; see page 119). Your first need is to replace the fluid; you can get adequate sodium in the food you eat. Popular recovery foods such as yogurt, muffins, pizza, and spaghetti have more sodium than

TABLE 6.1

Potassium in Popular Recovery Foods

A pound of sweat contains about 80 to 100 milligrams potassium. During two to three hours of hard exercise (expending 1,200 to 1,800 or more calories), you might lose 300 to 800 milligrams of potassium. The following chart ranks some fluids and foods for potassium content. In general, natural foods are preferable to commercial products. See tables 1.1 and 1.2 on pages 10 and 12 for a complete potassium list.

Food	Potassium (mg)	Serving
Potato	840	1 large (7 oz)
Yogurt	520	8 oz, low-fat
Orange juice	475	8 oz
Banana	450	Medium
Pineapple juice	335	8 oz
Raisins	300	1/4 cup
Beer	90	12 oz
Cranapple juice	70	8 oz
Gatorade	30	8 oz
Cola	5	12 oz can

Nutrition information from food labels and J. Pennington, 1998, *Bowes & Church's Food Values of Portions Commonly Used*, 17th ed. (Philadelphia: Lippincott).

you may realize. Sprinkle a little salt on your food or choose salty items such as pretzels, crackers, or soup (see table 6.2). Also, if you're prone to muscle cramping, experiment with adding extra salt to your training diet to see if that gives you relief. For the ordinary exerciser, salt depletion is unlikely, even though that is the electrolyte lost in the highest concentration. Even athletes who eat a low-salt diet tend to maintain sodium balance because they have low-salt sweat. The less salt they eat, the less they lose. The kidneys and sweat glands tend to conserve sodium when it is in short supply. But there are exceptions to this generality, and active people who exercise for more than four hours and sweat excessively should be sure to consume extra salt.

In extreme circumstances, such as during a century bike ride or a tennis tournament that lasts for more than four hours in the heat, you have a higher risk of becoming sodium depleted. To prevent this, be

TABLE 6.2

Sodium in Popular Recovery Foods

A pound of sweat contains about 400 to 700 milligrams of sodium. If you have adapted to exercising in the heat, you'll lose less sodium in sweat than the person who is not acclimatized. If you need salt, you'll crave it. Notice that it's easy to get sodium through foods that aren't salty, such as bread and bagels. Sports drinks are relatively low in sodium; the primary purpose of the sodium in sports drinks is to enhance the rate of fluid absorption and retention and maintain the desire to drink.

Recovery food	Sodium (mg)
Chicken Noodle Soup, 1 can Campbell's	2,225
Ramen Noodles, Maruchan, 1 packet	1,560
Pizza, 1/2 of 12 in. cheese	1,300
Macaroni and Cheese, Kraft, 1 cup	560
Spaghettios, 1 cup	890
Spaghetti sauce, 1/2 cup Ragu	820
Salt, 1 small packet	500
Bagel, 1 Lender's New York style	410
Cheerios, 1 cup	280
American cheese, Kraft, 1 slice (2/3 ounce)	260
Fruit yogurt (8 oz)	250
Pretzels, 1 Dutch Snyder's	240
Yogurt, Dannon blueberry, 1 cup	200
Saltines, 5	180
Bread, 1 slice Pepperidge Farm Hearty Slices	190
Potato chips, 20 Lays	180
Gatorade, 8 oz	110
PowerAde	70
Beer, 12 oz	15
Coke, 12 oz	10
Orange juice, 8 oz	5
Potential losses in a 2 hr workout	1,000–2,000

Data from food labels and J. Pennington, 1998, *Bowes & Church's Food Values of Portions Commonly Used*, 17th ed. (Philadelphia: Lippincott).

sure to consume salted fluids or foods during the event; don't drink just plain water. You should target about 250 to 500 milligrams of sodium per hour, the amount in 20 to 40 ounces (600 to 1,200 milliliters) of Gatorade, for example.

Many people who exercise extensively in the heat end up craving salt. Such cravings are your body's way of telling you that you need extra salt. You might want to sprinkle some salt on your recovery meal. The big appetite that likely accompanies this salt craving will help you consume more than enough sodium.

If you are tempted to replace sodium losses with commercially prepared fluid-replacement beverages, look closely at table 6.2 and note that most of these special sports drinks are sodium poor. Commercial fluid-replacement drinks are designed to be taken during intense exercise. They are very dilute, which helps them empty faster from the stomach. They are not the best recovery foods in terms of electrolyte content, carbohydrates, and overall nutritional value unless you drink large volumes.

Recovery and Alcohol

Alcohol and athletics seem to go hand in hand. Competitors gather at the pub after a team workout, celebrate victories with champagne, quench thirst with a cold beer. One might think that the detrimental effects of alcohol on performance would make athletes less likely to drink alcohol, but that is not the case. Even serious recreational runners drink more than their sedentary counterparts do.

If you are determined to drink alcohol as a part of your recovery diet, keep in mind the following facts:

- Alcohol is a depressant and, apart from killing pain, offers no edge for athletes. You can't be sharp, quick, and drunk.

- Late-night drinking that contributes to getting too little sleep can wreck the next day's training session. Drinks that contain congeners—red wine, cognac, whiskey—are more likely to cause hangovers than other alcoholic beverages. The best hangover remedy is to avoid drinking excessively in the first place, but if you have a hangover, drink fruit juice or broth.

- Alcohol is a poor source of carbohydrates. A 12-ounce can of beer has only 14 grams of carbs, as compared to 40 grams in a can of soft drink. You can get loaded with beer, but your muscles will not get carbo loaded—unless you consume pretzels, thick-crust pizza, or other carbo-rich foods along with the beer.

- Alcohol is absorbed directly from the stomach into the bloodstream, appearing within five minutes after you drink it. After a hard workout, alcohol on an empty stomach can quickly contribute to a drunken stupor. You'd be better off enjoying the natural high from exercise than being brought down by a few postexercise beers.

- Beer is often a significant source of postexercise fluids; athletes commonly consume larger volumes of beer than they might of water or soft drinks. But the alcohol in beer has a diuretic effect—the more you drink, the more fluids you lose. This process is unhealthy for recovery and often unhealthy for the next exercise bout.

  Although low-alcohol beer allows for proper rehydration, regular beer sends athletes running to the bathroom. One study showed that athletes who drank beer eliminated about 16 ounces (500 milliliters) more urine (over the course of four hours) than those who drink low-alcohol (2 percent) beer or alcohol-free beer (Sherriffs and Maughan 1997). For optimal rehydration, minimize alcohol intake.

- Your liver breaks down alcohol at a fixed rate—about four ounces (250 milliliters) of wine or one can of beer (750 milliliters) per hour. Exercise does not hasten that process, nor does coffee.

- Hot tubs, alcohol, and athletes are a bad combination. The hotter your body, the drunker you may feel. Alcohol impairs your ability to control your body temperature, and the high temperature of the hot tub heightens the response of the body to alcohol.

- Winter sports and alcohol are a dangerous combination. Don't drink while skiing. Après ski, if you choose to drink alcohol, alternate with soft drinks or juices for carbs and fluids.

- The calories in alcohol are easily fattening. People who drink moderately often consume alcohol calories on top of their regular caloric intake because alcohol stimulates the appetite. These excess calories promote body-fat accumulation, commonly in the trunk area—the well-known spare tire. If you are trying to maintain a lean machine, abstaining is preferable to imbibing.

- If you are determined to drink, drink moderately. The definition of moderate drinking is two drinks per day for men and one for women. And have at least one glass of water for every alcoholic drink you consume.

- Don't start drinking if you can't easily stop. Be conscious of your ability to keep alcohol consumption within socially and medically acceptable bounds.

How Much Alcohol Is Too Much?

The answer varies. What's too much alcohol for one person may be OK for another. In general, large, muscular athletes can handle more alcohol without untoward consequences than can smaller people. Women are more susceptible than men to the effects of alcohol. People who drink regularly can handle more alcohol than nondrinkers can.

Experts say it's not how much you drink but the extent to which drinking interferes with your life that determines whether you have a problem with alcohol. So besides counting drinks, try answering these questions honestly:

- Are you ever mad at yourself, knowing that alcohol keeps you from being who you really are?
- Are you tired of regretting your actions?
- If alcohol is not available, do you make it available?
- Do you change your plans so that you can have a drink?

An estimated 14 million Americans (more than 7 percent of adults) have serious problems with alcohol, but only about 10 percent of these seek help for their drinking problems. If you are a heavy drinker, or know one, you may not have a clue where to go for advice.

To turn the tide, you need to weigh the pleasures of alcohol against the pain and problems it causes and conclude that drinking isn't worth the price. You'd rather have a loving relationship and a successful career. A helpful resource for problem drinkers and their families is *Sober for Good: New Solutions for Drinking Problems—Advice From Those Who Have Succeeded* by Anne Fletcher. The book contains words of wisdom from 222 people who have resolved their drinking problems. See appendix B for additional information.

For every problem drinker, about five other people suffer as a result. If you are one of the sufferers, what can you say to your spouse or loved one who drinks too much? What won't work are nagging, humiliation, and trying to control your loved one's drinking by, let's say, dumping alcohol down the drain. Ultimately, the person has to want to quit for himself or herself, but your actions can help the person move in the right direction.

- The worst thing you can do is to do nothing. Rather, address the drinking problem directly and let the person know that you are aware of the problem. As one recovering alcoholic commented, "I thought I had everyone fooled."
- Don't make it easy for the problem drinker to keep drinking. For example, don't call in sick for anyone.
- Don't stop loving the person. Make it clear that the problem is the drinking, not the drinker. Your loved one is a good person with a bad problem, not a bad person.
- Don't nag, criticize, preach, or complain. Say what you feel: "I'm worried about you." Be loving but firm, and understand that the problem drinker may need to try several times before he or she gets and stays sober.
- Remind them that life can be ordinary or it can be great.

Recovery Vitamins

After exhaustive exercise, many people believe that extra vitamins are needed to replace what was depleted during exercise. To date, there is no research to support that belief. Vitamins are not used up during exercise; they are recycled, like spark plugs in a car.

Some people believe that vitamins can help repair the oxidative damage that occurs during exercise, which is thought to hinder muscle repair and enhance cancer risk. Hence, they take antioxidant vitamins (C, E, beta-carotene). A study with ultrarunners who took 1,500 milligrams of vitamin C for the week before a race suggests that they had higher blood levels of vitamin C compared with a group of peers who took no C, but this did not translate into benefits in terms of oxidative or immune changes. (The recommended intake is 75 to 90 milligrams, so this was an extremely high dose) (Nieman et al. 2002).

Another study with runners who took 1,000 milligrams of C and 1,000 IU of E for four weeks before a very hard 12-mile run indicated no reduction in the indicators of muscle damage (Dawson et al. 2002). Research supports the concept that the body can handle the stresses of exercise. That's where eating well on a daily basis is undoubtedly a wise investment in optimal recovery; supplements are not the answer!

Sick, Tired, or Overtrained?

Although proper nutrition can optimize recovery, even active people who eat well can become chronically fatigued for a variety of reasons, including excessive training, inadequate rest, or too little sleep. If you have a strenuous and prolonged training schedule in addition to other commitments and responsibilities, you may find yourself with too little time for proper eating, sleeping, and self-care.

Listed here are some symptoms associated with overtraining. If you are experiencing two or more of these symptoms, take heed.

- Unusually poor performance in training and competition
- Failure to improve performance despite diligent training
- Inability to perform better in competition than during practice
- Loss of appetite and body weight
- Insomnia
- Joint and muscle pains that have no apparent cause
- Frequent colds or respiratory infections
- Irritability and anxiety that may be accompanied by depression

(continued)

(*continued*)

Rather than overtrain to the point of chronic fatigue, you should take steps to prevent it. Eat a proper sports diet that provides adequate carbohydrates and protein, allow recovery time between bouts of intense exercise, and plan your schedule so that you get enough sleep at night. You should also try to minimize stress in your life and curtail disruptive activities that might drain your physical and mental energy reserves.

From W. Sherman and E. Maglischo, 1991, "Minimizing Chronic Fatigue Among Swimmers: Special Emphasis on Nutrition," *Sports Science Exchange* 4 (35). Gatorade Sports Science Institute.

Time to Rest

As I discuss in chapter 7, rest is an important part of your training program. Yet, some people feel guilty if they don't train every day. They fear becoming unfit, fat, and lazy if they miss a day of training. That scenario is unlikely. These compulsive exercisers overlook the important physiological fact that rest is essential for top performance. Rest enhances the recovery process, reduces risk of injury, and invests in future performance. To replace depleted glycogen stores completely, the muscles may need up to two days of rest with no exercise and a high-carbohydrate diet. True athletes plan days with no exercise. Compulsive exercisers, in comparison, push themselves relentlessly, and often pay the price of poorer performance.

The same athletes who avoid rest after an event also tend to overtrain while preparing for an event. Many athletes train for two or three hours per day, thinking that such a regimen will help them improve. That sort of training program, however, is unlikely to enhance performance. Research has shown that swimmers performed just as well on one 90-minute training session per day as they did with double workouts of two 90-minute sessions (Costill et al. 1991). Quality training is better than quantity training. Do not underestimate the power of rest.

Food Works!

By eating the appropriate foods and fluids before, during, and after exercise, you can significantly improve your stamina, endurance, and enjoyment of exercise. The following guidelines summarize the keys to optimal performance:

- Start your exercise program well fueled every day. The target intake is three to five grams of carbohydrate per pound (6 to 10 grams per kilogram) of body weight per day.

- Start your exercise program well hydrated every day. Your daily goal is to urinate every two to four hours clear or pale yellow urine.

- Consume adequate carbohydrates and fluids during exercise that lasts longer than 60 to 90 minutes. The target intake is 0.5 gram of carbohydrate per pound (about 1 gram per kilogram) of body weight (about 300 calories if you weigh 150 pounds) per hour of exercise, as tolerated, after the first 60 to 90 minutes and about eight ounces (250 milliliters) of fluid every 15 to 20 minutes. Your best bet is to know your hourly sweat rate (by weighing yourself before and after an hour of exercise) so you can take the guesswork out of trying to drink the right amount.

- After exhaustive exercise, recover with adequate carbohydrates and fluids. You should consume about 75 grams (300 calories) of carbohydrates every hour taken at 30-minute intervals for four to five hours. Drink until your urine is clear and copious.

- Allow adequate rest days for your muscles to refuel and recover. You should taper at least one week before competition, and each week during training you should schedule at least one day with no exercise and another easy day or a day off.

7

Eliminating Carbohydrate Confusion

Without question, wholesome carbohydrates are the best choices for fueling your muscles and promoting good health. People of all ages and athletic abilities should nourish themselves with abundant fruits, vegetables, and whole-grain foods, with adequate protein and health-ful fats balanced into the meals and snacks.

Unfortunately, confusion about carbohydrates—what they are and how much to eat—keeps people from properly balancing their diet. As one runner put it, "I know I should eat carbohydrates for muscle fuel, but which carbs are best? How much is too much? If I have carbs for break-fast, can I also have them at lunch—or is that fattening?" Like many active people, he was confused by this seemingly complex subject. The purpose of this chapter is to eliminate this confusion so you can make choices that best promote your health, desired weight, and performance.

Simple Sugars

The carbohydrate family includes both simple and complex carbohy-drates. The simple carbohydrates are monosaccharides and disaccharides (single- and double-sugar molecules). Glucose, fructose, and galactose are monosaccharides, the simplest sugars, and can be symbolized like this:

The disaccharides can be symbolized like this:

Three common disaccharides include table sugar (sucrose, a combination of glucose and fructose), milk sugar (lactose, a combination of glucose and galactose), and corn syrup (a combination of glucose and fructose commonly used in soft drinks). These are converted into glucose molecules before entering the bloodstream to provide fuel for the body.

Table sugar, honey, and corn syrup contain glucose and fructose but in differing amounts. Table sugar, which is 50 percent glucose and 50 percent fructose, is a disaccharide. With digestion, it breaks apart into two monosaccharides. The high-fructose type of corn syrup used in soft drinks breaks down to about 55 percent fructose and 45 percent glucose. Honey converts into 31 percent glucose, 38 percent fructose, 10 percent other sugars, 17 percent water, and 4 percent miscellaneous particles. All fruits and vegetables offer a variety of sugars in differing proportions. And all end up as glucose, the fuel used by your muscles and brain.

Some athletes mistakenly think that honey is nutritionally superior to refined white sugar. If you prefer honey because of the pleasant taste, fine. But it's not superior for health or performance. Sugar in any form—honey, brown sugar, raw sugar, maple syrup, or jelly—has insignificant amounts of vitamins or minerals, and your body digests any type of sugar or carbohydrate into glucose before using it for fuel.

A third type of sugar that has entered the sports market is the glucose polymer. Polymers are chains of about five glucose molecules. Sports drinks sweetened with polymers can provide more energy value with less sweetness than regular sugar provides.

Complex Carbohydrates

Complex carbohydrates, such as starch in plant foods and glycogen in muscles, are formed when sugars link together to form long, complex chains, similar to a string of hundreds of pearls. They can be symbolized like this:

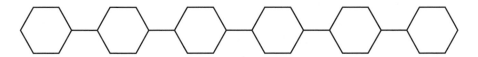

Plants store extra sugars in the form of starch. For example, corn, which is sweet when it's young, becomes starchy as it gets older. Its extra sugar converts into starch. In contrast to corn and other vegetables, fruits tend to convert starches into sugars as they ripen. A good example is the banana:

- A green banana with some yellow is 80 percent starch and 7 percent sugar.
- A mostly yellow banana is 25 percent starch and 65 percent sugar.
- A spotted and speckled banana is 5 percent starch and 90 percent sugar.

The potatoes, rice, bread, and other starches that you eat are digested into glucose, then are either burned for energy or stored for future use. Humans store extra glucose mostly in the form of muscle glycogen and liver glycogen. This glycogen is readily available for energy during exercise.

Sugars and starches have similar abilities to fuel muscles but different abilities to nourish them with vitamins and minerals:

- The carbohydrates in sugary soft drinks provide energy but no vitamins or minerals.
- The carbohydrates in polymer drinks provide energy but no vitamins or minerals, unless the drink is fortified.
- The carbohydrates in wholesome fruits, vegetables, and grains provide energy, vitamins, minerals, fiber, and phytochemicals— the fuel and spark plugs that your body's engine needs to function best.

Quick and Slow Carbs

Athletes used to be told to choose starchy complex carbohydrates such as bagels, potatoes, and bread for preexercise snacks because these foods were thought to contribute to a stable blood sugar level. Sugary simple carbohydrates, in contrast, were thought to trigger a sugar high followed by a sugar low and a debilitating hypoglycemic reaction (see chapter 5 to learn how this is not usually the case).

Today we know that the effect of a carbohydrate on blood sugar cannot be determined by whether it is a simple or a complex carbohydrate. Instead, the effect is determined by its glycemic response, or the ability of the food to contribute glucose to the bloodstream. Many factors influence the glycemic response of a food, including the amount eaten, fiber content, amount of added fat, and the way the food is prepared. By ranking foods according to their ability to elevate blood sugar, nutrition professionals have developed a glycemic index. A baked potato has a higher glycemic effect than a boiled potato; wheat made into bread has a higher glycemic effect than wheat made into pasta; plain sugar has a higher glycemic effect than sugar combined with fat, such as ice cream or cookies.

The glycemic index was originally designed to help people with diabetes closely control their blood sugars. Because people with diabetes tend to eat foods in meal combinations that buffer the individual glycemic responses, the glycemic index is less predictive for them. Athletes, however, tend to eat a singular food for a sports snack and can perhaps gain benefit from this ranking system to determine whether to eat a food before, during, or after exercise.

High-glycemic-index carbohydrates (potatoes, corn flakes, honey) quickly enter the bloodstream and are best eaten during or after exercise. Low- to moderate-glycemic-index foods (rice, pasta, bananas) slowly enter the bloodstream and are desirable before endurance exercise because they provide sustained energy. For example, in a study in which the subjects ate either 300 calories of carbohydrates from oatmeal (moderate GI) or puffed rice (high GI) for a preexercise meal 45 minutes before biking to exhaustion, they exercised for 165 minutes with oatmeal, 141 minutes with puffed rice, and 134 minutes with only water (Kirwan et al. 2001). But other similar studies fail to show an improvement (Wee et al. 1999). This result may relate to large individual glycemic responses to foods.

So, should you bother to fret about the glycemic effect of your preexercise meal or snack? In some situations, yes. For example, if you are unable to consume calories during endurance exercise (such as swimmers who have difficulty eating while exercising or people with finicky stomachs, who prefer to abstain from anything but water during exercise), eating a low-glycemic food might enhance your endurance and stamina. But if you will be consuming carbohydrates during exercise (sports drinks, gels, fruit), the energizing power of those snacks will be stronger than the effect of eating a low-glycemic food preexercise. The main point is to pay more attention to the benefits gained by fueling during exercise than fretting about the glycemic effect of a preexercise snack (Burke et al. 1998).

After exercise, if you need to rapidly recover within six hours for, let's say, the next game in a soccer tournament, your best bet is to eat high-glycemic foods and fluids. They quickly enter the bloodstream and enhance the rate of glycogen replacement.

Is White Bread Poison?

White bread offers lackluster nutrition, but it is not poison or a bad food. White bread can be part of an overall wholesome diet. That is, if you have bran cereal for breakfast and brown rice for dinner, your diet can healthfully accommodate a sandwich made on white pita for lunch.

The reputation of white bread for being unhealthful is partially because of its high glycemic effect. That is, 200 calories of white bread digests quickly and causes the blood glucose (blood sugar) to rise higher than would the same amount of a whole-grain, fiber-rich bread. High blood glucose triggers the body to secrete insulin to carry the sugar out of the blood. Insulin can stimulate the appetite, as well as fat deposition, and that's where white bread gets its bad reputation.

If you are physically fit, your muscles readily store the sugar from the digested bread as glycogen with the need of much less insulin than required by a sedentary person. Hence, active people can better handle high glycemic foods such as white bread and have less need to worry about the glycemic effect of the food. Yet, regardless of the glycemic effect, white bread fails to offer whole-grain goodness. So for that reason alone, you should try to eat more whole wheat, rye, and multigrain breads.

The list in table 7.1 ranks foods according to the glycemic response to 200 calories (50 grams) of carbohydrates per serving of the food. Although a person might eat one large 200-calorie baked potato in a sitting, most people do not eat 200 calories of, for example, rice cakes, carrots, honey, or table sugar at one time. Hence, the actual glycemic load of a food may differ from its ranking according to this list.

For overall health, foods with a low-glycemic effect tend to be wise choices. They are the wholesome, fiber-rich fruits, vegetables, and whole grains that are health protective and satiating. They can curb the appetite and help with weight management. Yet, because the glycemic response to a food varies from person to person as well as from meal to meal (depending on the combinations of foods eaten), you should experiment to learn what food combinations satisfy you personally and offer lasting energy.

TABLE 7.1

Glycemic Index of Popular Sports Foods

Food	GI	Food	GI
High GI (>70)		MET-Rx, vanilla	58
Glucose	100	Powerbar, chocolate	56-83
Corn flakes	92	Potato, boiled	56
Honey, Canadian	87	Rice, white long grain	56
Potato, baked	85	Rice, brown	55
Potato, microwaved	82	Boost, vanilla	53
Gatorade	78-89	Kidney beans, canned	52
Rice cakes	78	Orange juice	52
Jelly beans	78	Banana, overripe	52
Cheerios	74	Pumpernickel bread	50
Cream of Wheat, instant	74	Ensure, vanilla	48-75
Graham crackers	74	Peas, green	48
MET-Rx bar, vanilla	74	Lentil soup	44
Bread, white Wonder	73	Spaghetti, no sauce	44
Bagel, Lender's white	72	Candy bar, milk chocolate	43
Watermelon	72	Chickpeas, canned	42
Bread, whole wheat	71 (52-87)	Apple juice	40
Grape-Nuts	71	Strawberries	40
Moderate GI (40-70)		*Low GI (<40)*	
Sugar, white (sucrose)	68	PR-Bar, Ironman chocolate	39
Cranberry juice, Ocean Spray	68	Apple	38
Snickers	68	Pear	38
Stoned-wheat thins	67	All-bran cereal	38
Cream of Wheat, regular	66	Chocolate milk	34
Oatmeal	66	Fruit yogurt, low-fat	33
Mars Bar	65	M&Ms, Peanut	33
Couscous	65	Milk, skim	32
Powerade	65	Apricots, dried	31
Raisins	64	Banana, underripe	30
Coca-Cola	63	Lentils, boiled	30
Cytomax	62	Peach	28
Raisin Bran	61	Milk, whole	27
Muffin, bran	60	Barley	25
Corn	60	Grapefruit	25
Sweet Potato	59	Fructose	24

Data from food companies; K. Foster-Powell, S. Holt and J. Brand Miller, 2002, "International table of glycemic index and glycemic load values," *Am J Clin Nutr*, 76: 5-56; and Gretebeck R. et al., "Glycemic index of popular sports drinks and energy foods," *J Am Diet Assoc*, 2002, 102 (3): 415-416.

Additional information about the glycemic index can be found at www.mendosa.com/gilists.htm.

Stored Glucose and Glycogen

The average 150-pound (68-kilogram) male has about 1,800 calories of carbohydrates stored in the liver, muscles, and blood in approximately the following distribution:

Muscle glycogen	1,400 calories
Liver glycogen	320 calories
Blood glucose	80 calories
Total	**1,800 calories**

These limited carbohydrate stores influence how long you can enjoy exercising. When your glycogen stores get too low, you hit the wall—that is, you feel overwhelmingly fatigued and yearn to quit.

In comparison to the approximately 1,800 calories of stored carbohydrates, the average, lean 150-pound man also has about 60,000 to 100,000 calories of stored fat—enough to run hundreds of miles. Unfortunately for endurance athletes, fat cannot be used exclusively as fuel because the muscles need a certain amount of carbohydrates to function well. Carbohydrates are a limiting factor for endurance athletes.

During low-level exercise such as walking, the muscles burn primarily fats for energy. During light to moderate aerobic exercise, such as jogging, stored fat provides 50 to 60 percent of the fuel. When you exercise hard, as in sprinting or racing or other intense exercise, you rely primarily on the glycogen stores.

Biochemical changes that occur during training influence the amount of glycogen you can store in your muscles. The figures that follow indicate that well-trained muscles develop the ability to store about 20 to 50 percent more glycogen than untrained muscles (Costill et al. 1981; Sherman et al. 1981). This change enhances endurance capacity and is one reason why a novice runner can't just carbo load and run a top-quality marathon.

Muscle Glycogen per 100 Grams (3.5 oz) of Muscle

Untrained muscle	13 g
Trained muscle	32 g
Carbo-loaded muscle	35-40 g

Because of the unfounded fear that carbohydrates are fattening or that high protein intake is better for muscles, many athletes today are

Steps of Digestion: Food Into Fuel

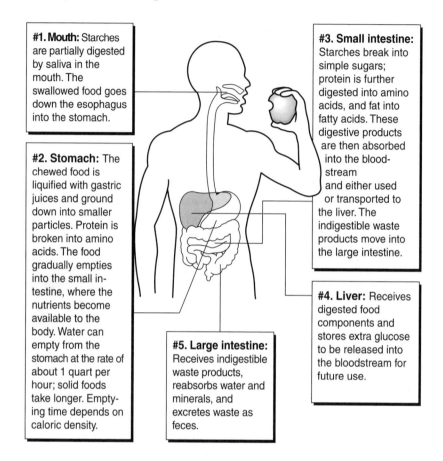

#1. Mouth: Starches are partially digested by saliva in the mouth. The swallowed food goes down the esophagus into the stomach.

#2. Stomach: The chewed food is liquified with gastric juices and ground down into smaller particles. Protein is broken into amino acids. The food gradually empties into the small intestine, where the nutrients become available to the body. Water can empty from the stomach at the rate of about 1 quart per hour; solid foods take longer. Emptying time depends on caloric density.

#3. Small intestine: Starches break into simple sugars; protein is further digested into amino acids, and fat into fatty acids. These digestive products are then absorbed into the bloodstream and either used or transported to the liver. The indigestible waste products move into the large intestine.

#4. Liver: Receives digested food components and stores extra glucose to be released into the bloodstream for future use.

#5. Large intestine: Receives indigestible waste products, reabsorbs water and minerals, and excretes waste as feces.

skimping on carbs. The resulting 40 percent carbohydrate diet can potentially hurt performance; it contrasts sharply to the 55 to 65 percent carb diet recommended by most exercise professionals.

A case in point is ice hockey. Ice hockey is an incredibly intense sport that relies on both muscular strength and power. During a game, carbohydrates are a primary fuel; muscle carbohydrate (glycogen) stores decline between 38 and 88 percent. Muscle glycogen depletion relates closely to muscular fatigue. A motion analysis of elite ice-hockey teams showed that the players with a high-carbohydrate (60 percent) diet skated not only 30 percent more distance but also faster than the players who ate their standard low-carbohydrate (40 percent) diet. In the final period of the game when a team either wins or loses, the high-carb group skated 11 percent more distance than they did in the first period; the low-carb group skated 14 percent less.

The researchers conclude that

1. low muscle glycogen at the start of the game can jeopardize performance at the end of the game;

2. three days between games (with training on two of those days) plus a 40 percent carbohydrate diet is insufficient to replace normal muscle glycogen stores (the players with the high-carb diet had 45 percent more glycogen); and

3. the differences in performance between the well-fueled players and those who ate inadequate carbohydrates was most evident in the last period of the game. Carbs work! (Ackermark et al. 1996).

Carbo Loading for Endurance Exercise

If you are preparing for an endurance event that lasts for more than 90 minutes—a competitive marathon, triathlon, cross-country ski race, or long-distance bike race—you should saturate your muscles with carbohydrates. But carbo loading means much more than stuffing yourself with pasta. Here is my nine-step carbohydrate-loading plan to help all endurance athletes fuel optimally for their events.

Carbo Load Daily

Your daily diet should be carbohydrate based and balanced with adequate protein (see chapter 8) and appropriate fat (see chapter 2). A daily 55 to 65 percent carbohydrate intake prevents chronic glycogen depletion and allows you not only to train at your best but also to compete at your best.

The philosophy that "if some carbohydrates are good, then more will be better" does not hold true for carbo loading. If you eat too much, you will likely experience intestinal distress and your muscles will be no better fueled than if you'd eaten an adequate amount (Rauch et al. 1995). The best target is about four grams of carbohydrate per pound (nine grams per kilogram) of body weight per day. By counting grams of carbohydrates you'll know if your sports diet hits this target.

Taper Your Training

Forget any plans for last-minute training sprees. Do your final hard training three weeks before race day and start tapering your training at least two weeks out. Although hard training builds you up, it also tears you down, and you need time to heal any damage that occurred during training and to completely refuel with carbohydrates. Some exercise scientists suggest you reduce your exercise time to 30 percent of normal, doing little exercise in the last 7 to 10 days before the event other than some short, intense speed intervals to keep you sharp (Houmard et al. 1990).

Correct tapering requires tremendous mental discipline and control. Most athletes are afraid to taper for such a long time. They are afraid they will get out of shape because they are exercising less. Worry not. The proof will come when you perform better—perhaps 9 percent better! Swimmers, for example, maximized their performance when they tapered for two weeks (Costill et al. 1985). Research suggests a 10- to 13-day taper can be better than a 7-day taper (Zarkadas, Carter, and Banister 1994).

Because you will be exercising less during the pre-event taper, you do not need to eat hundreds of additional calories when carbo loading. Simply maintain your standard intake (this should be about 3 to 5 grams of carbohydrate per pound of body weight, or 6 to 10 grams per kilogram). The 600 to 1,000 or so calories that you generally burn during training will be used to give your muscles extra fuel. If you save the calories that you might have burned during training, you can approximately double your glycogen stores and will be able to exercise harder during the third hour of your event (Rauch et al. 1995).

You'll know you have properly carbo loaded if you have gained two to four pounds (one to two kilograms), which is mostly water weight. With each ounce of stored glycogen, you store about three ounces of water. This water becomes available during exercise and reduces dehydration.

Rapid Loading

Some athletes prefer to not taper their exercise for two to three weeks before an endurance event; they are barely willing to take off one day for rest! To satisfy the needs of these intense athletes, researchers developed the following rapid-load program (Fairchild et al. 2002).

- One day before the event, the subjects exercycled very hard (130 percent $\dot{V}O_2$max) for two and a half minutes, and then in the last half minute they did an all-out effort to total exhaustion and depletion of muscle glycogen.

- As soon as tolerable, they started to consume a very high carbohydrate diet, targeting about 5 grams of carbohydrate per pound (10 grams per kilogram) of body weight, eaten over the course of the day. This means that an athlete who weighed 150 pounds (68 kilograms) needed to eat about 750 grams of carbs, which is the equivalent of 3,000 calories of carbohydrates. Because they were filling up on so many carbs, they had little room for fats or protein in that day's diet (only 10 percent of total calories, as opposed to a standard day with 45 percent of calories from protein and fat).
- Throughout the day they consumed carbo-loading beverages, juices, gels, and other forms of carbohydrate-dense products. By resting, the athletes gave their muscles the opportunity to superload using the abundance of carbs that flooded the system. The athletes were able to achieve levels of glycogen as high as those reached by athletes who carbo loaded for three to six days.

If this rapid-load protocol sounds enticing to you, be sure to practice it before the event. The drastic change in diet may lead to intestinal problems. Don't ruin your performance in the competition with adverse bathroom breaks!

Eat Enough Protein

Because endurance athletes burn some protein for energy, you should take special care to eat two small servings every day of protein-rich foods in addition to getting protein from two to three dairy servings. Even when carbo loading, your diet should include about 0.6 to 0.7 grams of protein per pound (1.3 to 1.6 grams per kilogram) of body weight. See chapters 1 and 8 for more protein guidelines.

Do Not Fat Load

To reduce your fat intake to 20 to 25 percent of your calories, have toast with jam rather than with butter, pancakes moistened with maple syrup rather than with margarine, and pasta with tomato sauce rather than with oil and cheese. A little fat is OK, but don't fat load.

To achieve a 55 to 65 percent carbohydrate diet, you have to trade some of the fat calories for more carbohydrates. For example, trade the fat calories in two pats of butter and a dollop of sour cream for a second plain baked potato. When you trade fat for more carbs, you need to eat a larger volume of food to obtain adequate calories. A one-pound box of spaghetti cooks into a mountain of pasta but provides only 1,600 calories. That's a reasonable calorie goal for a hefty premarathon meal, but it may be more volume than anticipated. See table 7.2 for a sample carbo-loading menu.

TABLE 7.2

Sample Carbo-Loading Menu

If you are preparing for a marathon or other endurance event, you should be sure to taper off your exercise and increase your carbohydrates. The following high-carb diet provides about 4 grams of carbs per pound (9 grams per kilogram) of body weight for a 150-pound (68-kilogram) marathoner. The menu includes adequate protein (0.8 grams per pound, or 1.8 grams per kilogram; see chapter 8) to maintain your muscles.

Breakfast

1 cup orange juice
1/2 cup Grape-Nuts
1 medium banana
1 cup 2% milk
1 english muffin
1 tbsp jelly
750 calories; 85% carbohydrates

Lunch

2 slices oatmeal bread
3 oz turkey breast with lettuce, tomato
8 oz apple juice
1 cup frozen yogurt
750 calories; 65% carbohydrates

Dinner

3 cups spaghetti (6 oz uncooked)
1 cup tomato sauce
2 oz ground turkey
1/4 loaf multigrain bread (4 oz)
1,300 calories; 70% carbohydrates

Snack

1 cup vanilla yogurt
6 fig bars
500 calories; 80% carbohydrates

Total: 3,300 calories; 75% carb (610 g), 15% protein (125 g), 10% fat (40 g)

Choose Fiber-Rich Foods

Fiber-rich foods promote regular bowel movements and keep your system running smoothly. Bran muffins, whole-wheat bread, bran cereal, fruits, and vegetables are some good choices. If you carbo load on too much white bread, pasta, rice, and other refined products, you're likely to become constipated, particularly if you are doing less training. See the section on fiber in chapter 2 for more information. If you are worried about diarrhea, you should avoid fiber-rich foods before an event.

Plan Meal Times Carefully

On the day before the event, you might want to eat your biggest meal at lunchtime so that the food will have more time to digest and pass through your system. Later, enjoy a normal-sized dinner and a bedtime snack. One runner discovered with dismay that the exceptionally hefty dinner she ate the night before a marathon was still sitting heavily in her system on marathon morning.

Drink Extra Fluids

To reduce your risk of becoming dehydrated, drink plenty of fluids before and during the event.

- Drink about four to eight extra glasses of water and juices during the two days before the event. You should have to urinate every two to four hours.
- Limit dehydrating fluids such as beer, wine, and other alcoholic beverages.
- On race morning, drink at least three glasses of water up to two hours before the event and one to two cups 5 to 10 minutes before race time.

Eat Breakfast on Event Day

Eating breakfast is important, but almost as important is choosing food you're familiar with. This approach will prevent hunger and help maintain normal blood sugar level. As part of your training, you should have practiced eating before races to learn which foods in what amounts work best for you. Don't try any new foods. That festive pancake breakfast may settle like Mississippi mud, and so may the expensive energy bar you've been saving for a special occasion.

Be Sensible About Your Selections

Do not carbo load on only fruit or you are likely to get diarrhea. Do not carbo load on only refined white bread products or you are likely to become constipated. Do not carbo load on beer or you'll become dehydrated. Do not do too much last-minute training or you'll fatigue your muscles. And do not blow it all by eating unfamiliar foods that might upset your system. Change your exercise program more than your diet.

Bonking

Whereas depleted muscle glycogen causes athletes to hit the wall, depleted liver glycogen causes them to bonk or crash. Liver glycogen feeds into the bloodstream to maintain a normal blood sugar level essential for "brain food." Despite adequate muscle glycogen, an athlete may feel uncoordinated, lightheaded, unable to concentrate, and weakened because the liver is releasing inadequate sugar into the bloodstream.

You already know that your muscles and brain require glucose for energy. What you may not be aware of is that although the muscles can store glucose and burn fat, the brain does neither. This means that for the brain to function optimally, you must consume food close enough to strenuous events to supply sugar to the blood so the brain has fuel. Athletes with low blood sugar tend to perform poorly because the poorly fueled brain limits muscular function and mental drive.

John, a 28-year-old runner and banker, faithfully carbo loaded his muscles for three days before his first Boston Marathon. On the evening before the marathon, he ate dinner at 5:00 and then went to bed at 8:30 to ensure himself a good night's rest. But, as often happens with anxious athletes, he tossed and turned all night (which burned a significant amount of calories), got up early the next morning, and chose not to eat breakfast, even though the marathon didn't start until noon. By noon, he had depleted his limited liver glycogen stores. He lost his mental drive about 8 miles into the race and quit at 12 miles. His muscles were well fueled, but energy was unavailable to his brain, so he lacked the mental stamina to endure the marathon.

John could have prevented this needless fatigue by eating some oatmeal, cereal, or other carbohydrate at breakfast to refuel his liver glycogen stores. Athletic success depends on both well-fueled muscles and a well-fueled mind.

The Best Source of Glycogen

A landmark study by exercise physiologist Dr. J. Bergstrom and his colleagues (1967) explains why carbohydrates are essential for high-energy athletic performance. The researchers compared the rate at which muscle glycogen was replaced in subjects who exercised to exhaustion and then ate either a high-protein, high-fat diet or a high-carbohydrate diet.

The subjects on the high-protein, high-fat diet (similar to the diet of folks who live on steak, eggs, hamburgers, tuna salad, peanut butter, and cheese) remained glycogen depleted for five days. The subjects on a high-carbohydrate diet totally replenished their muscle glycogen in two days. This result shows that protein and fats aren't stored as muscle fuel and that carbohydrates are important in replacing depleted glycogen stores.

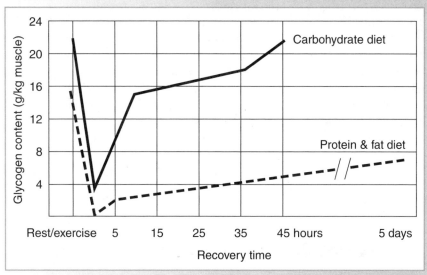

Reprinted, by permission, from J. Bergstrom, L. Hermansen, E. Hultman, B. Saltin, 1967, "Diet muscle glycogen and physical performance," *Acta Physiologica Scandinavia* 71:140.

If you are trying to stay away from carbs like bagels, pasta, and breads because you mistakenly believe carbohydrates to be fattening, think again. If you are dieting and exercising, you'll want to include carbs in your diet because carbohydrates are not fattening and you need them to fuel your muscles so that you can enjoy your exercise program.

Annie, a 28-year-old nurse practitioner and dedicated exerciser, learned the importance of recovery days and adequate carbohydrates through a sports-nutrition experiment. When she first came to see me, she insisted on training every day to get in shape for her first marathon. I recommended that she take at least one or two days off a week. Annie decided to experiment with her two-hour Sunday run to determine if her running improved with running less and eating better. She discovered she could train at her best when she did little or no training the day before her long run (to rest her muscles) followed by a day off after her long run (to refuel). She stopped forcing herself to do the obligatory daily training run any day when her muscles felt fatigued. Instead, she planned at least one or two rest days per week into her training schedule and started focusing on quality training rather than quantity training. Her running improved, as did her mental outlook and enthusiasm for her sport. She ran a personal best in the marathon, cutting seven minutes off her time.

Many athletes hesitate to exercise less because they are afraid of getting out of shape. If this sounds like you, remember that rest will enhance, not hurt, your performance. You won't lose fitness but rather will enhance your strength and endurance with better-fueled muscles. Athletes who underestimate the value of rest and instead train relentlessly set the stage for injuries, chronic glycogen depletion, chronic fatigue, and reduced performance. These athletes often hope that vitamin supplements, special sports foods, and other pills and potions will boost their energy. All they really need to perform better is less exercise.

If you are severely overtrained, you may need weeks, if not months, to recover. One study with swimmers showed that a two-and-a-half-week taper was inadequate to recover from the staleness acquired during a six-month season (Hooper et al. 1995). I've said it before and I'll say it again: Don't underestimate the value of rest!

Carbohydrates for Building Muscles?

"I know that for running I should eat carbohydrates to fuel my muscles. But for weightlifting, shouldn't I eat a lot of protein to build them up?"

Perhaps, like Steve, a 34-year-old runner who lifts weights, you are confused about what to eat for energy, strength, and top performance—carbohydrates or protein. This is what I recommend:

- Eat carbohydrate-rich breakfasts, such as oatmeal, rather than eggs.
- Focus your lunches and dinners on whole-grain breads, potatoes, brown rice, fruits, and vegetables. Wholesome carbohydrates should cover two-thirds of your plate.
- Eat fish, chicken, lean meats, low-fat cheeses, and other proteins as an accompaniment to lunch and dinner, not as the focus. Alternatively, you could eat carbohydrate-rich protein such as beans and rice, lentil soup, chili, hummus, and other vegetarian choices.

Carbohydrates are fundamental for both runners and bodybuilders, because unlike protein or fat, carbs are readily stored in your muscles for fuel during exercise. Adequate protein is important for building and protecting your muscles, but you should dedicate only one-third of your dinner plate to protein-rich foods. See chapter 8 for more information about protein requirements.

Recovery From Daily Training

As I mentioned in chapter 6, carbohydrates are important for refueling after competitive events. Carbs are also important on a daily basis for those who train hard day after day and want to maintain high energy. If you eat a low-carbohydrate diet, your muscles will feel chronically fatigued. You'll train, but not at your best.

The following chart illustrates the glycogen depletion that can occur when athletes eat an inadequate amount of carbohydrates and still try to exercise hard day after day (Costill, Bowers, Branam, et al. 1971). In this landmark study, on three consecutive days the subjects in this study ran hard for 10 miles (at a pace of 6 to 8 minutes per mile). They ate their standard meals: a diet that provided about 45 to 50 percent of calories from carbohydrates, not the 55 to 65 percent required in a top-performance sports diet. The subjects' muscles became increasingly glycogen depleted. Had the runners eaten larger portions of carbohydrates (and smaller portions of proteins and fats), they would have better replaced their glycogen stores and better invested in top performance.

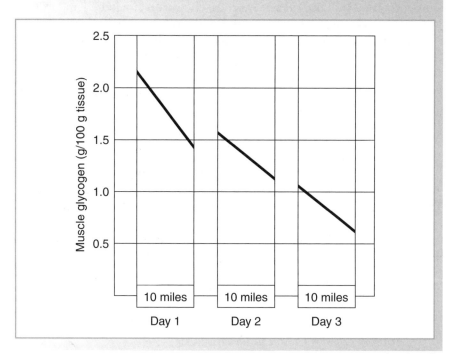

(continued)

(continued)

This study emphasizes the need not only for a daily carbohydrate-rich diet but also for recovery days with light or no training. If you are doing daily hard workouts, take heed: Your depleted muscles need at least one, if not two, days to refuel after exhaustive sessions. (If you are a casual exerciser who uses significantly less glycogen during, let's say, a half-hour walk or a gentle swim, recovery days are less essential.)

Are Carbohydrates Fattening?

Stacey, a personal trainer, wanted to eat carbohydrates for fuel but also wanted to maintain a lean weight. Like many weight-conscious athletes, Stacey considered carbohydrates to be fattening foods, and she was frustrated. "I don't keep crackers, bread, cereal, or bagels in the house, because when they are there, I eat them—too many of them! I want to lose weight, not gain it from all those fattening carbohydrates."

Fad diets preach the message that carbohydrates are fattening. Wrong! Carbohydrates are not fattening. *Excess calories* are fattening, in particular excess calories of fats are fattening—butter on bread, oil on pasta, mayonnaise on sandwiches, cheese on crackers. Fats provide 36 calories per teaspoon, compared with 16 for carbohydrates. But the conversion of excess carbohydrates into body fat is limited because you burn the carbs when you exercise. Your body preferentially burns the carbohydrates and stores the fats; the metabolic cost of converting excess carbohydrates into body fat is 23 percent. Excess dietary fats, on the other hand, are easily stored as body fat; the metabolic cost of converting excess dietary fat into body fat is only 3 percent of ingested calories (Sims and Danforth 1987).

If you are destined to be gluttonous, your better bet is to overeat pretzels (carbohydrates) rather than peanuts (fats). You'll fuel your muscles better, and the next day you'll have a high-energy workout with muscles well loaded with carbohydrates. But be aware that a continuous intake of excess calories from carbohydrates will eventually contribute to weight gain. When your glycogen stores are filled, the excess calories will be stored as body fat (Hill et al. 1992).

Rather than try to stay away from breads and bagels and other grains, remember these points:

- Carbohydrates are less fattening than fatty foods.
- You need carbs to fuel your muscles.
- You burn carbs off during hard exercise.

- Carbohydrates are a friendly fuel; the enemy is excess calories of fats.
- When dieting to lose weight, you should energize with fiber-rich cereal, whole-grain breads, potatoes, and other carbohydrate-dense vegetables but reduce your intake of the butter, margarine, and mayonnaise that often accompany them.

Some advertisements for sports foods claim that athletes should eat fewer carbs and more fat to burn more body fat and lose weight. Not true! No research to date shows that burning fat results in losing body fat. The only way to lose body fat is to create a calorie deficit.

Carbohydrate-Rich Foods

All too often I talk with athletes who think they eat a carbohydrate-rich diet when they really don't.

Eric, a 33-year-old store manager and triathlete, intended to carbo load the night before his first triathlon. Because of inadequate nutrition knowledge, he "carbo loaded" with a pepperoni pizza with double cheese. Little did he know that of the 1,800 calories in the large pizza, 1,200 were from the protein and fat in the double cheese and pepperoni. Only 35 percent of the calories, from the thin crust and tomato sauce, were from carbohydrates. No wonder he felt sluggish during the event.

I gave Eric a list of carbohydrates in common foods (see table 7.3) to post on his refrigerator. With this tool he learned to select high-carbohydrate foods.

In addition, I taught him how to make better selections based on the nutrition-facts panel on food labels. You, too, can use labels to guide your selections. The nutrition-facts panel lists the number of grams of carbohydrate, protein, and fat (and alcohol if present) per serving, as well as the calories per gram:

- 1 gram carbohydrate = 4 calories
- 1 gram protein = 4 calories
- 1 gram fat = 9 calories
- 1 gram alcohol = 7 calories

Using this information, you can make some simple calculations. To determine the number of carbohydrate calories in a food item, multiply the number of grams of carbohydrate by four (calories per gram). Next,

TABLE 7.3

Carbohydrates in Common Foods

To fuel your muscles, the foundation of every meal should be carbohydrate-rich foods. To determine your carbohydrate needs precisely, you can target 3 to 5 grams of carbohydrates per pound (7 to 11 grams per kilogram) of body weight (ACSM 2000).

For example, if you weigh 160 pounds (73 kilograms), this comes to 480 to 800 grams, or about 60 percent of a 3,200- to 5,300-calorie diet—a range of fuel appropriate for an active person of that weight. Note that this method of calculating carbohydrate needs works best for active athletes with high calorie needs, not for sedentary people.

Food labels are the handiest source of carbohydrate information. The following list of carbohydrate-rich foods can help you keep a tally.

Food	Amount	Carbohydrates (grams)	Total calories
Fruits			
Raisins	1/3 cup	40	150
Banana	1 medium	25	105
Apricots, dried	10 halves	20	85
Apple	1 medium	20	80
Orange	1 medium	15	65
Vegetables			
Spaghetti sauce, Prego	1/2 cup	22	120
Corn, canned	1/2 cup	15	70
Winter squash	1/2 cup	15	60
Peas	1/2 cup	10	60
Carrot	1 medium	10	40
Green beans	1/2 cup	5	20
Broccoli	1/2 cup	5	20
Zucchini	1/2 cup	2	10
Bread-type foods			
Hoagie roll	1	75	400
Bagel, Thomas's	1	57	300
Pita	1 average (3 oz)	46	240
Tortilla	1 large (2.5 oz)	36	220
English muffin	1	25	120
Bread, rye	1 slice	15	80
Waffle, Eggo	1	14	90
Saltines	5	10	60
Graham crackers	2 squares	10	70
Breakfast cereals			
Grape-Nuts	1/2 cup	47	210
Raisin Bran, Kellogg's	1 cup	45	190
Granola, low-fat	2/3 cup	45	210
Oatmeal, maple instant	1 packet	30	160
Cream of Wheat, cooked	1 cup	25	120

Food	Amount	Carbohydrates (grams)	Total calories
Beverages			
Apricot nectar	8 oz	35	140
Cranraspberry juice	8 oz	35	140
Apple juice	8 oz	30	120
Orange juice	8 oz	25	105
Cola	12 oz	39	155
Milk, chocolate	8 oz	25	180
Gatorade	8 oz	14	50
Beer	12 oz	13	145
Milk, 2%	8 oz	12	120
Grains, pasta, starches			
Baked potato	1 large	50	220
Baked beans	1 cup	50	260
Rice, cooked	1 cup	45	200
Lentils, cooked	1 cup	40	230
Stuffing, bread	1 cup	40	340
Spaghetti, cooked	1 cup	40	200
Ramen noodles	1/2 package	25	180
Entrees, convenience foods			
Macaroni and cheese, Kraft	1 cup	48	410
Bean burrito, frozen	5 oz	45	370
Spaghettios	1 cup	37	180
Lentil soup, Progresso	12 oz	33	210
Refried beans, canned	1 cup	32	200
Sweets, snacks, desserts			
Fruit yogurt	1 cup	50	225
Frozen yogurt	1 cup	44	240
Pop-Tart, blueberry	1	36	200
Fig Newton	1	11	55
Oreo	1	8	50
Honey	1 tbsp	15	60
Maple syrup	1 tbsp	13	50
Strawberry jam	1 tbsp	13	50
Cranberry sauce	1 tbsp	7	30

Nutrient data from food labels and J. Pennington, 1998, *Bowes & Church's Food Values of Portions Commonly Used*, 17th ed. (Philadelphia: Lippincott).

compare the carbohydrate calories to the total calories per serving to determine the percentage of calories that are from carbohydrates.

For example, a half-cup serving of a gourmet vanilla ice cream might have 200 total calories and 20 grams of carbohydrates.

$$19 \text{ g carb} \times 4 \text{ cal/g} = 76 \text{ cal from carbs}$$

$$76 \text{ cal carb} \div 220 \text{ total cal} = 35\% \text{ carbs}$$

Using food-label information, you can determine that ice cream contains relatively fewer carbohydrates than frozen yogurt does. For example, for every 100 calories of vanilla ice cream (two spoonfuls!), you get only 10 grams of carbohydrates. This is equal to 40 calories of carbohydrates, which is 40 percent of total calories. On the other hand, for every 100 calories of frozen yogurt (four spoonfuls), you get about 22 grams of carbohydrates. This is roughly 88 calories of carbohydrates and 88 percent of total calories.

Counting Carbohydrates

Your diet should be at least 55 percent carbohydrate for daily training and 55 to 65 percent carbohydrate before an endurance event. You can achieve a diet that is 55 to 65 percent carbohydrate by opting for more starches and grains and fewer fatty, greasy foods. Replace muffins with bagels, granola with muesli, alfredo sauce with tomato sauce on pasta. Note that a high-carbohydrate diet can and should include a small amount of fat. If you try to eat carbohydrates exclusively, you may end up with an unbalanced intake, a linear diet that differs from the balance and variety found with the Food Guide Pyramid.

Like many registered dietitians and sports nutritionists, I use a computer program that calculates the percentage of carbohydrate and fat in a diet so that athletes can see how their intake compares to the target goals of 55 to 65 percent carbohydrate, 20 to 30 percent fat, and 10 to 15 percent protein. Many of my clients are shocked at how easily fat creeps into their diets. For example, Peter, a health-conscious fitness exerciser, simply indulged in too many helpings of peanuts, almonds, and sunflower seeds, his favorite snacks. By trading them in for higher carbohydrate items—granola, raisins, dried apricots, and bananas—he easily boosted his carbohydrate intake to 68 percent. "You know, my training has improved since I made that switch. My muscles feel springier and I have greater endurance. I feel great. I'm glad I learned this simple solution to my needless fatigue!"

Learning about the composition of your training diet is important. I generally see more athletes carbohydrate depleted during training periods than before competitions. They take good care of their diets before an important event but often neglect it in the hubbub of daily life. Unfortunately, they can't compete at their best if they don't train at their best.

If you want to feel completely at peace with your diet and verify that you are eating the right balance of carbohydrates, protein, and fat, consult with a registered dietitian, evaluate your diet using a computer program or the Internet, or count grams of carbohydrates (and protein and fat) based on the needs of your body. Some simple meals based on store-bought foods with nutrition labeling that details the number of carbs in a food might be cereal, milk, and juice; a peanut butter and jelly sandwich and a yogurt; or spaghetti with jarred tomato sauce, cottage cheese, and frozen vegetables. Although gathering food-label information may seem a huge project, a one-day effort can be interesting and provide peace of mind because you'll know that you're making wise choices that invest in both health and performance—or give you incentive to make a few changes.

The Balancing Act

As I've mentioned before, although you want to maximize your intake of carbohydrates, you shouldn't cut all protein and fat from your sports diet. Yet if you stuff yourself with too much protein and fat, you'll end up with inadequate carbohydrates. Your best bet is to fuel up on a foundation of carbs and have fat as the accompaniment to the meal. That is, have a carbohydrate-rich pasta dinner with meat sauce as the topping.

Another mistake health-conscious athletes commonly make is reducing their fat intake without replacing those calories with adequate carbohydrates. Don, a basketball player, cut butter, mayonnaise, and chips from his diet and lost two pounds within a week of making this nutrition change; he neglected to replace the deleted fat calories with adequate carbohydrates. He should have eaten, for example, two potatoes to get the same amount of calories in the one potato drenched with butter and sour cream.

Athletes who choose very low-fat diets must eat large quantities of carbohydrates to get adequate calories. If they have big appetites, as do six-foot, 10-inch basketball players, they often tire of chewing before they are adequately fed! The focus of the diet should be on carbohydrates, but some healthful fats (nuts, peanut butter, olive oil) can still be part of each meal. Eating 3 to 5 grams of carbohydrate per pound (6 to 10 grams per kilogram) of body weight will saturate your muscles with carbohydrates. After that, you can eat the balance of the calories in lean protein and healthful fat.

Any way you look at them, carbohydrates of any type are important for athletes. If you're wise, you'll choose to eat primarily wholesome breads, grains, and cereals from the base of the Food Guide Pyramid, along with a strong intake of carbohydrate-rich fruits, vegetables, legumes, and dried beans. Save the sugary carbohydrates from the tip of the pyramid for occasional treats.

8

Protein and Performance

Traditionally, protein-rich foods have been synonymous with muscular athletes. The (misguided) theory is that if you eat a lot of protein, you will build a lot of muscle. But extra protein does not build extra muscle, exercise does—heavy weightlifting, push-ups, and other forms of resistance exercise that build and strengthen muscles.

Confusion exists about the best diet for building muscles. When you work out in the weight room at the gym, you likely hear you need to consume lots of tuna, chicken breasts, and egg whites, and drink protein shakes between meals, to be stronger. But when you hang around in the cardio area, you hear that carbohydrate-rich pasta, cereal, and grains should be the foundation of your meals. And you are left wondering: What's the right balance?

Carbohydrate-rich grains, fruits, and vegetables are indeed the best foundation for every type of training program. Even bodybuilders need a carbohydrate-based diet because carbohydrates are stored in the muscles for energy. You can't lift weights and demand a lot from your workout sessions if your muscles are carbo depleted. Protein-based diets low in carbohydrates provide inadequate muscle fuel for you to exercise hard enough to build to your potential.

The best sports diet contains adequate, but not excessive, protein to build and repair muscle tissue, grow hair and fingernails, produce hormones, boost your immune system, and replace red blood cells. Most people who eat moderate portions of protein-rich foods daily get more protein than they need. Any excess protein is burned for energy or, as a last resort, stored as glycogen or fat. Humans do not store excess protein as protein or amino acids, so we need to consume adequate protein each day. Daily protein is particularly important for dieters who are restricting calories, because protein is burned for energy when carbohydrates are scarce.

When it comes to protein intake, athletes seem to fall into two categories. First are those who eat too much—the bodybuilders, weightlifters, and football players who can't seem to get enough of the stuff. Those in the second group eat too little—the runners, triathletes, dancers, and weight-conscious athletes who never touch meat and trade most protein calories for more salads and veggies. Individuals in either group can perform poorly because of dietary imbalances.

Josh, for example, was a protein pusher. A college hockey player, he routinely snacked after practice on a big protein bar and a protein shake. That one snack satisfied his protein needs for the whole day! As an athlete, he has a slightly higher protein need than a sedentary person, but he overcompensated for that need with the generous servings of chicken and fish he devoured at meals, never mind his high-protein snack.

Peter, a vegetarian marathon runner who focused his intake on pasta meals, was a protein avoider. He consumed few protein-rich foods of any types—plant or animal products. He was humbled when he learned that his food intake was deficient not only in protein but also in iron (for red blood cells), zinc (for healing), calcium (for bones), and several other nutrients. No wonder he became anemic, suffered a lingering cold and flu, and performed poorly despite consistent training.

Defining Protein Needs

Research has yet to define the exact protein requirements of sports-active people because individual needs vary. People in the following groups have the highest protein needs:

- **Endurance athletes and others doing intense exercise.** About 5 percent of energy can come from protein during endurance exercise, particularly if muscle glycogen stores are depleted and blood glucose is low.
- **Dieters consuming too few calories.** The protein is converted into glucose and burned for energy instead of being used to build and repair muscles.

- **Growing teenage athletes.** They need enough protein for both growth and muscular development.
- **Untrained people starting an exercise program.** They need extra protein to build muscles.

In scrutinizing the protein needs of athletes, exercise scientists have found that athletes need only slightly more protein than other people do to repair the small amounts of muscle damage that occur with training, provide energy (in very small amounts) for exercise, and support the building of new muscle tissue.

In general, pinpointing exact protein requirements is a moot point because most athletes tend to eat more protein than they require just through standard meals. That is, within the recommendation of the food pyramid, a 150-pound (68-kilogram) recreational athlete who burns 3,000 calories can easily consume 10 to 15 percent of calories from protein. This amount is equal to 300 to 450 protein calories, or 75 to 110 grams of protein, which is 0.5 to 0.7 grams of protein per pound (1.0 to 1.5 grams of protein per kilogram) and more than the RDA (0.4 gram/pound; 0.8 gram/kilogram).

But individuals have a range of protein needs. The following are some safe and adequate recommendations for protein intake. These recommendations include a margin of safety and are not minimal amounts:

	Grams of protein	
	Per pound of body weight	Per kilogram
Current RDA for sedentary adult	0.4	0.8
Recreational exerciser, adult	0.5-0.7	0.8-1.5
Endurance athlete, adult	0.6-0.7	1.2-1.6
Growing teenage athlete	0.7-0.9	1.5-2.0
Adult building muscle mass	0.7-0.8	1.5-1.7
Athlete restricting calories	0.8-0.9	1.8-2.0
Estimated upper requirement for adults	0.9	2.0
Average protein intake of male endurance athletes	0.5-0.9	1.2-2.0
Average protein intake of female athletes	0.5-0.8	1.1-1.7

Data compiled from American College of Sports Medicine, American Dietetic Association, and Dietitians of Canada Joint Position Statement. Nutrition and Athletic Performance. *Medicine and Science in Sports and Exercise* 32 (12): 2130-2145, 2000; R. Maughan and L. Burke, editors. *Sports Nutrition* (part of the Handbook of Sports Medicine and Science series, an IOC Medical Commission Publication) Malden, MA: Blackwell Publishing, 2002; Institute of Medicine. *Dietary Reference Intakes for Energy, Carbohydrate, Fiber, Fatty Acids, Cholesterol, Protein and Amino Acids*. Food and Nutrition Board, Washington, DC: National Academy Press, 2002.

In contrast to the belief that if a little more protein is good, a lot more will be better, no scientific evidence to date suggests that protein intakes exceeding 0.9 grams of protein per pound (2.0 grams per kilogram) will provide an additional advantage (Lemon 1995). Nor is there evidence that taking a protein supplement on top of an adequate diet (0.5 gram of protein per pound, or about 1 gram per kilogram) will enhance muscle strength or size (Godard, Williamson, and Trappe 2002).

Calculating Your Protein Needs

Figuring your protein needs is easy. To learn if you are meeting your protein needs in your current diet, follow two easy steps. First, identify yourself in a category from the previous list that recommends the amount of protein needed by a variety of people. For example, if you are a 140-pound (64-kilogram) bike racer, you would fit the category of an "endurance athlete, adult" and would need about 85 to 100 grams of protein per day:

$$140 \text{ lb} \times 0.6 \text{ g/lb} = 84 \text{ g protein}$$

$$140 \text{ lb} \times 0.7 \text{ g/lb} = 98 \text{ g protein}$$

Second, keep track of your protein intake by listing everything you eat and drink for one 24-hour period. For example, the nutrition facts on the label of a six-ounce can of tuna might tell you it contains 15 grams of protein and two and one-half servings per can. So, if you eat the whole can, you're getting about 40 grams of protein.

Table 8.1 lists the amount of protein in some common foods. The information on food labels can provide additional information. Most fruits and vegetables have only small amounts of protein, which may contribute a total of 5 to 10 grams of protein per day, depending on how much you eat. Butter, margarine, oil, sugar, soda, alcohol, and coffee contain no protein, and most desserts contain very little.

An easier way to assess whether you are getting adequate, but not excessive, protein in your daily diet is to use this rule of thumb: 16 ounces (two cups, or 500 milliliters) of milk or yogurt plus two small servings of protein-rich foods meets the daily protein requirement. Combined with the small amounts of protein in other foods that round out the meals, this should suit the needs of a healthy 150-pound adult. Here's a sample of one day's worth of protein-rich foods for an active adult. Of course, you'll need to eat other foods to round out your calorie and nutritional requirements.

Breakfast	1 cup milk on cereal
Lunch	2 oz sandwich filling (tuna, roast beef, turkey)
	1 cup yogurt
Dinner	4 oz meat, fish, poultry, or the equivalent in lentils or other beans and legumes

TABLE 8.1

Protein in Common Foods

Although animal products provide high quality protein, you don't have to eat beef to get plenty of protein. You can eat a variety of plant proteins. Note that you need to eat a generous portion (more calories) of beans and other plant protein to equal the protein in animal foods. (See chapter 1 for more information about protein.)

Animal sources	Grams of protein per standard serving	Grams of protein per 100 cal (amount)
Egg white	3.5 / 1 large egg	20 / 6 egg whites
Egg	6 / 1 large	8 / 1.3 eggs
Cheddar cheese	7 / 1 oz	6 / 0.9 oz
Milk, 1%	8 / 8 oz	8 / 8 oz
Yogurt	11 / 1 cup	8 / 6 oz
Cottage cheese	15 / 1/2 cup	15 / 1/2 cup
Haddock	27 / 4 oz cooked	21 / 3 oz
Hamburger	30 / 4 oz broiled	10 / 1.5 oz
Pork loin	30 / 4 oz roasted	10 / 1.5 oz
Chicken breast	35 / 4 oz roasted	18 / 2 oz
Tuna	40 / 6 oz	20 / 3 oz
Plant sources		
Almonds, dried	3 / 12 nuts	3.5 / 14 nuts
Peanut butter	4.5 / 1 tbsp	4.5 / 1 tbsp
Kidney beans	6 / 1/2 cup	6 / 1/2 cup
Hummus	6 / 1/2 cup	3 / 1/4 cup
Refried beans	7 / 1/2 cup	7 / 1/2 cup
Lentil soup	11 / 10.5 oz	6.5 / 6 oz
Tofu, extra firm	11 / 3.5 oz	12 / 4 oz
Baked beans	14 / 1 cup	7 / 1/2 cup

Data from food labels and J. Pennington, 1998, *Bowes & Church's Food Values of Portions Commonly Used*, 17th ed. (Philadelphia: Lippincott).

Growing teens and others with high-protein needs can get additional protein and calcium by drinking another two cups of milk.

Note that you have a daily need for protein. As I mentioned before, some people eat protein-rich foods only once or twice per week and live on salads and pasta for most of their meals. They cheat themselves of an optimal training diet.

Too Much Protein

Contrary to what most people think, too much protein can create problems with health and performance. Jasper, an aspiring bodybuilder, chowed down on chicken and beef yet avoided pasta and potatoes, much to the detriment of his athletic aspirations. He tired easily and asked me if this high-protein diet might be hurting his performance. Here's what I told him:

- If you fill your stomach with too much protein, you won't be fueling your muscles with carbohydrates.

- Anyone who eats excess protein may need to urinate more frequently, because protein breaks down into urea, a waste product eliminated in the urine. Frequent trips to the bathroom may be an inconvenience during training and competition, to say nothing of increasing the risk of becoming dehydrated and burdening the kidneys.

- A diet based on animal protein tends to be expensive. You can save money by eating smaller portions of beef, lamb, pork, and other animal proteins. Use that money to buy more plant proteins (beans, lentils, tofu) and more fruits, vegetables, grains, and potatoes.

- A diet high in protein can easily be high in fat (juicy steaks, bacon and eggs, pepperoni pizza, and so on). For the sake of your heart and for improved athletic performance, you should reduce your intake of the saturated fats found in animal proteins. This kind of diet may also reduce your risk of certain cancers.

I encouraged Jasper to reduce his meat portions at dinner to one-third of his plate and to fill two-thirds with potatoes, vegetables, and whole-grain bread. Within two days, he noticed an improvement in his energy level. He then changed his breakfast from bacon and eggs to cereal and a banana, and lunch became chili or pasta rather than burgers. His diet gradually became a winner. "I'm amazed," he now says, "at the power of food. Eating carbohydrate-based foods that fuel my muscles definitely enhances my sports performance!"

Healthful Meat Choices

"I rarely eat meat except when I'm at home," commented Christina, a college student who lived off campus and was responsible for her own food. "I like meat, but it seems to spoil before I get around to cooking it for dinner." She cooked mostly pasta and consequently wondered if she consumed too little protein.

If you, like Christina, think you eat too little protein and the accompanying nutrients iron and zinc, and you are willing to eat animal proteins, eating a small amount of lean red meat two to four times per week can enhance the quality of your sports diet. Here are some tips to keep in mind for health-promoting, low-fat meat eatery:

- Take advantage of the deli. For precooked meats, buy rotisserie chicken or slices of lean roast beef, ham, and turkey in the deli section at the grocery store.
- Buy extralean cuts of beef, pork, and lamb to reduce your intake of saturated fats. Forgo cuts with a marbled appearance and trim the fat off steaks and chops before cooking them.
- Get rid of more fat. After browning ground beef, drain it in a colander and rinse it with hot water to remove the fat before adding it to spaghetti sauce.
- At a cafeteria, request two rolls when you order one hamburger. Use one roll to absorb the grease. Throw it away and then eat the second roll with the degreased burger.
- Integrate meat into a meal as an accompaniment. Add a little extralean hamburger to spaghetti sauce, stir-fry a small piece of steak with lots of veggies, serve a pile of rice along with one lean pork chop, make a savory potato-rich stew with a little lean lamb, or buy deli roast beef for sandwiches made on hearty bread.

Protein and the Vegetarian

Many active people choose not to eat animal protein. Some just eat no red meat; others eat no chicken, fish, eggs, or dairy foods. They may think that animal protein is hard to digest, bad for the health, unethical to eat, or harmful to the environment. Whatever their reason for abstaining, they often overlook the fact that they still need to eat adequate protein to maintain good health. (And a balanced vegetarian diet is indeed a good investment in good health.)

The trick to eating a balanced vegetarian diet is to make the effort to replace beef with beans. If you eliminate meat, you need to add a source of plant protein. You can easily get adequate protein to support your sports program by including kidney beans, chickpeas, peanut butter, tofu, nuts, and other plant proteins in your daily diet. Some nonmeat eaters, however, simply fuel up only on carbohydrates and neglect their protein needs. The following is a typical example of one athlete's protein-deficient diet.

Peter, a 150-pound (68-kilogram) runner, consumed only 6 percent of his calories from protein, equal to 0.3 grams of protein per pound

(0.7 grams per kilogram), or half the recommended intake for athletes. A normal day of eating for Peter looked something like this:

Meal	Protein (g)*	Calories
Breakfast		
1 large bagel	4	400
2 cups orange juice	2	220
Lunch		
2 large bananas	3	300
12 oz tropical fruit drink	—	240
1 bran muffin	4	300
Dinner		
3 cups cooked pasta	20	660
1 cup tomato sauce	2	100
24 oz sweetened iced tea	—	300
Snack		
1 cup dried fruit	5	480
Total	40	3,000

*Recommended protein intake: 90 to 135 grams of protein (0.6 to 0.9 grams of protein per pound of body weight)

To improve his protein intake, he simply needed to add peanut butter to the bagel, replace the fruit drink with yogurt, add beans or tofu to the spaghetti at dinnertime, and mix in some nuts with the dried fruit for a snack. All these changes were easy to make; Peter just had to be more responsible with balancing his diet.

The Vegetarian Female Athlete

Female athletes commonly choose to eat a meatless diet. They may refer to themselves as vegetarians, but many fit into the non-meat-eater category. That is, they eat too much fruit, too many salads, and abundant jellybeans—but no beans, tofu, yogurt, or plant sources of protein. This protein deficiency, along with an overall calorie-deficient diet, is associated with medical problems, specifically loss of regular menstrual cycles.

Vegetarian Females and Amenorrhea

Some athletic women, in their obsession to lose weight, consume a very low-calorie and low-protein vegetarian diet. This drastic reduction in food intake can lead to amenorrhea; that is, they stop having regular menstrual periods. Research suggests that amenorrheic athletes have a four and one-half times higher risk for suffering a stress fracture than do regularly menstruating athletes (Clark, Nelson, and Evans

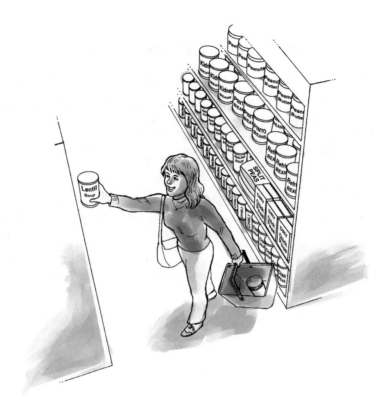

1988; Nativ 2000). Eating a balanced diet with adequate calories can enhance resumption of menses, provide adequate protein for building and protecting muscles, and enhance overall health.

Jessica, now a healthy gymnast, used to live on melon for breakfast, a salad for lunch, and steamed vegetables with brown rice for dinner. Once or twice a week, she'd sprinkle a few garbanzo beans on a salad or add some soy cheese to the vegetables. She thought her vegetarian diet was great, when in fact it was deficient in several nutrients. At one point she suffered a stress fracture that healed very slowly. She had spindly arms and legs with tiny muscles (despite her exercise program), and her menstrual period was absent, a sign of an unhealthy body.

Jessica needed to understand that a well-balanced sports diet includes adequate protein—either small portions of lean beef, pork, and lamb or generous portions of tofu, beans, and nuts. (Because plant proteins are less concentrated than animal proteins, you must eat larger portions to get the same amount of protein.) Dark meats are also important sources of two minerals—iron and zinc.

Iron and Zinc in Foods

Iron. Iron is a necessary component of hemoglobin, the protein that transports oxygen from the lungs to the working muscles. If you are iron deficient, you are likely to fatigue easily upon exertion. The recommended iron intake for men is 8 milligrams, for women 18 milligrams until menopause, and for women thereafter 8 milligrams. This target iron intake is set high because only a small percentage is absorbed. The best iron sources are animal products and fish; the body absorbs far less iron from plant foods.

Zinc. The mineral zinc is part of more than 100 enzymes that help your body function properly. For example, zinc helps remove carbon dioxide from your muscles when you exercise. Zinc also enhances the healing process. Because the zinc from animal protein is absorbed better than zinc from plants, vegetarian athletes are at risk of eating a zinc-deficient diet.

The recommended intake for zinc is 8 milligrams for women and 11 milligrams for men. Like the target for iron, this target is also set high and may be hard to consume. But athletes who sweat heavily and incur zinc losses through sweat should try to hit the target intake.

	Iron (mg)	Zinc (mg)
Animal sources[1]		
Alaskan king crab, 4 oz	1	9
Beef, 4 oz top round	3	6
Turkey, 4 oz breast	2	2
Swordfish, 4 oz	1	2
Pork loin, 4 oz	1	3
Oysters, 6 medium raw	5	75(!)
Shrimp, 12 large	2	1
Chicken thigh, 4 oz	1.5	3
Fish, 4 oz haddock	1	0.5
Tuna, 3 oz light canned	1	1
Egg, 1 large	1	0.5
Fruit and juice		
Prune juice, 8 oz	3	0.5
Apricots, 5 halves dried	0.8	0.2
Dates, 10 dried	1	0.2
Raisins, 1/3 cup	1	0.1
Vegetables and legumes[2]		
Refried beans, 1 cup	4	3
Spinach, 1/2 cup cooked	3	1
Tofu, 3 oz firm	1	2
Peas, 1/2 cup	1	1
Broccoli, 1/2 cup	0.5	0.3
Dairy		
Skim milk, 1 cup	0.1	1.0
Cheddar cheese, 1 oz	0.2	1.0

	Iron (mg)	Zinc (mg)
Grain		
Cereal, Total, 3/4 cup	18	15
Raisin Bran, Kellogg's, 1 cup	4.5	1.5
Cream of Wheat, 1 cup cooked	9	trace
Wheat germ, 1/4 cup	2	1.5
Pasta, 1 cup cooked, enriched	2	1
Bread, 1 slice enriched	1	0.2
Brown rice, 1 cup cooked	1	1.2
Other		
Molasses, 1 tbsp blackstrap	3.5	0.2

1. Animal sources of iron and zinc are absorbed best (except for iron from eggs).
2. Vegetable sources of iron and zinc are poorly absorbed.

Nutrient data from food labels and J. Pennington, 1998, *Bowes & Church's Food Values of Portions Commonly Used*, 17th ed. (Philadelphia: Lippincott).

Athletes and Anemia

Athletes who are at highest risk of suffering from iron-deficiency anemia include the following:

- Female athletes who lose iron through menstrual bleeding.
- Vegetarians who do not eat red meat (the best dietary source of iron) or iron-enriched breakfast cereals.
- Marathon runners, who may damage red blood cells by pounding their feet on the ground during training.
- Endurance athletes, who may lose iron through heavy sweat losses.
- Teenage athletes, particularly girls, who are growing quickly and may consume inadequate iron to meet expanded requirements.

Even marginal iron deficiency (found in about 12 percent of women in the United States) can hurt athletic performance. Hence, you want to eat iron-rich foods each day. You can boost your iron intake in several easy ways:

- Eat lean cuts of beef, lamb, pork, and the dark meat of skinless chicken or turkey three to four times per week.
- Select breads and cereals with the words "iron-enriched" or "fortified" on the label. This added iron supplements the small amount that naturally occurs in grains. Eat these foods with a source of vitamin C (for example, orange juice with cereal, tomato on a sandwich), which may enhance iron absorption.

- Use cast-iron skillets for cooking. These vessels offer more nutritional value than stainless-steel cookware! The iron content of spaghetti sauce simmered in a cast-iron skillet for three hours may increase from 3 to 88 milligrams for each half-cup (120 milliliters) of sauce.

- Don't drink coffee or tea with every meal, particularly if you are prone to being anemic. Substances in these beverages can interfere with iron absorption. Drinking them an hour before a meal is better than drinking them afterward.

- Combine poorly absorbed vegetable sources of iron (nonheme iron, 10 percent absorption rate) with animal sources (heme iron, 40 percent absorption rate). For example, eat broccoli with beef, spinach with chicken, chili with lean hamburger, and lentil soup with turkey.

If you are diagnosed with iron-deficiency anemia, you will need to take iron supplements, typically in the form of ferrous sulfate or ferrous gluconate. You will need about four months of supplementation to resolve the problem.

Be aware, though, that iron overload, a genetic condition that happens in about 1 in every 250 people and can be associated with arthritis and diabetes, is also a concern. Men and postmenopausal women are most susceptible because they have relatively low iron requirements. They should not take iron supplements unless recommended by their physicians. The best way to identify iron overload is by having your blood tested for serum ferritin to measure the amount of iron stored in the body. A level of 200 micrograms or higher signals danger.

The Balanced Vegetarian Diet

Without question, a diet based on plant foods can contribute to good health. A plant-based diet tends to have more fiber, less saturated fat and cholesterol, and more phytochemicals—active compounds that may play an important role in preventing and treating diseases such as cancer. Foods rich in phytochemicals include not only fruits and vegetables but also the protein-rich foods common to a plant-based diet: nuts, legumes, dried beans, and peas.

But some vegetarians (who for health reasons choose to not eat red meat) often turn to cheese for protein. They thrive on cheese-filled omelets, cheesy lasagna, salads frosted with shredded cheese, and slices of whole-grain bread piled high with cheese. They are unaware, though, that cheese has far more saturated fat than lean meats and that eating a cheese sandwich is, in that respect, worse than a lean roast-beef sandwich without mayonnaise. As I have mentioned before, lean meat, eaten in small portions as the accompaniment to lots of carbohydrates, is not the health culprit it is deemed to be. Refer to table 2.1 on page 30 for the amount of fat and cholesterol in some meats.

Tofu (soybean curd) and other soy products, such as soy burgers and soy milk, are excellent healthful additions to a meat-free diet. They not only contain a source of high-quality protein that is equivalent in value to animal protein but also have properties that may protect against heart disease and cancer. If you make the effort to include soy foods in your diet, the more likely you are to lower the bad cholesterol, increase the good cholesterol, and delay cancer tumor growth. As little as four ounces (120 grams) of tofu, one-third cup (30 grams) of soy flour, or one cup of soy milk (240 milliliters) per day can bring positive health changes.

If you want to omit animal protein from your diet, or if you already do, you are making a potentially healthful lifestyle change. The trick is to choose a balanced vegetarian diet and choose enough vegetable proteins to satisfy your protein requirements. Doing this can be easier for a man who is eating 3,000 or more calories than for a woman dieter who eats half that amount. Even vegetarians who dislike cooking can easily select a balanced diet that contains the right amount of protein. See table 8.2 for a sample cook-free vegetarian meal plan.

Lisa, a vegetarian dieter who would spend an hour a day working out at the gym, thought she was eating adequate protein when she included one tablespoon of peanut butter (only 4 grams of protein) on a slice of whole-wheat toast for breakfast, a half cup (120 grams) of hummus (6 grams of protein) with pita at lunch, and one-quarter cake of tofu (only 9 grams of protein) at dinner. These 19 grams of protein fell far short of the daily 50 to 70 grams of protein she needed. No wonder she wasn't building muscle the way she wanted!

When Lisa recognized that her diet was deficient in plant proteins, she traded in calories from protein-poor pita, pasta, and fruits for more calories from higher protein nuts and beans. This boosted her intake of the amino acids she needed to build muscles. She had better workouts and felt better overall.

Milk, other dairy foods, fish, poultry, meat, and all animal sources of protein contain all eight or nine essential amino acids and are often referred to as complete proteins. The protein in soy foods such as tofu, tempeh, and soy milk are also complete proteins. The protein in rice, beans, pasta, lentils, nuts, fruits, vegetables, and other plant foods are incomplete because they have low levels of some of the essential amino acids. Therefore, vegetarians must know how to combine incomplete proteins to make them complete. Vegetarians who drink milk can easily do this by adding dairy to each meal, such as by combining milk with oatmeal or sprinkling grated low-fat cheese on beans. The strict

TABLE 8.2

Easy Vegetarian Meals With No Cooking!

This cook-free menu is appropriate for an active, 150-pound (68-kilogram) lactovegetarian (that is, a vegetarian who drinks milk and eats dairy foods) who might need about 2,800 calories per day. Including low-fat dairy foods is one trick for balancing a simple vegetarian diet. Low-fat milk, yogurt, and cheeses are convenient, quick, easy, and popular protein sources.

Food	Protein (g)	Calories
Breakfast		
1 cup orange juice	2	110
2 cups bran flakes	8	240
1 medium banana	1	100
1 1/2 cups low-fat milk	12	150
Lunch		
2 peanut butter sandwiches	30	700
1 apple	1	100
2 cups milk	16	200
Snack		
1 cup fruit yogurt	10	250
Dinner		
1 medium pizza	70	1,000
Total:	150	2,850

Note: The 150 grams of protein accounts for 20 percent of the 2,850 calories and allows 1 gram of protein per pound (2.2 grams per kilogram) of body weight. This is slightly higher than the recommended sports diet with 15 percent of calories from protein, or 0.6 to 0.9 grams of protein per pound (1.3 to 2.0 grams per kilogram) of body weight. This menu demonstrates that lactovegetarians can easily get adequate protein with wise food choices.

vegetarian needs to choose complementary vegetable proteins that are high in the particular limiting amino acid.

In times past, vegetarians were told to eat the complementary proteins together at each meal. We now know that eating them over the course of the day is equally effective. Nevertheless, the following combinations work well together:

Grains and Milk Products

- Cereal plus milk
- Pasta plus cheese
- Bread plus cheese

Grains, Beans, and Legumes

- Rice plus beans
- Pita plus split-pea soup

- Tortillas plus beans
- Cornbread plus chili with kidney beans
- Brown bread plus baked beans

Legumes and Seeds
- Chickpeas plus tahini (as in hummus)
- Tofu plus sesame seeds

Following these guidelines, vegetarian athletes can plan their diets to be sure they consume an adequate amount of complete proteins every day. One key is to eat a wide variety of foods to optimize the intake of a variety of amino acids.

Note that although most vegetarians can get the right amount of protein, they may lack iron and zinc, minerals found primarily in meats and other animal products. Pure vegans, who eat only plant foods, also need to be sure they get adequate riboflavin, calcium, and vitamin B-12, either through a supplement or from carefully selected food sources. See the list of vegetarian Web sites in appendix B for additional information.

Protein and Amino Acids

The need for protein is actually a need for amino acids. All proteins are made up of amino acids that your body needs to build tissue, hence their nickname "building blocks." There are 21 of these amino acids, and every protein in your body is made up of some combination of them. Your body can make some amino acids itself, but eight of them (nine for children), called the essential amino acids, must come from the foods you eat.

Taking extra amino acids, such as large doses of ornithine or arginine, will not make your muscles bigger or stronger. To date, no scientific evidence indicates that individual amino acids have a bodybuilding effect. Your body needs all the essential amino acids to make new muscles. Real food provides the proper balance of all the amino acids, works well, and costs less than amino acid supplements. Real food, along with regular exercise, can help you achieve your athletic goals.

Protein Powders and Bars

According to the advertisements in bodybuilding magazines, protein supplements are essential for optimal muscle development. If you have been hanging around the power gyms, you've undoubtedly heard intense conversations about some of these products with tantalizing names such as MegaMass and Muscle Builder. The protein-praising bodybuilders who come to me for advice often lug gym bags bulging with assorted pills, powders, and potions. They wonder if these supplements are better than the protein in standard food, if they are worth the price, and if they work. Some are avid believers in the stuff, and others are skeptical.

Patrick, an 18-year-old high school student, marveled at the three pounds (1.3 kilograms) he had gained in one month since he started drinking a protein shake before bed. But he had simultaneously enlarged his eating and exercise program. I suspect that the wholesome meals and consistent training made more of a difference than the protein supplement did.

Jake, a 33-year-old bus driver, took a protein drink after every workout and with every meal. He gained bulk and felt stronger. Were the improvements because of the extra calories in his diet or because of the expensive protein drink? I would guess it was the extra calories.

Bulking up is a matter of dedicating yourself to extra exercise and extra calories, not to extra supplements. No scientific evidence supports the idea that protein or amino acids in supplements are more effective than protein in ordinary foods. If you are struggling to develop bigger muscles, change your body image, and improve your strength, I address how to gain weight healthfully in chapter 10. This chapter addresses the role of protein in the gaining process. Heed the following tips:

- **Exercise, not extra protein, is the key to developing bigger muscles.** In theory, if you want to gain one pound (0.5 kilograms) of muscle per week, you need only 14 extra grams of protein per day, the amount in two ounces of meat—a mere forkful (Bernadot 1992)! By eating a small amount of protein in your preexercise snack (milk with cereal, a yogurt with granola, half a turkey sandwich), you can optimize the muscle-building process (Rasmussen et al. 2000). See "Recovery Protein" in chapter 6 on page 127.

- **Beware of extra fat.** If you are currently eating large amounts of protein-rich foods such as cheese omelets, fried chicken, and cheeseburgers, you may be consuming an excessive amount of calories from saturated fat that can easily become stored as body fat, not as bulging biceps.

- **Expensive muscle-building supplements are not the answer.** The amount of protein in these formulas is often less than that which you might easily get through foods, but at two to four times the price. In addition, real foods provide a nice package of vitamins, minerals, and other nutrients that are often missing in engineered food.

Protein source	Cost	Protein (g)	Cost/g protein
Met-Rx Big 100 Bar	$2.50	26	9.5¢
PowerBar ProteinPlus	$1.95	24	8.0¢
Tuna, 6 oz can	$0.99	30	3.5¢
Skim milk, 1 qt	$0.75	32	2.5¢
Peanut butter, 2 tbsp	$0.15	7	2.0¢

Few athletes need to spend money on protein supplements. Even vegetarians can get enough protein through foods. I recommend commercial protein supplements in only a few medical situations, such as with malnourished patients with AIDS or cancer. Protein supplements are also helpful for my clients with anorexia who claim to be vegetarian (a politically correct way of eliminating yet another source of calories from their diets) but commonly are just fat-phobic non-meat eaters. For example, one "vegetarian" student refused to eat animal products and also disliked tofu and beans. Her only acceptable source of protein was a fat-free protein supplement. This case contrasts to the 160-pound (73-kilogram) protein fanatic who eats a six-egg-white omelet for breakfast, a can of tuna for lunch, and two chicken breasts for dinner and drinks skim milk by the quart, totaling more than 160 grams of high-quality protein. And he wonders whether he needs a supplement. He's already getting more than one gram of protein per pound of body weight. He needs more carbs for optimal muscle fueling, not more protein!

Food Works!

People who are interested in building muscles and gaining weight commonly turn to protein for a sports-nutrition edge. Protein is just one part of a muscle-building program. You also need adequate carbs to fuel your muscles, adequate calories to provide the energy to build muscles, and adequate muscle-building exercise to stimulate muscular growth. Because most athletes get plenty of protein through standard foods and the typical American diet, buying special protein supplements is generally a needless expense.

If you have concerns about the adequacy of your diet and wonder if it offers adequate protein, your best bet is to meet with a sports nutritionist who is a registered dietitian. This professional can give you personalized information and allay your fears. To find a local RD, go to www.eatright.org and put your zip code into the referral network, or call 800-366-1655.

PART II

Balancing Weight and Activity

Finding a Healthy Body Fat Level

When you look in the mirror or at people at the mall, you see that nature wants humans to have some body fat. In fact, the reference 24-year-old woman is about 27 percent fat and the reference 24-year-old man is about 15 percent fat. Some of us have more fat than others— undesired bumps and bulges, spare tires around our waists, and fat on our thighs.

Society preaches that thinner is better, and consequently many of my clients yearn to have a fat-free image. Women strive to be sleek, slender, and slim. Men want to be bulky, muscular, and trim. While a certain amount of leanness is desirable for health and performance, obsessions about body fatness are unhealthy. One man did 1,000 sit-ups each day, hoping to get rid of the fat on his abdomen. A woman spent hours on the stair stepper, hoping to eliminate the fat on her thighs. Both came to me asking to have their body fat measured, and both were shocked to learn that they were leaner than they thought.

Scantily clad athletes commonly see themselves as being too fat, but rarely too thin. Measuring body fat can thus offer a helpful perspective about where a person is in the scheme of fatness. For my clients who know they are overfat, body-fat measurement is a positive tool that allows them to quantify loss of body fat and gain of muscle as they embark on their diet and exercise program. The purpose of this chapter is to talk about bodies, body fat, and body fatness, discuss the different methods of body fat measurement, and offer perspectives about how fatness is less important than health. Even overfat people can be fit, healthy, and at peace with their bodies.

Body Fat: Why Do We Have It?

Although excess body fat is excess baggage that slows us down, we need a certain amount of fat for our bodies to function normally. Fat, or adipose tissue, is an essential part of our nerves, spinal cord, brain, and cell membranes. Internal fat pads the kidneys and other organs; external fat offers a layer of protection against cold weather. For the reference man, essential fat comprises about 4 percent of body weight, that is, 6 fat pounds for a 150-pound man (2.7 fat kilograms for a 68-kilogram man). In comparison, the reference woman has about 12 percent essential fat, that is, 15 fat pounds for a 125-pound woman (6.8 fat kilograms for a 57-kilogram woman). Table 9.1 further describes the various levels of body fatness.

Women store essential fat in their hips, thighs, and breasts. This fat is readily available to nourish a healthy baby if a woman becomes pregnant. If you are a woman fighting the battle of the bulging thighs, you may be fighting a losing battle. The activity of the enzymes that store fat in women's thighs and hips is very high compared with the enzyme activity in other fat storage areas in women and to fat storage in the hips and thighs of men. Moreover, the activity of the enzymes that release the fat is low, making it difficult to lose fat in these areas. The easiest time for women to lose fat in this area is during the last

TABLE 9.1

Defining Body Fatness by Percentage of Fat

Classification	Image	Males	Females
Very low fat	Skinny	7-10	14-17
Low fat	Trim	10-13	17-20
Average fat	Normal	13-17	20-27
Above normal fat	Plump	17-25	27-31
Very high fat	Fat	>25	>31
Essential fat		3-5	11-13

Adapted, by permission, from Getchell and Anderson, 1982, *Being fit: a personal guide* (New York, NY: John Wiley and Sons, Inc.).

trimester of pregnancy and breastfeeding. At those times, the activity of the fat-storing enzymes drops and the activity of the fat-releasing enzymes increases. Nature, again, is protective of a woman's ability to care for her offspring.

Body Fat and Exercise

Myths and misconceptions are abundant surrounding the role of exercise in weight management. Here's a true or false quiz to test your knowledge about body fat and exercise.

1. If you start an exercise program, you'll lose body fat.

False. To lose body fat you have to create a calorie deficit for the entire day. That is, you have to burn off more calories than you consume. Exercise can help contribute to the calorie deficit, but exercise is often overrated as a way to reduce body fat. Exercise is better used as a tool to help prevent weight gain and to maintain weight loss. Exercise helps relieve stress (which can reduce stress eating), helps you feel good about yourself, boosts your metabolism, and increases the desire to feed yourself healthfully.

Many people do successfully lose weight by adding exercise. That happens because they start a total health campaign that includes not only adding activity but also subtracting some calories. After they work out, they tend to feel great, they've relieved stress, and they have less desire to unwind after a hectic day by munching through a bag of chips as they had done before starting the exercise program.

But some of my clients complain to me that they have lost no weight despite hours of working out. That often happens because they are rewarding themselves afterward with generous amounts of calories that replace all they burned off. They may have exercised for 30 minutes and burned off 300 calories, but then they consumed 300 calories of "recovery food" in 3 minutes. Despite popular belief, appetite tends to keep up with your exercise load (except in extreme conditions). The more you exercise, the hungrier you will eventually become and the more likely it is that you will eat enough to replace the calories you burned off. Nature does a wonderful job of protecting your body from wasting away, particularly if you are already lean with little excess fat to lose.

Another factor that influences the effectiveness of exercise as a means to lose weight relates to the toll of exercise on your total daily activity. That is, some avid exercisers put all their effort into exercising hard for one or two hours per day but then do little spontaneous activity the rest of the day (Thompson et al. 1995). For example, a group of moderately obese college-age students who participated in a 16-month aerobic exercise program had similar daily energy expenditures before starting and at the end of the program. The students seem to have become more sedentary at other times of the day (Bailey, Jacobsen, and Donnelly 2002). This pattern is common among both casual and serious exercisers, many of who claim to maintain weight despite their hard workouts.

If you do want to use exercise to promote weight loss, perhaps the most effective type of exercise is exercise that builds muscle. Unlike aerobic exercise that burns calories primarily during the exercise session but very few thereafter, strength training builds muscles that boost your metabolism throughout the entire day and night. Muscle tissue actively burns calories. The more muscle mass you have, the more calories you burn. In a study with men and women ages 50 to 70 who strength trained three days per week for 12 weeks, metabolic rate increased 15 percent and participants lost four pounds (1.8 kilograms) of fat without actively dieting (Nelson et al. 1994).

2. **To lose body fat, do low-intensity, fat-burning exercise.**

False. To lose fat, you have to create a calorie deficit for the day. You can do this by adding on exercise of any type, eating less, or combining the two. Just be sure that by the end of the day you have eaten fewer calories than you needed. That way, you'll dip into the stored body fat and burn it for energy.

Some people think that the key to body-fat loss is doing fat-burning exercise or low-intensity exercise that uses more fat than muscle glycogen for fuel. Wrong. No studies have shown that burning fat during exercise affects loss of body fat (Zelasko 1995). But because you can sustain low-intensity exercise for longer than you can high-intensity workouts, you can easily burn off more calories in, let's say, 60 minutes of slow jogging (600 calories) than in 10 minutes of fast running (150 calories).

High-intensity exercise may actually contribute to a lower percentage of body fat (Yoshioka et al. 2001). Research on 1,366 women and 1,257 men suggests that those who did high-intensity exercise tended to have less body fat than those who did lower-intensity fat-burning exercise (Tremblay, Despres, Leblanc, et al. 1990). The big concern about doing high-intensity exercise relates to the higher risk of injury. If you choose to exercise harder, be sure to exercise wisely—warm up, stretch, and don't do too much, too soon.

3. **Men are more likely to lose weight with exercise than are women.**

True. In one study with previously sedentary, normal-weight men and women who participated in an 18-month marathon training program, the men increased their intake by about 500 calories per day and the women increased by only 60 calories, despite having added 50 miles per week of running. The men lost about six pounds (2.7 kilograms) of fat; the women lost less than five pounds (2.3 kilograms) of fat, despite their larger calorie deficit (Janssen, Graef, and Saris 1989). Similarly, other studies suggest that normal-weight women fail to lose significant amounts of fat when they add exercise.

In a study with previously sedentary, overweight males and females (average ages 22 to 24 years) who did fitness exercise five times a week for 16 months with no dietary restrictions, the men lost 12 pounds (5.4 kilograms) and body fat dropped from 27 to 22 percent. They failed to eat enough to compensate for the extra calories burned. The women, however, had no significant weight or body-fat changes; their appetites kept up with their calorie expenditure (Kirk, Donnelly, and Jacobsen 2002).

In terms of evolution, nature wants women to have fat and be fertile; men are supposed to be lean hunters. Given that extreme amounts of exercise can be interpreted as a famine (because of the high calorie deficit), "food efficiency" may develop, particularly in women who maintain a chronic energy deficit.

4. **To reduce the fat around the stomach and hips, you should incorporate sit-ups into your exercise program.**

False. Spot reducing sounds like a great idea. But the truth is that you can't reduce through vigorous exercise only the fat cells in one localized area of your body. When you lose fat, you lose it everywhere, not just from the part of your body you are working most vigorously. Moreover, you need to create a calorie deficit for the entire day to reduce body fat. Muscle movement itself does not result in loss of body fat. For example, the man who did 1,000 sit-ups every day trying to burn off the fat in his abdomen certainly built strong abdominal muscles, but he failed to create a calorie deficit and lose abdominal fat.

5. **If you become injured and are unable to exercise for a week, your muscles will turn into fat.**

False. Muscle does not turn into fat, nor does fat turn into muscle. Muscle and fat are separate entities and not interchangeable. Perhaps you've noticed a fat layer on roast beef or pork chops. A similar fat layer occurs in humans. The fat tissue is a layer of fat-filled cells that covers the muscles. Muscle is the protein-rich tissue that performs exercise. When you exercise, you build up muscle tissue. When you consume fewer calories than you expend, you reduce the fat layer.

If, because of injury or illness, you are unable to exercise, your muscles may lose their tone, but they won't turn into fat. Unexercised muscle tissue actually shrinks in size. For example, Joe, a skier, broke his leg and was shocked to see how scrawny his leg muscles looked when the cast was removed five weeks later. Once Joe started exercising again, he rebuilt the muscle to its original size.

If you overeat (as often happens with inactive athletes who are bored, depressed, and hopeful that chocolate-chip cookies will cure all ailments), you will become fatter. I often counsel wounded football players who gain 10 to 20 pounds (4.5 to 9.0 kilograms) after an injury. They continue to eat lumberjack portions although they need fewer calories. The extra fat takes up more space than the muscle, and the players feel and look flabby.

Feeling frustrated and disappointed when you are injured is normal. Share your feelings with others who understand. Think positive and visualize your injury getting better every day. Find the positive aspect. Time off from exercise can mean more time for friends, family, and other hobbies.

When injured, some very thin athletes do migrate to their natural weight, that is, the weight they would naturally maintain without rigorous exercise and restricted calories. For example, a 13-year-old gymnast perceived herself as getting fat when she suffered a knee injury. She was simply catching up and attaining the physique that was appropriate for her age and genetics.

6. **Cellulite is a special kind of fat that appears after a person has repeatedly gained and lost weight.**

False. Cellulite is a fad description of the bulging orange-peel appearance of fat that sometimes appears on the hips, thighs, and buttocks. Although much is written about cellulite, little is understood about it. Some medical professionals believe that the bumpy, dimpled appearance of cellulite may result from restrictions of connective tissue separating fat cells into compartments. If you overeat and fill the fat cells, the compartmental restrictions may cause the fat to bulge.

Women are afflicted by cellulite more than men are because their skin is thinner and their fat compartments are larger and more rounded. Also, women tend to deposit fat in their hips, thighs, and buttocks, areas in which cellulite appears easily. In contrast, men tend to deposit fat around their waists.

Some medical specialists suspect that a genetic predisposition toward cellulite may exist. If a mother has cellulite, the daughter is likely to acquire it as well. Cellulite generally appears as a person ages, because the skin loses its elasticity and becomes thinner.

Did you pass the quiz?

If you are exercising to lose weight, I encourage you to separate exercise and weight. Yes, you should exercise for health, fitness, stress relief and, most important, for enjoyment. I discourage you from exercising to burn calories. Under those conditions, exercise feels like punishment for having excess body fat. This type of disagreeable exercise fails to become part of a lifelong health-promotion plan.

Your job is to find an exercise program that has purpose and meaning so that you will enjoy incorporating exercise into your daily schedule. Consider these examples:

- Jim bought a dog and is now walking the dog three miles per day.
- David enjoys gardening in the summer and walking in the woods in the winter.
- Gretchen, a busy executive, takes a 30-minute walk at lunch to relieve stress and process her feelings.
- Sherri commutes to work by bicycle.

Although exercise without creation of a calorie deficit fails to result in weight loss, we do know that exercise is important in maintaining weight loss. People who burn off 1,000 to 2,000 calories per week tend to be leaner and healthier than sedentary people. Again, you want to find an exercise program that has purpose and meaning so that you will enjoy incorporating exercise into your daily schedule for the rest of your life.

Women, Body Fat, and Menopause

It's no secret that women aged 45 to 50 constantly complain about fat gain and a thickened waist. Based on their stories, one could assume perimenopausal (the years surrounding menopause) fat gain is inevitable. Despite popular belief, however, women do not inevitably gain fat with menopause. Yes, they commonly gain fat that settles in and around the abdominal area, but the changes are not due to the hormonal shifts of menopause. Rather, the fat gain is primarily associated with reduced metabolic rate, less activity, and a calorie imbalance.

When women (and men) age, they tend to lose muscle mass (unless they do regular strength training). Because muscle drives the metabolic rate, less

(continued)

(continued)

muscle means a lower metabolic rate and fewer calories burned. In addition, if a woman is feeling chronically fatigued because of "night sweats," poor sleep, and the hormonal shifts of menopause, she may lack the desire to exercise. This perpetuates more muscle loss and extends the drop in metabolism.

Menopause also occurs during a time when a woman's lifestyle becomes less active. That is, if her children have grown up and left home, she may find herself sitting and reading rather than running up and down stairs carrying endless loads of laundry. By the time she is 50ish, she may also be more affluent and have more money to spend on restaurant eating, vacations, and cruises. And she may be attending more business meetings that involve abundant food. The combination of easy access to delicious food, lower activity level, and the attitude that "I'm tired of dieting and depriving myself of tasty food" that may accompany 35 or more years of restrictive eating can contribute to the excess calories that settle around the waist. But don't blame menopause! A study of 485 women ages 42 to 50 suggests that the women on average gained the same amount of weight whether or not they had gone through menopause (Wing et al. 1991).

The best way to prevent weight gain is to exercise and maintain an active lifestyle. The optimal exercise program includes both aerobic exercise (to enhance cardiovascular fitness) and strengthening exercise (to preserve muscles and bone density). The book *Strong Women Stay Slim* by Miriam Nelson (Random House 1999) is a good resource for helping women develop a health-protective exercise program.

Body Image: Waiting for the Perfect Body

Jessica, a competitive high school swimmer, was sensitive about her bulky body and described herself as feeling fat. As I measured her body fat, she anxiously awaited the decisive moment. "You are actually very lean, Jessica," I said. "You simply have a lot of muscle and a big bone structure. You have very little excess fat."

Visual appearance and body weight are deceptive for athletes who tend to compare themselves with their teammates. We come in all different sizes and shapes, most of which are genetically determined. Although you can change your body to a certain extent by losing fat or building muscle, you can't do a complete makeover. Even if you lose the excess baggage, sometimes you still won't end up with the body you want.

If you are a woman who has large thighs (like all the women in your family), or if you are a man who hates your "love handles" (that all the men in the family also have), you need to be realistic in your expectations. You can trim the fat on your thighs or around your waist a bit by creating a calorie deficit, but you are unlikely to get it to vanish. Rather than obsess about your body flaw, I recommend that you let go of your dissatisfaction with your body, accept yourself for the sincere and caring person you are, and focus on the things in life that really matter. You can waste a lot of mental energy fretting about undesired body fat.

Again, we come in sizes and shapes unique to our genetic makeup. Just as some of us have thick hair, others have thin hair. Some of us have blue eyes, and others have brown eyes. No one seems to care about hair thickness or eye color, but the media have made us all care about body fatness. As a result, too many self-conscious people feel inadequate because of repeated failures at transforming themselves into a shape they aren't meant to be.

To put into perspective how irrelevant body shape or size is, think about a person who has been most influential in your life. Does that person's weight modify your relationship with him or her in any way? Likely not. I suspect that there are few (if any) people in your life for whom your feelings are based solely on their appearance.

Remember that your value as a partner, colleague, or lover does not depend on your physical appearance. Your beauty comes from the inside. Your concern about how you look can be a mask for how you feel about yourself. People who obsess about their imperfect bodies commonly have low self-esteem. Somehow, they feel that they are not good enough.

What's Your Body Type?

Like it or not, you are born with a specific body shape that is yours for life. Most people do not exactly fit one description. For example, a tall, muscular basketball player might fall into the continuum between an ectomorph and a mesomorph.

Health professionals describe the standard body types by these categories:

- Ectomorph—relatively long legs and arms, narrow fingers and toes, and delicate bone structure (long-distance runner)
- Mesomorph—heavy bone and muscle development, broad hands, and a muscular chest (football player)
- Endomorph—round and soft, often with slender wrists and ankles and relatively small facial features (sumo wrestler)

Fashion designers prefer to describe body shapes by these categories:

- Pear—normally has narrow shoulders, a small chest, and an average waist; fat concentration is usually in the hips and thighs
- Apple—usually has a round tummy, with no visible waistline; fat concentration is in the waist; limbs are thin

(continued)

(continued)

- Inverted triangle—usually has broad shoulders and narrow hips; fat concentration is generally in the chest
- Hourglass—broad hips and chest and a small waist; fat concentration normally in the chest and hips

Are You Imagining the Wrong Body?

Because of today's appearance consciousness, you undoubtedly hold an image of what you are supposed to look like. Yet few people naturally possess their desired physique. Most of us are ordinary mortals, complete with bumps, bulges, fat, and fleshiness. Women, in particular, have a natural roundness and softness that tends to become rounder and softer with aging.

In general, about one-third of all Americans are truly dissatisfied with their appearance, women more than men. A woman will most commonly complain about her thighs, abdomen, breasts, and buttocks. A man expresses dissatisfaction with his abdomen, upper body, and balding scalp. Sometimes the problem is imaginary (such as when the anorexic skater complains about her fat thighs); sometimes it is real and ranges from a mild complaint about love handles that hang over the running shorts to a major preoccupation with thunder thighs that results in relentless dieting and exercise.

Even lean athletes, men and women alike, are not immune from the epidemic of body dissatisfaction despite their fitness. Many perceive themselves as having unacceptable bodies, and out of desperation they develop eating disorders. The best predictor of who will develop an eating disorder relates to who struggles most with body image.

What you look like on the outside should have little to do with how you feel on the inside. But in reality, many people think like this:

1. I have a defect (fat thighs) that makes me different from others.
2. Other people notice this difference.
3. My looks affect how these people see me—as repulsive and ugly.
4. I'm bad, unlovable, inadequate.

This type of thinking is common among young dancers experiencing body changes as they blossom from girls into women and develop hips and thighs, runners feeling pressure to be thinner, exercise leaders who think every student scrutinizes their bulges, and numerous other people who think they have imperfect bodies.

Distorted Body Images: Not for Women Only

Since the birth of the Barbie doll, women have become increasingly obsessed about their looks. Today, men are also becoming more obsessed and feel pressure to acquire a lean and muscular look. The GI Joe doll is one example of why the obsession is becoming more common. In 1964, if GI Joe were an actual man, he would have a 44-inch (112-centimeter) chest and 12-inch (30-centimeter) biceps. Today, if the GI Joe Extreme doll were an actual man, he would have a 55-inch (140-centimeter) chest and 27-inch (68-centimeter) biceps. His biceps would be almost the same size as his waist.

We should not be surprised, then, that body dysmorphic disorder (BDD)—preoccupation with an imagined defect in appearance or an excessive concern for a slight physical defect—is on the rise, even in men. Men suffering from BDD feel socially anxious, believing that everyone around them is seeing their flaws and judging their appearance.

Muscle dysmorphia, a subtype of BDD, affects men who are obsessed with thoughts that they are too small and do not have enough muscle mass. Many of these men spend extraordinary hours at the gym and take dangerous steroids and other drugs to bulk up. As one man commented, "Why should I be Clark Kent when I can be Superman?" (Olivardia 2002).

Learn to Love Your Body

If you are dissatisfied with your body, you might think the solution is to lose weight, pump iron, or do thousands of sit-ups. This "outside" approach to correcting body dissatisfaction tends to be inadequate. Concern about what you look like is really a mask for how you feel about yourself, your self-esteem. Given that about 25 percent of your self-esteem is tied to how you look, you can't feel good about yourself unless you like your body and feel confident with how you look. Weight issues are often self-esteem issues, a feeling of "I'm not good enough."

The best approach to resolving your body shape issues is to learn to love the body you have. As I mentioned before, much of what you look like, your size and shape, is genetically determined. You can slightly redesign the house that nature gave you, but you can't totally remodel it, at least without paying a high price.

If you are struggling with your body image, you need to think back to identify when you first got the message that something was wrong with your body. Perhaps it was a parent who lovingly remarked that you looked good but that if only you'd lose a few pounds you'd look even better. Maybe it was the siblings who teased you about your flabby thighs, or the relative who molested you. (Sexual abuse is a common cause of body hate.) Then you need to take the following steps to be at peace with your body and learn to like yourself:

- Rename your disliked body part (that is, rename "ugly jelly belly" a more loving "round tummy").
- Identify the parts of your body that you like.
- Give yourself credit for your attractive body parts with positive talk.

Making Peace With Your Body

If you find yourself obsessing about the look of your body, give yourself permission to live your life in a healthier way. Here's a Declaration of Independence From Weight Obsessions, taken from EDAP, the Eating Disorders Awareness and Prevention Program.

I declare, from this day forward, I will choose to live my life by the following tenets. In doing so, I declare myself free and independent from the pressures and constraints of a weight-obsessed world.

- I will accept my body in its natural size and shape.
- I will celebrate all that my body can do for me each day.
- I will treat my body with respect, give it enough rest, fuel it with a variety of foods, exercise it moderately, and listen to what it needs.
- I will choose to resist our society's pressures to judge myself and other people on physical characteristics like body weight, shape, or size. I will respect people based on their depth of character and the impact of their accomplishments.
- I will refuse to deny my body of valuable nutrients by dieting or using weight loss products.
- I will avoid categorizing foods as either "good" or "bad." I will not associate guilt or shame with eating certain foods. Instead, I will nourish my body with a balance of foods, listening and responding to what it needs.
- I will not use food to mask my emotional needs.
- I will not avoid participating in activities that I enjoy (e.g., swimming, dancing, enjoying a meal) simply because I am self-conscious about the way my body looks. I will recognize that I have the right to enjoy any activities regardless of my body shape or size.
- I will believe that my self-esteem and identity come from within!

Signature: _____ Date: _____

Courtesy of the National Eating Disorders Association.
www.NationalEatingDisorders.org

Don't dwell on the negative but instead love all the good things your body does for you. It rides bikes, lifts weights at the gym, goes canoeing, and lets you have fun. How could you enjoy sports without your body? Remember that a healthy body can come in all types of sizes and shapes. You can even be fat and fit.

To start improving your relationship with your body, close your eyes and imagine that you have your desired body. Visualize the confident carriage, verbal expression, and body language you would use. Open your eyes and assume those characteristics. With practice, you'll come to learn that appearance is only skin deep and that your real worth is the love, care, and concern that you offer your family and friends. You'll be able to muster the courage to face intimidating situations. You can even put on that bathing suit and feel at peace!

Don't Play the Numbers Game

Some people give too much power to the number on the bathroom scale. Jean, a dedicated exerciser, resorted to keeping her scale in the trunk of her car because it too easily ruined her day. Paul, a marathoner, said, "One morning I got so mad at the scale. It told me I'd gained three pounds, and I'd been starving myself for half a week. I angrily jumped up and down on it until it broke. That's the last time I've weighed myself!" Paul can laugh now when he recalls that story, but he wasn't laughing at the time.

If you worry about your weight, I advise against weighing yourself daily. You'll likely refer to yourself as being good when the pounds drop and bad when they go up. Nonsense. You are the same lovable person, regardless of a pound or two either way.

A scale measures not only fat but also muscle gain, water, food, intestinal contents, the coffee you drank just before weighing yourself, and so on. The scale may give you irrelevant information. For example, if you increase your exercise program, decrease your food intake, build up muscle, and lose fat, the scale may indicate that your weight has remained the same. You will feel thinner, look thinner, and your clothes will be looser, but you will not gain the psychological rewards if you depend on the scale. Scales can also be inaccurate.

Some athletes play games with the scales and fool only themselves. For example, runners, racquetball players, and other athletes who perspire heavily often prefer to weigh themselves after a hard workout. During exercise, they may have lost five pounds (two kilograms)—five pounds of sweat, not fat.

The only time to weigh yourself (if you insist) is the first thing in the morning. Get up, empty your bladder and bowels, and then step on the scale before you eat or drink anything. You'll be weighing your body, pure and simple. If you weigh yourself at the end of the day, you'll also be weighing your dinner, beverages, and other foods in your intestines.

Also remember that weight is more than a matter of willpower. Weight, like height, is largely under genetic control. When it comes to height, you have likely accepted the fact that you can't force yourself to grow six inches. But when it comes to weight, you may demand your body to lose an inappropriate number of pounds.

Certainly, if you are overfat, you can reduce to an appropriate level of body fatness. Weighing yourself weekly on the scale can provide positive reinforcement. But if you are already a lean athlete who is struggling to drop those final five pounds below an appropriate weight, you may feel like a failure and question your self-worth: "Why can't I do something as simple as lose five pounds?"

Some athletes are in a difficult situation when it comes to meeting the weight demands of their sport. For example, wrestlers, rowers, ballet dancers, and figure skaters participate in a sports system that does not accommodate athletes as designed by nature. This circumstance raises ethical concerns. Should genetically stocky people be discouraged from ballet, figure skating, gymnastics, and other sports that favor thinness? Should rowers be encouraged to drop 15 pounds (7 kilograms) to reach a lower weight class? The governing bodies of such sports need to understand that weight is more than a matter of willpower and somehow accommodate the fact that health and fitness are more important than weight.

How Much Should I Weigh?

Although only nature knows the best weight for your body, the following guidelines offer a method to estimate the midpoint of a healthy weight range (plus or minus 10 percent, depending on whether you have large or small bones). This rule-of-thumb guide does not apply to everybody—especially muscular bodybuilders.

Women: 100 pounds for the first five feet of height, 5 pounds per inch thereafter (45 kilograms for the first 152 centimeters, 0.9 kilograms per centimeter thereafter).

Men: 106 pounds for the first five feet of height, 6 pounds per inch thereafter (48 kilograms for the first 152 centimeters, 1.07 kilograms per centimeter thereafter).

For example, a woman who is five feet, 6 inches (167 centimeters) could appropriately weigh 100 + 30 = 130 pounds (45 + 14 = 59 kilograms), with a range of 117 to 143 pounds (53 to 65 kilograms). A man who is five feet, 10 inches (178 centimeters) could appropriately weigh 106 + 60 = 166 pounds (48 + 28 = 76 kilograms), with a range of 149 to 183 (68 to 83 kilograms).

Although athletes commonly want to be leaner than the average person, heed this message: If you are striving to weigh significantly less than the weight estimated by this guideline, think again. Pay attention to the genetic design for your body and don't struggle to get too light. The best weight goal is to be fit and healthy rather than sleek and skinny.

If you are significantly overweight, your initial target should be to lose just 5 to 10 percent of your current weight. If you weigh 200 pounds (90 kilograms), losing just 10 to 20 pounds (5 to 10 kilograms) is enough to improve your health status and significantly reduce your risk of heart disease, diabetes, and high blood pressure. Although you may want to lose more fat for cosmetic reasons, you should know that losing the initial few pounds is a meaningful accomplishment.

Body Fat Measurements: Fact or Fiction?

When I counsel athletes who have a poor concept of an appropriate weight, I measure their body fat rather than rely on a scale and height and weight charts. The fat measurement helps put in perspective the proportion of an athlete's body that is muscle, bone, essential fat, and excess fat. The scale provides a meaningless number because it doesn't indicate the composition of the pounds. Although some pounds are desirable muscle weight, others are less desirable fat weight. Obviously, the muscle weight contributes to top athletic performance in most sports. The fat weight is the bigger concern, because excess fat can slow you down.

Believe me, judging from the tension that radiates from the body of a weight-conscious athlete, I believe that getting your body fat measured ranks high on the list of anxiety-provoking life experiences. This number unveils the truth. Hulky football players are often humbled to learn that 20 percent of their brawn is flab. Some of the weight they lug around is fat, not solid, steely muscle. Weight-conscious gymnasts are often thrilled to learn that they are leaner than they thought they were.

If you want to have your body fat measured, you'll certainly want to have it done correctly by a qualified health professional to eliminate any possibility of being told that you are fatter than you really are. Inaccurate readings can send people into a tizzy. If you later want to be remeasured, try to have it done by the same person using the same technique to ensure greater consistency.

These are four common methods to estimate percent body fat:

- Underwater weighing, which sounds intriguing and traditionally has been considered the most accurate method
- The BodPod, which uses a method similar to underwater weighing, except that the body displaces air instead of water
- Skinfold calipers, which are more convenient, less sensational, and relatively accurate
- Bioelectrical impedance analysis (BIA), which is a snazzy, computerized method that includes special scales and hand-held instruments and is relatively accurate if you are hydrated appropriately

When it comes to measuring body fat, no simple, inexpensive method is 100 percent accurate. Underwater weighing, air displacement, calipers, and electrical impedance all have potential inaccuracies. The following information evaluates these options to help you decide the best way to estimate your ideal weight, should you want to quantify the fats of life.

Keep in mind that body-fat measurements should include a conversation about an appropriate weight for your body. That is, if you are far leaner than other members of your genetic family but still have a higher percentage of fat than you desire, you may already be lean for your body. For example, a five-foot, six-inch (168-centimeter) walker lost 50 pounds (23 kilograms), from 200 to 150 (91 to 68 kilograms), and wanted to reach a seemingly appropriate weight goal of 130 pounds (59 kilograms). Because she couldn't seem to lose beyond 150 without severely restricting her intake, I measured her body fat. She was 28 percent fat, at the higher end of average but far leaner than anyone else in her family. I suggested that she be at peace with this healthier weight and remember that she was currently thin for her body.

Underwater Weighing

With underwater weighing, the subject exhales all the air in his or her lungs and then is weighed while submerged in a tank of water. Despite popular belief, this technique does not measure body fat. Instead, it measures body density, which translates mathematically into percent fat. During the translation, however, significant error can creep into the picture. The equations for translating density into fat are most appropriate for the standard male. This excludes many thin runners and muscular bodybuilders. The same equations can be inappropriately used for girls on the high school swim team, 50-year-old marathoners, and professional football players.

Body density differs among all types of athletes, and age, gender, and race affect it. Children and senior citizens differ from each other in body density. The anorexic ballerina with osteoporotic, low-density bones is far different from the standard male and may receive an inaccurate estimate of percentage of fat unless the difference in density is accounted for using a population-specific equation.

Errors with underwater weighing also stem from the inexperience of the person being weighed. If you've never been submerged into a weighing tank, you are likely to be nervous and may not completely exhale all the air in your lungs before going under the water. This will affect the density reading. Exercise physiologists have estimated that as little as two cups (a half liter) of air can affect body-fat measurements by as much as 3 to 5 percent. Intestinal gas can also disrupt the accuracy, as can poorly calibrated equipment. Many portable underwater weighing systems (the kinds that show up at road races, health fairs, and runners' expos) may lack the precision of a weighing system used in a research laboratory.

If you are looking for a perfect measurement tool, underwater weighing has sources of error. But so do the other methods.

Bod Pod

The Bod Pod Body Composition System (Life Measurement, Inc., Concord, California) is a big, podlike chamber with a top that swings open and a seat inside. The person sits inside, scantily clad (standard clothing takes up space and alters the reading). The technician closes the top of the Bod Pod and then takes air-pressure measurements that determine body volume from air displacement. These measurements are then translated into percent body fat, using a principle similar to underwater weighing. The accuracy is similar to that of underwater weighing; they agree within 1 percent (Fields, Goran, and McCrory 2002). Because the Bod Pod is quick, comfortable, easy, and less stressful than the underwater weighing method, it is gaining in popularity in both health clubs and research settings. The Bod Pod is user friendly and can easily accommodate elderly people, children, and obese people.

Skinfold Calipers

Skinfold calipers are large pinchers that measure the thickness of the fat layer on specific body sites. Health professionals well trained in the technique are the most qualified to use this method. Active people often obtain their measurements from students or novice technicians who may be using imprecise or poorly calibrated calipers at crowded health fairs or fitness events. A hasty measurement an inch above or below the established pinch point can add 5 to 15 millimeters of fat to the measurement. Those little millimeters can translate inaccurately into a high body-fat reading.

I often get phone calls from frenzied athletes who were hastily measured at a health fair and were told that they are overfat when they suspect that they're really not. When I carefully remeasure them in my quiet office, I can get a much better reading. I can also use my professional judgment to determine if the number I get seems reasonable for that person. The eyeball method is fairly reliable.

Individual fat patterns also contribute to inaccurate calculations. For example, one female skier had inherited abnormally fat arms. Many conversion formulas use an arm measurement. According to one calculation that used this measurement, the skier's body was 28 percent fat. Another method, which adjusted for the fat arms, produced an estimate of 19 percent fat. That's quite a variation.

Even accurate measurements commonly translate into erroneous information because of inappropriate conversion equations. To be most accurate, the measurements from a runner, wrestler, bodybuilder, or gymnast should be plugged into sport-specific conversion equations. Such equations are seldom used for the average athlete. In harried situations, such as at some health fairs, the technicians are unlikely to take the time to switch formulas. They may even forget to convert from the equation for a male to one for a female. One rushed technician incorrectly used a man's formula on a woman. The unfortunate woman ended up with a measurement of 8 percent more fat than she really had and a depressed state of mind. She had frustrations about her weight until she decided to have her fat remeasured under conditions that were more peaceful.

As you can see, the accuracy of body-fat measurements using calipers depends on the precision of the technician, the accuracy of the caliper, and the appropriateness of the conversion equations. Repeated measurements by different technicians using different calipers and different equations can yield widely different results.

Skinfold caliper measurements can be used to measure changes in body fatness. I often record on a monthly basis the measurements of people losing a significant amount of weight through regular exercise. By comparing the numbers (either as measurements in millimeters or converted into percent fat), the dieters can monitor changes. People recovering from anorexia also appreciate repeat skinfold measurements as a way to see that they are rebuilding muscle, not just gaining fat. This use of calipers may not give a 100 percent accurate picture, but it shows trends, particularly when the same technician measures the dieter each time, using the same calipers and same conversion equations.

Bioelectrical Impedance

Body composition is commonly measured by using bioelectrical impedance analysis, a computerized system that sends an imperceptible electrical current through the body. The amount of water in the body affects the opposition to the flow of the current (impedance). Because water is only in fat-free tissue, the current flow can be translated into percent body fat.

Measuring body composition by bioelectrical impedance is a simple procedure that takes just minutes to perform. The whole-body machine (with electrodes attached to the wrists and ankles) is portable, easy to use, and popular at road races and health fairs. Other models that assess regional body composition come in the form of scales (leg to leg, such as the Tanita scale) and the hand-held Omron model (arm to arm).

Although it is a popular method, estimating body fatness by electrical impedance can be problematic, particularly among athletes. Because of the nature of the conversion equations, the body fatness of lean athletes is sometimes overestimated, and the fatness of overweight people is sometimes underestimated. If you measure yourself after you exercise, you'll likely have a lower percentage of fat compared with the preexercise measurement because hydration affects the measurement (Demura et al. 2002). You will get an inaccurate reading if you are dehydrated, so don't bother to be measured after hard exercise or after you've had any alcoholic beverages.

Other factors that may affect the accuracy of the measurement include ethnic background, premenstrual bloat, food in the stomach, and carbo-loaded muscles (water is stored along with the carbohydrates). The calculations are based on the assumption that the standard person is 73 percent water. Research has shown that young people tend to be 77 percent water and older folks 71 percent. If you are improperly positioned during the test (say, with part of your arms touching your body), you will also get an inaccurate reading. This error can easily happen in crowded exhibitions.

With the development of new sport-specific equations, accuracy is improving. Testing of the Omron hand-held model indicates that it gives a reasonably accurate (within 3.5 percent) measurement 65 percent of the time with women and 70 percent of the time with men (Gibson, Heyward, and Mermier 2000). The Tanita scale assessments in a group of healthy males are similar to those produced by underwater weighing (Cable et al. 2002).

What's the Use?

Until researchers find the definitive method to measure body fat, here's my advice. Consider body-fat measurement as a comparative measurement to reflect changes in your body as you lose fat, gain muscle, shape up, and slim down. Don't expect more accuracy than is possible (see table 9.2). The standard error is plus or minus 3 percent. Hence, if you are measured at 15 percent, you might be 12 percent or 18 percent. That doesn't take into account another 3 percent biological error because of individual variations in body fatness.

Your best bet is to see how the measurements change over time. Have the same person measure you at bimonthly intervals over the year. Calipers and electrical impedance are generally the most available and least expensive methods. Although not 100 percent accurate, they provide enough information to help you assess trends in your body-fat changes. But the measurements likely tell you nothing you didn't already know from looking at yourself in the mirror or from the fit of your clothing.

TABLE 9.2

Variability in Body-Fat Measurement

Just as weighing yourself on different scales results in different pound values, having your body fat measured by different people using different methods results in different body-fat numbers. This study done on 57 white males (with an average age of 22) demonstrates the significant variability that occurs even under scientific conditions (Stout et al. 1994).

Measurement method	Average reading (% fat)	Range (% fat)
Underwater weighing	15.0	4.4-34.5
Calipers	12.5	4.5-26.5
Futrex 5000	14.0	4.5-32.5
Futrex 1000	18.5	10.0-37.0
BIA	18.0	9.0-31.0

Data from J. Stout, J. Eckerson, T. Housch, G. Johnson, and N. Betts, 1994, "Validity of body fat estimations in males," *Med Sci Sports Exerc* 26(5): 262.

Words of Wisdom

I strongly recommend that instead of entrusting your fate to an unreliable number, you listen to your body. Each person has a set-point weight at which the body tends to hover. You may slightly overeat one day and slightly undereat the next, but your weight will stay more or less the same. If you drop below this natural weight, your body will start to talk to you. You may fight a nagging hunger, become obsessed with food, and feel chronically fatigued. On the other hand, if you are above your set point, you will feel uncomfortable and flabby.

My experience in counseling athletes of all ages and weights indicate that you likely do know your comfortable weight zone. As Tricia, a five-foot, two-inch masters swimmer, acknowledged, "I can diet down to 110 pounds, an appropriate weight for the average person of my height. But I don't stay there. My body is most comfortable between 117 and 120. That's heavier than most people my height, but that's what's normal for me and where I fit in with the rest of my family. Everyone is heavyset."

She had learned through years of unsuccessful dieting that she would never be able to fit her ideal image of perfectly thin. She has now accepted her build and recognizes that she can healthfully participate in sports regardless of the few extra pounds. Weight, after all, is more than a matter of willpower, and happiness is not based on thinness.

10

Bulking Up Without Adding Fat

To listen to all the ads for diets and diet foods, one might think that the only people who struggle with weight concerns are those who want to lose weight. Yet a significant number of people, primarily teenage boys and young men, struggle to gain weight. In a survey of 400 young men ages 13 to 18 years (grades 7 to 12), 25 percent had deliberately tried to gain weight in the past 12 months (O'Dea and Rawstorne 2001). They wanted to bulk up by building bigger muscles so that they could be stronger, have a better body image, improve their sports performance, and better protect themselves in sports with physical contact (football, soccer, rugby, hockey, boxing).

For those struggling to gain weight, eating can be a task, food a medicine, and the food bills an economic drain. Many skinny athletes turn to doughnuts, cookies, ice cream, and fatty and fried foods to help them pump in calories, less expensively but unhealthfully. They often wonder about weight-gain drinks, thinking ordinary food is not good enough. That is not the case.

If you are feeling self-consciously thin, hate your skinny image, and seem to eat nonstop in hopes of putting a little meat on your bones, the information in this chapter, along with the protein information in chapter 8, can give you the knowledge you need to reach your goal healthfully.

Increasing Your Weight

Theoretically, to gain 1 pound (0.45 kilograms) of body weight per week, you'd need to consume an additional 500 calories per day above your typical intake. Some people are hard gainers and require more calories than other people do to add weight. For example, in one landmark research study (Sims 1976), 200 prisoners with no family history of obesity volunteered to be gluttons. The goal was to gain 20 to 25 percent above their normal weights (about 30 to 40 pounds) by deliberately overeating. For more than half a year, the prisoners ate extravagantly and exercised minimally. Yet only 20 of the 200 prisoners managed to gain the weight. Of those, only 2 (who had an undetected family history of obesity or diabetes) gained the weight easily. One prisoner tried for 30 weeks to add 12 pounds to his 132-pound frame, but he couldn't get any fatter.

A similar response was seen in another study with identical twins who were overfed by 1,000 calories for 100 days. The weight gain varied considerably. Some twins gained only 9.5 pounds (4.3 kilograms), whereas others gained 29 pounds (13.2 kilograms). Each twin pair gained a similar amount of weight, suggesting strong genetic control (Bouchard 1990).

This discrepancy mystifies researchers. What happened to the excess calories that didn't turn into fat? Some say the body adjusts its metabolism to help maintain a predetermined genetic weight (Leibel, Rosenbaum, and Hirsch 1995). Others look at increases in fidgeting, changes in body posture, and greater activity in daily life (Levine 1999).

If you are a hard gainer, take a good look at your genetic endowment. If other family members are thin, you probably have inherited a genetic predisposition to thinness. You can alter your physique to a certain extent with diet, weight training, and aging, but you shouldn't expect miracles. Marathoner Bill Rodgers will never look like bodybuilder Charles Atlas, no matter how much eating and weightlifting he does!

Among my clients, I've observed that hard gainers are good fidgeters. They twiddle their fingers, swing their legs back and forth while sitting, and seem unable to sit still. All this involuntary movement burns calories. In comparison, the people who complain about their inability to lose weight generally sit calmly. I tell the fidgeters to mellow out. Chronic fidgeting can burn an extra 300 to 700 calories per day.

Extra Protein to Build Muscles?

Most people who want to bulk up believe that the best way to gain weight is to lift weights (true) and eat a very high-protein diet (false). Although you do want to eat adequate protein (see chapter 8), your body doesn't store excess protein as bulging muscles. The pound of steak just doesn't convert into bigger biceps. You need extra calories, and those calories should come primarily from extra carbohydrates rather than extra protein. Carbohydrates fuel your muscles so that the muscles can perform intense muscle-building exercise. By overloading the muscle not with protein but with weightlifting and other resistance exercise, the muscle fibers increase in size.

To date, research indicates that protein powders and amino acid supplements are a fruitless expense when it comes to gaining muscle weight (Godard, Williamson, and Trappe 2002). They offer nothing that you cannot obtain from standard foods. The only reason these supplements supposedly work for some athletes is that the protein beverage provides additional calories. One can just as easily eat another sandwich to get those calories.

You are most likely to gain weight if you consistently eat larger-than-normal meals. I often counsel skinny athletes who swear they eat huge amounts of food. For example, Peter, a swimmer, swore that he ate at least twice what his friends did. But he ate only two meals per day. Because he swam both before and after school, he lacked time to enjoy a hearty breakfast and afternoon snack. He found time to eat only lunch and dinner. Granted, he did eat a lot at those meals, but that merely compensated for the lack of breakfast and snacks.

Peter gained three pounds (1.4 kilograms) within three weeks after he started to eat three meals per day and an additional snack on a consistent basis. "I now look at food as my weight-gain medicine and have chosen to become more responsible and plan ahead so I have food with me at the right times. There are days when I'm rushed and almost forget about gathering my breakfast on the go—two energy bars with two cups of yogurt that I eat on my way to school. I've learned to put a big note on my swim bag and that helps me remember to pack my sports breakfast. I'm enjoying the benefits—more energy, less morning hunger, plus a few pounds extra weight."

Keith, a six-foot, four-inch high school basketball player, expressed a different complaint about his efforts to gain weight. He felt embarrassed whenever he ate with his friends because he'd eat twice what they did. A large pizza was no challenge. When I calculated his calorie needs, he began to understand why he wasn't gaining weight. He needed about 6,000 calories per day to maintain his weight, plus more to gain weight. The pizza was 1,800 calories. Two pizzas would have been more appropriate.

I told Keith to feed his body what it needed and stop comparing his food intake with that of his shorter friends. I suggested that he explain to any teasers that his body was like a limousine that needed more gas to go the distance.

Boosting Your Calories

If you have a busy schedule, finding the time to eat can be the biggest challenge to boosting your calories. You might need to pack a stash of portable snacks in your gym bag if you do most of your eating outside the home. To take in the extra calories needed to gain weight, you can eat frequently throughout the day, if that fits your lifestyle. Plan to have food on hand for every eating opportunity or try these tips:

- Eat an extra snack, such as a bedtime peanut butter sandwich with a glass of milk.
- Eat larger-than-normal portions at mealtime.
- Eat higher calorie foods.

If you eat foods that are compact and dense (for example, granola instead of puffed rice), more calories can fit into your stomach with less volume.

When you make your food selections, keep in mind that fats are the most concentrated form of calories. One teaspoon of fat (butter, oil, margarine, or mayonnaise) has 36 calories; the same amount of carbohydrate or protein has only 16 calories. Most protein-rich foods contain fat (such as the cream in cheese, the grease in hamburgers, or the oil in peanut butter), so these foods tend to be high in calories. But some of these fats are bad for your health: the saturated fat in cheese, beef, chicken skin, butter, and bacon. Try to limit your intake of the bad fats and focus on the healthful fats, such as peanut butter, walnuts, almonds, olive oil, and oily fish like salmon and tuna. You should still be eating the basic high-carbohydrate sports diet described in chapters 1 and 7; you'll be adding extra unsaturated fats to that foundation. Eating too many fatty foods can not only clog your arteries but also leave your muscles unfueled.

Boost Those Calories!

These choices alone in one day will boost your calories by 890!

When food seems like a medicine and every calorie counts, boost your intake by choosing higher-calorie foods. Small changes in your diet can make big changes in your weight.

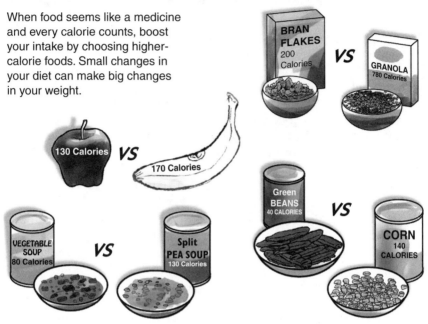

The following foods and beverages can help you healthfully boost your calorie intake:

Cold cereal. Choose dense cereals (as opposed to flaked and puffed types), such as granola, muesli, Grape-Nuts, and Wheat Chex. Top with nuts, sunflower seeds, or raisins, bananas, or other fruits.

Hot cereal. Cooking with milk instead of water adds calories and nutritional value. Add still more calories with mix-ins such as powdered milk, margarine, peanut butter, walnuts, sunflower seeds, wheat germ, ground flax meal, and dried fruit.

Juices. Apple, cranberry, cranapple, grape, pineapple, and most of the juice blends (such as mango-orange-banana) have more calories than grapefruit, orange, or tomato juice. To increase the calorie value of frozen orange juice, add less water than the directions indicate.

Fruits. Bananas, pineapple, mangos, raisins, dates, dried apricots, and other dried fruits contain more calories than watery fruits such as grapefruit, plums, and peaches. Enjoy fruit smoothies.

Milk. To boost the calorie value of milk, add one-quarter cup of powdered milk to one cup of 2 percent milk. Or try malt powder, Ovaltine, Carnation Instant Breakfast, Nestle's Quik, and other flavorings.

Mix these up by the quart to have them waiting for you in the refrigerator. You can also make blender drinks such as milk shakes and fruit smoothies. Fixing these kinds of drinks is far less expensive than buying the canned liquid meal supplements that are typically just milk-based formulas with added vitamins. Plus, they taste better.

Toast. Spread with generous amounts of peanut butter, margarine, jam, or honey.

Sandwiches. Select hearty, dense breads (as opposed to fluffy types) such as sprouted wheat, honey bran, rye, and pumpernickel. The bigger and more thickly sliced, the better. Spread with a moderate amount of margarine or mayonnaise. Stuff with tuna, chicken, hummus, or other fillings. Peanut butter and jelly makes an inexpensive, healthful, and high-calorie choice.

Soups. Hearty lentil, split-pea, minestrone, and barley soups have more calories than brothy chicken and beef types, unless the broth is chock full of veggies and meat. To make canned soups (such as tomato or chowder) more substantial, add evaporated milk in place of water or regular milk, or add extra powdered milk. Garnish with margarine, parmesan cheese, and croutons. If you wish to reduce your sodium intake, be sure to choose the reduced-sodium soups or homemade varieties.

Meats. Beef, pork, and lamb tend to have more calories than chicken or fish, but they also tend to have more saturated fat. Eat them in moderation and choose lean cuts. To boost calories, sauté chicken or fish in canola or olive oil and add wine sauces and bread-crumb toppings.

Beans, legumes. Lentils, split-pea soup, chili with beans, bean burritos, limas, and other dried beans are not only calorie dense but also packed with protein and carbohydrates. Hummus (made with chickpeas) is an easy snack or sandwich filling.

Vegetables. Peas, corn, carrots, winter squash, and beets have more calories than green beans, broccoli, summer squash, and other watery veggies. Top with margarine, slivered almonds, and grated low-fat cheese. Add calories by stir-frying veggies in olive oil instead of steaming them.

Salads. What may start out being low-calorie lettuce can quickly become a substantial meal by adding cottage cheese, garbanzo beans (chickpeas), sunflower seeds, assorted vegetables, chopped walnuts, raisins, tuna fish, lean meat, croutons, and a liberal dousing of salad dressing made with heart-healthy oil, preferably olive or canola.

Potatoes. Add margarine and extra powdered milk to mashed potatoes. Although you might be tempted to add lots of sour cream and gravy for extra calories, think again. You'd also be adding saturated fats that are unhealthful for your heart. Reduced-fat sour cream and low-fat gravies would be better alternatives.

Desserts. By selecting desserts with nutritional value, you can enjoy treats as well as nourish your body. Try oatmeal-raisin cookies, fig bars, chocolate pudding, stewed fruit compotes, low-fat frozen yogurt, apple crisp, or other fruit desserts. Blueberry muffins, cornbread with honey, banana bread, and other sweet breads and muffins can double as dessert. (See the recipe section beginning on page 361 for ideas.)

Snacks. A substantial afternoon or evening snack is an excellent way to boost your calorie intake. If you don't feel hungry, just think of the food as the weight-gain medicine that you have to take. Some healthful snack choices include fruit yogurt, low-fat cheese and crackers, peanuts, sunflower seeds, almonds, granola, pretzels, english muffins, multigrain bagels (with low-fat cream cheese and jelly), bran muffins, pizza, peanut butter crackers, milk shakes, instant breakfast drinks, hot cocoa, fruit smoothies, bananas, dried fruits, and even sandwiches. Think "second lunch" and "second dinner."

Alcohol. Moderate amounts of beer and wine can stimulate your appetite and add extra calories, particularly when consumed with snacks such as peanuts and popcorn. Because alcohol offers little nutritional value, do not substitute it for juices, milk, or other wholesome beverages. Never drink alcohol shortly before an event. It has a dehydrating effect and can blunt your reflexes, create problems with hypoglycemia, and hurt performance.

The sample menus in table 10.1 implement some of these suggestions. You can see how smart choices can accumulate into hefty calorie intake and help you meet your weight goals.

TABLE 10.1

Sample Weight Gain Menus

The trick to gaining weight is to eat larger than normal portions consistently for three meals per day and one or two snacks. These sample menus suggest healthful high-calorie, carbohydrate-rich sports meals.

Approximate calories		Approximate calories	
Breakfast			
16 oz orange juice	200	16 oz pineapple juice	280
6 pancakes	600	1 cup granola	500
1/4 cup syrup	200	1/4 cup raisins	120
1 pat margarine	50	16 oz low-fat milk	200
8 oz low-fat milk	100	1 large banana	130
Total:	1,150	Total:	1,230

(continued)

TABLE 10.1 *(continued)*

Approximate calories		Approximate calories	
Lunch			
4 slices hefty bread	400	1 7-inch pita pocket	240
1 6.5 oz can tuna	200	6 oz turkey breast	300
4 tbsp lite mayo	150	2 tbsp lite mayo	80
1 bowl lentil soup	250	2 cups apple juice	250
16 oz low-fat milk	200	1 cup fruit yogurt	250
2 oatmeal cookies	150	1 medium muffin	300
Total:	**1,350**	**Total:**	**1,420**
Dinner			
1 medium cheese pizza	1,400	1 breast chicken	300
16 oz lemonade	200	2 large potatoes	400
Total:	**1,600**	2 pats margarine	100
		1 cup peas	100
		2 biscuits	300
		2 tbsp honey	100
		16 oz low-fat milk	200
		Total:	**1,500**
Second lunch			
2 slices hearty bread	200	1 large N.Y.-style bagel	450
2 tbsp peanut butter	200	3 oz lite cheese	250
3 tbsp jelly	150	16 oz crangrape juice	350
12 oz low-fat milk	150	**Total:**	**1,050**
2 tbsp chocolate powder	100		
Total:	**800**		
Total for day: 4,900 calories		**Total for day:** 5,200 calories	
• 60% carbohydrate (745 g)		• 65% carbohydrate (832 g)	
• 15% protein (193 g)		• 15% protein (180 g)	
• 25% fat (121 g)		• 20% fat (123 g)	

Balancing Your Weight-Gain Diet

The best weight-gain diet follows the fundamental guidelines for healthy eating as described by the Food Guide Pyramid. Because your muscles become saturated with glycogen when fed 3 to 5 grams of carbohydrate per pound (7 to 11 grams per kilogram) of body weight and your body uses less than 1 gram of protein per pound (2.2 grams per kilogram) under growth conditions, your primary dietary goal is to satisfy these requirements for carbohydrates and proteins. Then you can choose the balance of the calories from a variety of (preferably healthful) fats or carbohydrates.

For example, Alex, a high school football player, wanted to gain weight. He was five feet, 10 inches (178 centimeters), weighed 140 pounds (64 kilograms), and wanted to gain 15 to 20 pounds (7 to 9 kilograms). I calculated that he was maintaining his weight on about 3,000 calories per day, and I recommended that he eat about 20 percent more to gain weight and try to hit the following targets.

Calories (increase by 20 percent):

$$20\% \times 3,000 \text{ cal} = \text{about } 600 \text{ more cal} = 3,600 \text{ total}$$
$$= 4 \text{ meals at } 900 \text{ cal each}$$

Carbohydrate (target 3 to 5 grams of carbohydrates per pound [about 6 to 10 grams per kilogram] or about 55 to 65 percent of calories from grains, fruits, vegetables, and other carbs):

$$4 \text{ g carb/lb} \times 140 \text{ lb} = 560 \text{ g carb} = 2,240 \text{ cal carb} = 62\% \text{ cal carb}$$

Protein (target 0.7 to 0.9 grams of protein per pound [1.5 to 2.0 grams per kilogram] or about 12 to 15 percent of calories from lean meats, beans, nuts, and low-fat dairy products):

$$0.8 \text{ g protein/lb} \times 140 \text{ lb} = 112 \text{ g protein}$$
$$= 448 \text{ cal protein} = 12\% \text{ cal protein}$$

Fat (target the balance [25 to 30 percent of calories] primarily from healthful fats in peanut butter, nuts, and olive and canola oil):

$$26\% \times 3,600 = 936 \text{ cal fat} = 104 \text{ g fat}$$

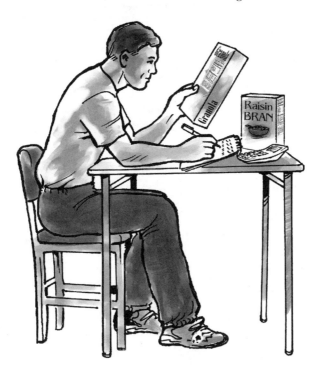

I taught another client, Martin, how to read food labels to learn more about the composition of the foods he was eating. He was surprised to learn that he could get most of his protein requirement with one six-ounce (170 grams) can of tuna (40 grams of protein) at lunch, two chicken breasts at dinner (80 grams of protein), and one quart (one liter) of low-fat milk (40 grams of protein) throughout the day. He no longer felt compelled to suffer through egg-white omelets for breakfast and buy expensive protein bars for snacks. Instead, he ate balanced carbohydrate-based meals, such as tuna on a hefty whole-grain sub roll and 16 ounces (500 milliliters) of milk at lunch, and chicken, two baked potatoes, a hefty salad, and more milk at dinner.

The simpler way to gain weight is to look at your day and figure out where you could eat more food. Steve, a volleyball player, described to me what he typically ate and together we listed ways he could consume more, without much effort, at certain times of the day. For example, Steve typically ate:

Typical intake	Calorie booster	Added calories
Breakfast		
1 bagel	Another bagel	+300
2 tbsp peanut butter	Another 2 tbsp peanut butter	+200
8 oz orange juice	Another 8 oz of orange juice	+100
Lunch		
One sandwich	Another half sandwich	+200
8 oz of milk	Another 8 oz of milk	+100
One cookie	A second cookie	+100
Snack		
Nothing	Granola bar	+200
	Cranapple juice	+200
Dinner		
Lasagna	Apple	+100
Salad		
Bread		
Milk		

By adding more to his meals and snack, he could potentially pump his intake by 1,500 calories! Granted, that is a lot of additional food. He might not eat all of that every day, but at least he knew how to get more calories with little fuss or effort. He just needed to be responsible and set aside enough time to eat the extra calories.

Patience Is a Virtue

By taking the prescribed 500 to 1,000 additional calories per day, you should see some weight gain. Be sure to include muscle-building resistance exercise (weight workouts, push-ups) to promote muscular growth rather than just fat deposits. Consult with the trainer at your school, health club, or gym for a specific exercise program that suits your needs. You might also want to have your body fat routinely measured, to be sure that your weight gain is indeed mostly muscle, not fat. Untrained men might gain about 3 pounds (1.4 kilograms) of muscle per month initially. The rate of gain in well-trained athletes is slower.

If you don't gain weight, look at your family members to see if you inherited a naturally trim physique. If everyone is thin, accept your physique and concentrate on improving your athletic skills. Rather than drain your energy fretting about being too thin, capitalize on being light, swift, and agile. You will likely be able to surpass the heavier hulks that lack your speed.

Also keep in mind that most people gain weight with age. If you are still growing or are in your 20s, your turn to bulk up may still come. All too often, scrawny young athletes fatten up once they get out of school and start working. That's why I hesitate to encourage my clients to force feed themselves. Doing so upsets the natural appetite regulatory mechanisms, and people lose the natural ability to stop eating when they are content. Such was the case with Wes, a 30-year-old photographer and former football player. He reported with a sigh, "I was skinny all through high school. In college, my football coach insisted that I gain weight by eating extra buttered bread, piles of french fries, and mounds of ice cream. I developed quite a liking for these foods. I continued to eat them even after I'd reached my weight-gain goals. Voila—look at me now! I'm 60 pounds overweight and can barely walk, to say nothing of playing football. I long for those days when I was lean and mean."

With a no-fatty-snacks food plan, Wes did lose weight over the course of a year. That fall, he coached an after-school football program. He carefully advised the thin kids to be patient, eat healthfully, and develop smart, lifelong eating habits.

I offer you the same advice. To gain weight, you need to choose larger portions of healthful foods at meals and snacks, eat on a regular schedule—no skipped or skimpy meals—and be responsible. You have to work hard to eat your fill consistently.

Questions From Parents of Skinny Kids

If you are the parent of a skinny kid, you undoubtedly want to help your child add weight healthfully—without eating tons of ice cream, supersized fast-food meals, and expensive (as well as questionable) nutritional supplements. The following are some answers to the questions parents commonly ask about how to support appropriate weight gain in growing kids.

Q. My 16-year-old son insists that I buy him protein powders and weight gain drinks so he can bulk up. Are these necessary?

A. No. The single most important nutrient your son needs is extra calories to perform the muscle-building exercise as well as build muscle. Most of these extra calories should come from carbohydrates (not protein supplements), because the carbs will fuel his muscles and allow him to have the energy he needs to perform the muscle-building exercise. I recommend replacing mealtime water with extra juice and low-fat milk as a simple way to boost calories.

Note that even with no exercise, just eating extra calories stimulates muscular growth. That is, sedentary people gain one pound of muscle with every three pounds of total weight that creeps on.

Q. My 12-year-old son is shorter than many of the girls his age. He feels embarrassed and asked me about protein supplements. Would they help him grow faster?

A. No amount of extra protein will speed the growth process. Boys generally grow fastest between the ages of 13 and 14. After this growth spurt, he will have enough male hormones to add muscle mass and start to grow a beard ("peach fuzz"). This growth spurt lasts longer in boys than in girls, and after the growth spurt boys continue to grow slowly until about age 20.

Q. My 13-year-old son wants to start lifting weights to bulk up for football. Should he?

A. Weightlifting (with light weights and a well-supervised program to prevent stress on immature bones and ligaments) can help your son grow stronger and help prevent injuries. But it will not contribute to bulkier muscles until he has enough male hormones to support muscular development. Boys bulk up after they have finished their growth spurt. Remind him that patience is a virtue!

Q. Is creatine a safe way to gain weight?

A. Creatine is a naturally occurring compound found in meat and fish. (Vegetarians tend to have lower creatine levels than meat eaters.) Creatine is also available in powder and pills. The muscles use creatine phosphate to generate energy for 1 to 10 seconds of intense work (such as occurs with weightlifting, wrestling, ice hockey and sprinting).

In people who respond to creatine supplements, their muscles may perform better during these brief, all-out exercise bouts (Terjung et al. 2000). By being able to lift heavier weights, for example, the muscles can become bigger, an attractive prospect to many teenage boys. But not everyone responds. In a study with 21 subjects, 4 were classified as nonresponders (Kilduff et al. 2002).

The research to date suggests no physical harm from creatine if it is taken in the recommended doses. Anecdotal reports suggest that cramping, nausea, and higher rate of injuries occur among athletes who take creatine, but scientific research has yet to substantiate this idea. The initial weight gain commonly seen with creatine is due to water gain, but in the long term, the gain may be attributed to muscle mass.

To date, no sports medicine organization has recommended the use of creatine in individuals under the age of 18. Although no evidence suggests that creatine is unsafe when taken by healthy adults as directed, it is a relatively new sports supplement and has not been extensively tested in growing children. And as with all sports supplements, the quality of the product is poorly controlled. What you buy may not be what you get. As with any supplement, I always remind my clients, "Buyer beware!"

The key question is whether creatine supplements contradict the spirit of fair play in sports. The answer is hotly debated.

Q. My 14-year-old son is uncomfortable with his scrawny physique. He's heard that creatine will help him gain weight and asked me to buy some for him. What should I tell him?

A. As a 14-year-old, your son is at an impressionable age. For him to start taking a muscle-building, performance-enhancing substance at his age establishes a risky attitude that could lead to the desire to take other dangerous substances down the road. Your job is to encourage him to do his best and discourage a win-at-all-cost attitude. Although you need to be truthful about possible benefits from the use of creatine, you can also send a strong message that discourages the use of creatine in young bodies that are still growing. Remind your son that there is no shortcut to excellent performance; it takes hard work. Tell him that you think the use of this substance is a poor choice for him and other members of his team.

11

Losing Weight Without Starvation

Flabby thighs and big butts haunt many active people. Hence, many people exercise primarily to burn calories and trim excess body fat. Although some exercisers successfully lose weight and attribute that loss to their exercise programs, others express frustration that they don't shed an ounce of fat despite consistent workouts. As Karen, a teacher and young mother complained, "I've been going to the gym for a month now and I haven't even lost one pound. I must be doing something wrong." Her husband, Peter, had the opposite response. "Since I've started going to the gym, I've painlessly dropped five pounds in the past month." Yes, gender differences exist when it comes to exercise and weight loss.

The purpose of this chapter is to help all people learn how to lose body fat by appropriately dealing with the American food supply. You'll learn how to eat wisely, improve your health, have energy to enjoy exercise, and lose excess body fat without feeling denied or deprived. Yes, despite popular belief, you can lose weight without dieting.

Because I'm a dietitian, most people assume that I put people on diets. I don't. I teach people how to eat healthfully and appropriately.

People who go *on* a diet simply go *off* a diet. They have a high chance of not only regaining all the lost weight but also regaining proportionately more fat than muscle. That represents a lot of wasted (or is that waisted?) effort.

Diet is a four-letter word, of which the first three letters spell *die*. Dieting conjures up visions of cottage cheese, grapefruit, rice cakes, and shredded wheat with skim milk. Diets have actually contributed to America's weight problem, because diets are associated with extreme hunger. The body rebels against hunger and the state of starvation by binge eating, more commonly known as blowing the diet, and the dieter gains weight despite extreme efforts to lose weight.

To lose weight healthfully and to successfully keep it off without dieting, you must pay attention to the following:

- **How much you eat.** There is an appropriate portion of any food.
- **When you eat.** Enjoy big breakfasts rather than big dinners.
- **Why you eat.** Eat when your body needs fuel, not when you are simply bored, stressed, or lonely.

The upcoming section includes numerous food-management tips to help you achieve your weight-loss goals. But before attempting a weight-loss program, you first might want to have your body fat measured (see chapter 9). By knowing what percentage of your weight is excess body fat, you'll have a valid perspective for setting an appropriate weight goal. All too often I counsel active people who weigh more than they desire, but their weight is primarily muscle with little excess fat. No wonder they struggle with trying to reduce. They have no excess body fat!

Learning How To Eat

If diets worked, then everyone who has ever gone on a diet would be thin. That's not what happens. Most dieters are heavy. Hence, the way to lose weight for the long haul is to learn how to eat healthfully and appropriately. In chapter 1 I talked about using the Food Guide Pyramid to guide healthful food choices. In this chapter I'll build on that information to help you choose the right portions at the right times so that you can lose weight without feeling denied or deprived. I'll teach you nutrition skill power, which is more powerful than the willpower you might yearn for. Such was the case with Roberta, a 42-year-old computer programmer, mother of two teenagers, and fitness runner.

"If only I had more willpower, I could lose weight," Roberta complained. "I've been trying to lose these same 8 to 10 pounds for 12, yes 12! years. I'm the diet queen!" Feeling completely helpless, Roberta came to me as a last resort to help her achieve her weight goals.

When reviewing her dieting history, I noticed that Roberta would diet by trying to exist on fruit for breakfast, salads for lunch, yogurt for a snack, and fish with vegetables for dinner. Her intake was spartan, to say the least, and it included a limited variety of food. I asked, "When you are not dieting, what do you eat?" She quickly listed her favorite foods (what she fed her children): cereal for breakfast, peanut butter and jelly sandwich for lunch, spaghetti for dinner. Every time she went on her diet to lose weight, she denied herself these favorite foods. She went to extremes to keep cereal and peanut butter out of her sight so that she wouldn't eat them. She deemed them too much temptation for her weak willpower, so she had her kids hide them from her.

I encouraged Roberta to stop looking at food as being fattening and instead enjoy satisfying meals. Eating good food, after all, is one of life's pleasures. Given that she had liked cereal, breads, and pasta since childhood, she was naive to think she could stop liking them. Instead of trying to keep these foods out of her life, I encouraged her to eat them more often. I pointed out that her standard diet foods (fruit, salad, and fish) had no power over her because she gave herself permission to eat them whenever she wanted. I encouraged her to eat cereal every day for breakfast (and even lunch, dinner, and snacks) to take the power away from that food, and I simultaneously taught her how to manage eating cereal in an appropriate portion.

If you, too, struggle with weight issues, you need to learn how to manage your favorite foods, not how to deny yourself of them. By enjoying appropriate portions of whatever you'd like to eat, as often as you'd like, you no longer need willpower to avoid them. Nutrition skill power, not willpower, enhances permanent weight loss without denial and deprivation.

One skill that enhances your ability to eat appropriate food portions is to eat mindfully (not mindlessly). That is, chew the food s-l-o-w-l-y, taste it, and savor each mouthful. By doing so, you'll need far less quantity to be satisfied, and you'll be content to eat a smaller portion. By mindfully eating your favorite foods, you will also diffuse the urge to do last-chance eating. (You know, "Last chance to eat peanut butter and jelly sandwiches before I go back on my diet. I'd better have another one!") You can enjoy more peanut butter (or whatever) when your body becomes hungry again. Nutrition skill power wins in the end.

A second skill that enhances weight loss is to choose more fruits, vegetables, unrefined grains, and fiber-rich foods that have low glycemic response, that is, that have the smallest effect on blood glucose (see chapter 7). Carbs with a low glycemic index (GI) promote weight loss by promoting satiety and delaying a return of hunger, which contributes to eating less in subsequent meals. High-glycemic carbs (that is, sugary sweets) produce the opposite effect. They trigger the release of more insulin, which can induce hunger and favor storage of fat.

Calorie for calorie, low-glycemic fruits, veggies, and whole grains are more satiating than are high-glycemic sodas, lollipops, and gummy bears. You still need to limit calories, but you can feel fuller on calories from low-glycemic foods. By regularly choosing low-GI carbs, you'll not only lose weight more easily but also maintain that weight loss more easily. Furthermore, the diet is rich in the foods that can reduce your risk of cancer, heart disease, and hypertension and are consistent with the U.S. dietary guidelines for healthy eating.

One Size Does Not Fit All

Time and again, I hear people complain, "I know what I should do to lose weight. I just don't do it." Lack of control over food has humbled these knowledgeable dieters. The truth is that successful weight reduction isn't as easy as it sounds, because one diet does not fit everyone. That's why professional advice, individually tailored to a person's lifestyle and food preferences, is far more successful than packaged programs or self-inflicted diets.

If you want to lose weight for the last time, I recommend that you get personalized, professional guidance from a registered dietitian (RD). This health professional has fulfilled specific educational requirements, has passed a registration exam, and is a recognized member of the nation's largest organization of nutrition professionals, the American Dietetic Association. Because some states lack specific standards defining who can rightfully call himself or herself a dietitian or nutritionist, you can protect yourself from frauds and nutrition gurus by seeking guidance from RDs.

Here are some ways to locate your local registered dietitian:

- Use the American Dietetic Association's referral network, available either by calling 800-366-1655 or by accessing www.eatright.org for a list of registered dietitians in your zip code. Find a dietitian who specializes in your specific concern: weight control, eating disorders, sports nutrition, cholesterol reduction, or whatever.

- Look in the Yellow Pages under dietitian or nutritionist and select a name followed by *RD*.

- Call the outpatient nutrition clinic at your community hospital.

- Ask your physician for a recommendation or inquire at a local sports-medicine clinic or health club.

- Call your state's dietetic association (see your phone book).

Counting Calories—Correctly

Most of my clients are afraid to eat real meals. They believe that eating, let's say, a cheese sandwich makes people fat. Eating diet foods, like rice cakes and carrots, feels safer. The problem is that the self-created diets commonly allow too few calories and too limited a selection of (boring) foods. The dieter ends up becoming too hungry. As a result he or she blows the diet and regains any lost weight, plus more.

I calculate for my clients an appropriate calorie budget, so that they know how much is OK to eat to maintain or lose weight. Just as you know how much money you can spend when you shop, you might find it helpful to know how many calories you can spend when you eat. (A calorie, or more correctly, a kilocalorie, is a measure of energy. It is the amount of heat needed to raise one liter of water by one degree Celsius.) To get an accurate assessment of your calorie needs, you should meet with a registered dietitian. Or, you can make a ballpark estimate of your calorie needs by using the following formula:

1. To estimate your resting metabolic rate (see table 11.1)—the amount of calories you need simply to breathe, pump blood, and be alive—multiply your healthy weight by 10 calories per pound (or 22 calories per kilogram). If you are significantly overweight, use an adjusted weight, a weight about halfway between your desired weight and your current weight. That is, if you weigh 160 pounds but at one time normally weighed 120 pounds, use 140 as your adjusted weight.

   Example: Roberta weighed about 130 pounds but could healthfully weigh about 120 pounds. Hence, she needed approximately 1,200 calories (120 × 10) simply to do nothing all day except exist.

TABLE 11.1

Resting Metabolic Rate

Some people think they deserve to eat only if they exercise, but that's not the case. You need hundreds of calories every day simply to live. Here's how a 150-pound (69-kilogram) man burns calories while resting in bed all day.

Organ	Calories per day	Percentage of resting metabolic rate
Brain	365	21
Heart	180	10
Kidney	120	7
Liver	560	32
Lung	160	9
Other tissues	370	21

2. Add more calories for daily activity apart from your purposeful exercise. If you are moderately active throughout the day, add about 50 percent of your resting metabolic rate (RMR). If you are sedentary, add 20 to 40 percent; if very active, add 60 to 80 percent of your RMR.

Example: Roberta was moderately active throughout the day with her two kids and her job. She burned about 600 calories (50 percent × 1,200 calories) for activities of daily living. Her totals were the following:

$$1,200 \text{ RMR} + 600 \text{ cal daily activity}$$
$$= 1,800 \text{ cal per day (without purposeful exercise)}$$

3. Add more calories for purposeful exercise (see table 11.2). For example, when Roberta went to the health club, she exercised aerobically for about 45 minutes and burned about 400 calories on the treadmill. Hence, this was her total calorie need:

$$1,200 \text{ cal RMR} + 600 \text{ cal daily activity} + 400 \text{ cal purposeful exercise}$$
$$= 2,200 \text{ total cal per day}$$

4. To lose weight, subtract 20 percent of your total calorie needs. Roberta deserved to eat about 2,200 calories per day to maintain her weight. Subtracting 20 percent of 2,200 calories (20 percent × 2,200 = about 400 calories) left her with about 1,800 calories for her reducing diet.

In the past Roberta had tried to reduce on 1,000 to 1,200 calories per day. She was skeptical about my proposed reducing plan of 1,800 calories. "If I can't lose weight on 1,000 calories, why would I lose weight on 1,800?" she questioned. I reminded her that when she cut back too much, she'd get too hungry and blow her diet. She also lost muscle, slowed her metabolism, and consumed too few of the nutrients she needed to protect her health and invest in top performance. I reminded her that slow and steady weight loss stays off; quick weight loss rapidly reappears. A reasonable weight-loss target is 0.5 to 1 pound (0.23 to 0.45 kilograms) a week for a person who weighs less than 150 pounds (68 kilograms); 1 to 2 pounds a week for heavier bodies.

The theory of "the less you eat, the more fat you will lose" contains little practical truth. Generally, the less you eat, the more you blow your diet and overeat because of extreme hunger. For example, if you knock off only 100 calories at the end of the day (the equivalent of two Oreos or a spoonful of ice cream), you'll theoretically lose 10 pounds (4.5 kilograms) of fat a year because 1 pound of fat equals 3,500 calories. If you eat 500 fewer calories per day than you normally do, you should lose

TABLE 11.2

Minutes of Continuous Activity Necessary to Expend 300 Calories Based on Body Weight

	Body weight (lb)													
	120	130	140	150	160	170	180	190	200	210	220	230	240	250
Conditioning exercises														
Cycling														
Stationary	66	61	57	53	50	47	44	42	40	38	36	35	33	32
Outdoor (leisure)	83	76	71	66	62	58	55	52	50	47	45	43	41	40
Walking (level)														
2.5 mph	110	102	94	88	83	78	73	70	66	63	60	58	55	53
3.0 mph	94	87	81	76	71	67	63	60	57	54	52	49	47	45
3.5 mph	83	76	71	66	62	58	55	52	50	47	45	43	41	40
Water aerobics	83	76	71	66	62	58	55	52	50	47	45	43	41	40
Lap swimming	41	38	35	33	31	29	28	26	25	24	23	22	21	20
Yoga	83	76	71	66	62	58	55	52	50	47	45	43	41	40
Resistance exercise	55	51	47	44	41	39	37	35	33	31	30	29	28	26
Dancing														
Aerobic dance	55	51	47	44	41	39	37	35	33	31	30	29	28	26
Low-impact aerobic dance	66	61	57	53	50	47	44	42	40	38	36	35	33	32
Ballroom dance (fast)	60	56	52	48	45	42	40	38	36	34	33	31	30	29
Ballroom dance (slow)	110	102	94	88	83	78	73	70	66	63	60	58	55	53
Lifestyle activities														
Golf (walking)	73	68	63	59	55	52	49	46	44	42	40	38	37	35
Raking the lawn	83	76	71	66	62	58	55	52	50	47	45	43	41	40
Lawn mowing														
Walking power mower	73	68	63	59	55	52	49	46	44	42	40	38	37	35
Riding mower	132	122	113	106	99	93	88	84	79	76	72	69	66	63
Vacuuming or sweeping	132	122	113	106	99	93	88	84	79	76	72	69	66	63

Reprinted from Ribisl, P. "A Slim Chance in a Fat World: Beating the Odds on Weight Control." ACSM's Health & Fitness Journal 6 (4): 33.

1 pound per week. Now think of the number of times you've tried to knock off 1,000 calories per day and have ended up gaining weight.

Remember, though, that weight loss is not always mathematical. Nature makes weight loss harder for people who try to get below their set-point weight (Leibel, Rosenbaum, and Hirsch 1995). If you have no excess fat to lose, nature will cause your body to conserve energy. I've had thin clients who eat far less than they deserve yet maintain weight.

Once you've established your total daily calories, divide them evenly throughout the day. Some people like having six small meals: breakfast, snack, lunch, snack, dinner, snack. Others, like Roberta, find that four meals per day work well for them.

I adhere to the philosophy that people should eat at least every four hours. That is, if you have breakfast at 7:00, you'll be hungry for lunch at 11:00. Yes, you could hold off until noon to eat, but your body will be happier if you honor your hunger. Hunger, after all, is simply a request for fuel. By eating lunch at 11:00, you'll be hankering for a second lunch at 3:00. I call this afternoon meal a second lunch, because if I were to call it a snack it would likely become cookies or chips. As a second lunch, it becomes an apple with peanut butter, or soup and crackers, or cereal and a banana.

Roberta was initially skeptical of this four-meal plan; meals, after all, are "fattening." She complained, "I'm afraid I'll get fat from eating so much at breakfast and two lunches." I reminded her that the purpose of the daytime meals is to ruin her appetite for dinner. By eating more during the day, she would then be less hungry that evening, have more energy to exercise from 5:00 to 6:00 P.M., and be able to eat less (diet) at night.

If you hold the fear that meals are fattening, think again and remember these ideas:

- You won't gain weight from eating a substantial breakfast or lunch. You'll have more energy to exercise and burn calories. Even if you were to eat too much at those meals, you could compensate by eating less at night.

- If you skimp on daytime meals and develop a deep hunger, you'll be likely to overeat at night because of the strong physiological drive to eat.

- You'll end up eating fewer calories, even though the breakfast and lunch and second lunch may be larger than before. You'll simply trade in the evening blown-diet calories for wholesome foods earlier in the day.

- If you are not hungry at night, you can skimp at dinner and simply eat soup or salad. But don't have just soup or salad for lunch. It's not enough.

Become familiar with the calorie content of the foods you commonly eat and then spend your calories wisely. That is, include at least three of the five food groups at each meal (see chapter 1) and two kinds of foods per snack. Too many dieters repetitively eat a single food, such as cottage cheese, for a meal. This practice limits their intake of the variety of vitamins, minerals, and other nutrients offered by a range of foods.

Roberta was an expert calorie counter. In fact, she expressed fear about becoming neurotic about counting calories. I reminded her to count calories loosely (0, 50, or 100) and to consider them a general guideline and helpful tool to determine how much (rather than how little) food she could appropriately eat.

More important, she needed to start listening to her body and learn what, let's say, 600 calories feels like. She could then use that feeling for future reference. For example, she could tell the right amount to eat at a restaurant by listening to her body's message of being pleasantly fed. Calorie counting can be a helpful bridge to get you in touch with the ability of your body to tell you how much is OK to eat so that you feel satisfied. You can and should quickly replace calorie counting with listening to your body's signals for hunger and satiety. Calorie counting should not become an obsession.

Nine Steps to Successful Fat Loss

Now that you know how many calories you can eat to lose body fat gradually, you need to learn how to eat those calories appropriately. Here are nine steps for successful fat loss.

Write It Down

Keep accurate food records of every morsel and drop for three days, if not more. (Research suggests that people who keep food records tend to lose weight effectively.) Record why you eat. Are you hungry, stressed, or bored? Include the time and amount you exercise as well. Evaluate your patterns for potentially fattening habits such as skimping at breakfast, nibbling all day, overeating at night because you've become too hungry, entertaining yourself with food when you're bored, or rewarding yourself with chocolate when you're stressed.

Pay careful attention to your mood when eating. Roberta discovered that at times a hug and human comforting could have better nourished her than food did. She acknowledged that eating a tub of popcorn diverted her loneliness or anxiety but did nothing to resolve the problem that triggered her eating.

If you eat for reasons other than to obtain fuel, you need to recognize that food should only be fuel. Like a drug, food should not be abused. Food becomes dangerously fattening when it is eaten for entertainment, comfort, or stress reduction. And no amount of any food will solve your problems.

Frontload Your Calories

If you eat lightly during the day and excessively at night, experiment with having a bigger breakfast and lunch and a lighter dinner. See chapters 3, 4, and 5 to review how eating earlier in the day prevents you from becoming too hungry, losing control, and overeating in the evening.

Roberta was surprised that I thought her diet breakfast of cereal with skim milk was too skimpy. She thought that diets were supposed to start at breakfast. I told her to start her diet at dinner. She needed more energy to get through her active day.

Eat Slowly

Overweight people tend to eat faster than their normal-weight counterparts do. Because the brain needs about 20 minutes to receive the signal that you've eaten your fill, slow eating can save you many calories. No matter how much you consume during those 20 minutes, the satiety signal doesn't move any faster. Try to pace your eating time so that you eat less and avoid the discomfort that often occurs after rapid eating. For example, choose soup for a first course before dinner at a restaurant. Hot soup takes time to eat and decreases the appetite for the entree. You'll be content to have a lighter meal.

Roberta had the bad habit of inhaling her meals in a matter of minutes. She'd eat nonstop, without enjoying the pleasures of the meal. I encouraged her to put her fork down frequently, taste the food, and eat it mindfully. You should pay attention to what you are eating. Remember: The best part about food is its taste. If you aren't taking time to enjoy the taste of food, you are missing one of the pleasures of life.

Because Roberta had eaten quickly for most of her life, I suggested that she practice slowly eating at least one meal per day and then build that up to two, then three meals. She discovered that lunchtime became more enjoyable once she gave herself permission to relax and enjoy both the meal and mealtime. She felt less tempted to eat dessert, because the slowly savored lunch satisfied her appetite.

Eat Your Favorite Foods

If you deny yourself permission to eat what you truly want to eat, you are likely to binge. But if you give yourself permission to eat your desired foods in diet portions, you will be less likely to blow your reducing plan. That is, if chocolate glazed doughnuts are among your favorites, then have one once or twice a week. Simply determine how many calories are in the doughnut and spend your calorie budget accordingly. When eating this treat, remember to chew it slowly, savor the taste, and fully enjoy it. You'll free yourself from the temptation to devour a dozen doughnuts in one sitting.

Roberta's downfall was chocolate-chip cookies. "I can go for four days without a cookie fix, but then I inevitably end up eating two great big ones." I encouraged Roberta to plan having a cookie lunch at least twice per week to prevent those unnecessary binges. When she did that, she discovered that she had less desire for cookies for treats because she did not feel denied or deprived. Eating bigger meals also helped abate the cookie cravings. By preventing herself from getting too hungry, she lost interest in sugary treats.

Avoid Temptation

Out of sight, out of mind, and out of mouth! If you spend a lot of free time in the kitchen, you might consider relocating to the den when you want to relax, where food is less likely to be available. At parties, socialize in the living room, away from the buffet table and away from the snacks. At the market, skip the aisle with the cookies.

Roberta used to take walks that went by the bakery. No wonder she'd succumb to temptation! I suggested that she walk down another street. This became the simple solution to what had been a major problem. She also learned to enter her house through the front door and go immediately upstairs to change her clothes and unwind from the day. Previously, she had entered the house through the kitchen door. She would then habitually open the refrigerator and graze for a few minutes while making that transition from working to being at home.

Keep a List of Nonfood Activities

When you are bored, lonely, tired, or nervous, you need to have some strategies in mind that have nothing to do with eating. For example,

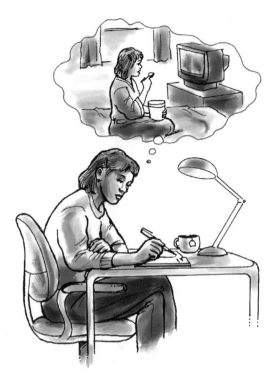

you might want to call a friend, write a letter, take a bath, water the plants, listen to music by candlelight, work on a puzzle, go for a walk, take a nap, play with your kids, or meditate. Food is designed to be fuel, not entertainment, not a reward for having survived another stressful day.

When Roberta felt tired and stressed, she would treat herself to food. I encouraged her to ask herself before indulging, "Am I hungry? Or am I tired and stressed?" If the answer was that she was tired, she talked herself into going to bed early. If the answer was that she was stressed, she learned to recognize that no amount of food would resolve the stress so she shouldn't even start to eat. Making a phone call to her best friend or writing a page in her journal became her slimming alternatives.

When you overeat because you are stressed, you are only trying to be nice to yourself. Food alters your brain chemistry and may put you in a happier mood—for the moment, that is. In the end this inappropriate coping skill will leave you even more stressed and depressed from the weight gain. Learning how to manage stress without food is the obvious solution.

Instructors from the Mind/Body Medical Institute in Boston suggest taking three deep, slow breaths—breathe in peace, breathe out stress—to dissipate stress. Meditation can also be helpful. Calm your mind by sitting in a comfortable position and focusing on the word ocean. Slowly inhale on "O" and exhale on "cean." Soon the calm vision of ocean waves will help soothe your nerves, and perhaps save you some calories.

Make a Realistic Eating Plan

You don't have to lose weight every day. Rather, every day you can choose to lose, maintain, or even gain weight. For example, if you face a hectic schedule and wonder how you will survive the stresses of the day, give yourself permission to fuel yourself fully and have a maintain-weight day. You'll need the energy to cope. If you are going to an elegant wedding and want to enjoy the full dinner, go right ahead! A gain-weight day from time to time is part of normal eating. Your body will simply be less hungry the next day, and you'll be able to compensate by eating a little less.

Roberta had always considered a diet to be a nonstop event that would last for weeks or months until she reached her goal weight. I invited her to see weight reduction as being a daily choice that depends on the stress level of the day. I also recommend that she plan on a treat once a week. Just as people need a day off from work, dieters need a day off from dieting. Roberta acknowledged, "Knowing that I can enjoy going out to eat on Friday night helps me stay with my reducing program the rest of the week."

Schedule Appointments for Exercise

If you have trouble following a consistent exercise program, scheduling the time to exercise in your appointment book can be helpful. You want to exercise regularly to tone muscles, relieve stress, and improve your health, but you should not overexercise. If you exercise too much, you will likely end up injured, tired, and irritable. As I mentioned before, exercise should be for fun and fitness, not simply for burning off calories. Be sure that you enjoy yourself.

Roberta would sometimes punish herself with extrahard workouts—more time on the stair stepper or longer, faster walks to burn more calories. Although she did expend 500 to 600 calories per session, she'd end up so hungry that by the end of the day she would inevitably replace those calories, plus more. I encouraged her to stop using exercise as punishment for having extra body fat. She should exercise to improve her health and performance. I reminded her that the *e* in *exercise* stands for enjoyment. Remember, exercise only contributes to weight loss if it culminates in a calorie deficit at the end of the day.

My clients commonly ask, "How much exercise is enough?" Enough for what? For overall health and fitness, the American College of Sports Medicine (ACSM Position Stand 1998) recommends accumulating at least 30 minutes of moderate physical activity most days of the week (about 150 calories per day, or 1,000 calories per week). The classic Harvard Alumni Health Study found that the lowest death rates from cardiovascular disease occurred among those who burned more than 1,000 calories per week (Sesso, Pfaffenbarger, and Lee 2000). The Institute of Medicine recommends 60 minutes each day of moderate physical activity (2,000 calories per week) to prevent weight gain and optimize health (Couzin 2002).

Think Fit and Healthy

Every morning before you get out of bed, visualize yourself being fitter and leaner. This picture will help you start the day with a positive attitude. If you tell yourself that you are eating more healthfully and are successfully losing weight, you will do so more easily. Positive self-talk is important for your well-being.

Roberta constantly reminded herself that she'd rather be healthier and leaner than allow herself to overeat. She took smaller portions. She made a daily eating plan and stuck to it. On her way home after work, she visualized herself eating a pleasant (but smaller) dinner, chewing the food slowly, savoring the taste, relaxing after dinner with a book rather than cookies, and successfully following her food plan. By practicing this scene before she arrived home, she discovered that she was better able to carry through with her good intentions.

Roberta also reminded herself that when she ate well, she felt better and exercised better. She also felt better about herself. After years of unsuccessful dieting, she liked feeling successful, perhaps even more than feeling thinner.

Fad Dieting

Every dieter wants to lose weight quickly, and a fad diet that promises instant success is appealing. Unfortunately, fad diets tend to work for only a short time, and dieters tend to regain the weight quickly. Have you ever met a person who has lost weight on a fad diet and has kept it off? Likely not! Eating works when you eat healthfully, in moderation. Dieters need to learn how to *manage* food—not how to eliminate foods.

Zone Diet: This 40-30-30 plan prescribes 40 percent of calories from carbohydrates, 30 percent from protein, and 30 percent from fat, the philosophy being eating fewer carbs will reduce insulin and consequently fat storage. The truth is, excess calories (of any type) promote fat storage, not excess carbohydrates. (If carbs are fattening, why are not the people in rice-eating countries fat—such as the natives in Japan and China?)

The Zone Diet was the fad response to high-carb–low-fat diets that failed to achieve weight loss promises. The seeming success of the Zone demonstrates that a strong intake of protein and fat can enhance weight reduction because these types of foods are more satisfying than fat-free foods. When you feel less hungry, you can more easily eat fewer calories and thereby lose weight.

The bad news is that athletes generally need more than 40 percent carbs to fuel their muscles for top performance. You cannot expect to do repeated days of hard exercise without having carbs be the foundation of each meal. If you are a casual exerciser, you may be able to exercise OK with a reduced carb intake. But do you really want to live your life calculating 40-30-30 meals? As one dieter said, "I didn't know if my meal would equate to 40-30-30, so I just didn't eat it." No wonder he lost weight!

Dr. Atkins' Diet Revolution: Based on high-protein, high-fat foods, this diet eliminates carbohydrates to the extent the body goes into ketosis. Ketosis is an abnormal condition in which the carbohydrate-depleted body resorts to fueling the brain with ketones (a fuel created when protein is burned for energy). Ketosis kills the appetite, which makes it easier to lose weight. But take heed: People who are in ketosis have bad-smelling breath.

Like the Zone Diet, this plan blames insulin and carbs as being fattening, and that is not the case (as explained above). And although this high-protein plan promotes the concept that you can eat all you want, just how many chicken breasts and cans of tuna can you eat for days in a row? The lack of variety contributes to food boredom and reduced calorie intake . . . to say nothing of reduced phytochemicals, fiber, and other health-protective food components from the lack of fruits and vegetables.

Many people swear by a modified Atkins diet, which simply eliminates potato, rice, pasta, breads, and other starches, but (thankfully) includes fruits and vegetables. If you are a recreational exerciser, you may be able to get enough carbs from fruits and vegetables for fitness workouts from a modified Atkins diet. But the question arises: Do you never want to eat another potato or bagel for the rest of your life?

The goal of losing weight is to learn how to eat smaller portions of the foods that you always have (and always will) like. Diets that deny favorite foods have a very limited life. Plus, the dieter ends up feeling guilty if he or she "cheats" and has a potato. In my value system, food is not a moral issue and eating is not cheating. Is living with guilt and self-anger for having eaten a potato conducive to optimal health? Doubtful!

Ultra Slim-Fast Plan: By drinking this canned beverage at breakfast and lunch, and then eating a normal dinner, the pounds supposedly drop off. Clearly, a 150-calorie can of Slim-Fast offers fewer calories than does a standard meal, but the reality is that *you* work, not Ultra-Slim Fast. And the reality is, you will have to work VERY hard to eat less dinner when your body is starving for more calories.

The better bet than a 150-calorie starvation meal is to eat at least 500 calories at breakfast and lunch, if not more. (See the information on how to calculate your personal calorie needs on page 221.) Adequate daytime meals provide needed fuel so your body does not shut down, conserve energy, and leave you feeling lifeless and unable to enjoy an afternoon workout. I'd say, if you insist on Slim Fast, have it for dinner (along with a generous serving of vegetables)—but not for breakfast and lunch!

Double-Duty Exercise Program: Doubling your workouts to burn more calories and melt away body fat may sound like a good idea. But what often

(continued)

(continued)

happens is that the more you exercise, the more you'll want to eat. You may burn an extra 400 calories but then succumb to eating 500. Or, if you fail to eat more, your body will conserve energy in response to this perceived "famine" caused by the huge calorie deficit. In addition, you can easily end up injured, exhausted, and sick with a cold or the flu. Exercise should be for enjoyment, not punishment.

Fat-Burning Thermogenic Program: Thermogenic weight-loss supplements are indeed popular. The primary ingredient in any of the thermogenic products is ephedrine, ephedra, or Ma Huang. These are powerful stimulants—so powerful that they not only boost the metabolic rate and contribute to (short-term) weight loss but also kill people. At least 70 deaths and 1,400 adverse events have been linked to ephedrine-containing products. Weight loss is not worth dying for. My advice is stay away from these products!

An extensive list of reviews of fad diets from A to Z is available at www.chasefreedom.com.

Weight-Loss Myths and Truths

Weight reduction is more complex than adding exercise and eliminating dietary fat. Confusion abounds among athletes, exercisers, and obesity researchers themselves about the best way to lose body fat. The one-diet-fits-all approach to losing weight is not appropriate; different people have different histories. Some overweight people are genetically heavy; others are genetically lean. Some are men; others are women. Some are recently overfat; others have been fighting the battle of the bulge for years. Some have taken comfort in food since childhood; others have recently turned to food to smother tough emotions. These factors contribute to the complexities of weight loss.

Despite the complex nature of weight loss, people are forever searching for a simple method to shed excess body fat. The following section addresses some of the questions people commonly ask about weight reduction.

Myth: Carbohydrates are fattening.
Truth: No! Excess calories are fattening. Calories come from carbohydrates (4 calories per gram), proteins (4 calories per gram), alcohol (7 calories per gram), and fats (9 calories per gram).

Excess calories from fats are the main dietary demons. Your body can easily store excess dietary fat as body fat, whereas you are more likely to burn off excess calories of carbohydrates. Butter, margarine, oil, mayonnaise, salad dressing, and grease are obvious fats. Fats are also hidden in meats, cheeses, peanut butter, nuts, and other protein foods. Although some fats are healthier than others, all fats are equally fattening.

Excess calories from alcohol also quickly add up and can easily inflate your body fat stores, as can the calories from the high-fat munchies that commonly accompany alcohol. But calories from carbohydrates are excellent for muscle fuel. Your body preferentially burns them for energy rather than stores them as fat.

Myth: High-protein, low-carbohydrate diets are the best choice if you want to lose weight.

Truth: If you want to lose weight, your best bet is to eat smaller portions at dinner and create a calorie deficit for the day. The fundamental type of calories eaten, either protein or carbohydrate, seems to have less importance. In one eight-week study, subjects who ate 1,600 calories of either a high-protein diet (30 percent protein, 40 percent carb) or a high-carb diet (15 percent protein, 55 percent carb) lost the same amount of weight (Luscombe et al. 2002).

A high-protein, low-carbohydrate diet seemingly works because of several factors:

1. The dieter loses water weight. Carbs hold water in the muscles. For each ounce of carbohydrate you stored as glycogen, your body simultaneously stores three ounces of water. When you deplete carbs during exercise, your body releases the water and you experience a significant loss of weight that's mostly water, not fat.

2. People eliminate many calories when they eliminate carbohydrates. For example, you might eliminate not only the baked potato (200 calories) but also two pats of butter (100 calories) on top of the potato, and this creates a calorie deficit.

3. Protein tends to be more satiating than is carbohydrate. That is, protein (and fat) lingers longer in the stomach than does carbohydrate. Hence, having high-protein (and fat) eggs and bacon for breakfast stays with you longer than does a high-carb bagel with jam. By curbing hunger, you have fewer urges to eat and can more easily cut calories, at least until you start to crave carbs and binge eat.

The overwhelming reason that high-protein, low-carbohydrate diets do not work is that dieters fail to stay on them for a long time. They may lose weight, only to regain it. The trick to losing weight is to learn how to deal with the American food supply so that you won't regain the weight. Remember: You should never start a food program that you do not want to maintain for the rest of your life. Do you really want never to eat breads, potatoes, or crackers again?

Myth: If you eat fat, you will get fat.
Truth: If you eat excess calories you will get fat. Weight control relies on a calorie budget, not only on a fat-gram budget. Fat loss occurs when you burn off more calories than you eat. If you require 2,400 calories per day to maintain your weight but eat only 2,000 calories, you will lose body fat. The kind of calories that you eat may be of less consequence. If you choose to spend 300 of your 2,000 calories on high-fat peanut butter instead of fat-free bagels, you can still lose body fat. Fatty foods that fit into your calorie budget are not inherently fattening (Alford, Blankenship, and Hagen 1990; McManus et al. 2001). Look at your friends. I'll bet that you know of several people who eat fat but are not. You can appropriately eat 25 to 30 percent of your calories from fat.

Some people eat large portions of fat-free foods thinking that fat free means calorie free. Bad idea! Excess calories, regardless of the source, will ultimately be stored as fat (Hill et al. 1992). Dieters who try to fool the dieting system by eating only fat-free foods fool only themselves. For example, Sharon, a personal trainer, reported that she'd been known to eat a whole box of fat-free pretzels for a snack. Paul, a bodybuilder, routinely polished off a half gallon of fat-free frozen yogurt, and Nancy, a swimmer, used to eat at least six fat-free bagels per day. No wonder they all complained that they hadn't lost weight even though they avoided foods containing fat. They were eating too many calories. To lose body fat, they needed to create a calorie deficit.

The advice to eat no fat and lose body fat tends to work best for overweight people who eliminate fatty foods and lose weight because they eat fewer calories. For example, instead of having 700 calories of bacon, eggs, and buttered toast for breakfast, Elliott switched to 400 calories of cereal and banana as part of a conscious effort to lose 50 pounds (23 kilograms), and he successfully dropped weight because of the continued calorie deficit.

In contrast, when already lean people eat a low-fat diet, they commonly feel driven to eat more calories of carbohydrates to compensate for the reduction in fat calories. Weight reduction becomes increasingly hard if you strive to be lighter than nature designed (Leibel, Rosenbaum, and Hirsch 1995). For example, Paula, who wanted to lose three pounds (1.4 kilograms) but was already at her set-point weight, reported that she craved bread, pretzels, and other low-fat foods. I recommended that Paula include some fat in her diet so that she could eat a wider variety of food and enjoy better dietary balance (her extremely low-fat diet was lacking in protein, iron, and zinc), feel more satisfied (foods with fat provide a pleasant feeling of fullness), and be more at peace with food.

Her fat-free food plan created guilt feelings whenever she succumbed to eating a food with fat. For example, she declined a piece of birthday cake because it contained fat. She said that she would have felt too guilty if she had eaten some. I reminded Paula that other people enjoyed the cake and didn't get fat from eating it. Clearly, she was confusing appropriate eating with her desire to be in control. This desire to control fat had little to do with weight and more to do with rigidity.

Because only excess fat calories are fattening, you can eat fat as a part of your calorie budget. Note that many lean athletes eat fat and are thin. You can too, as long as you don't overeat total calories. Just as fat free does not mean calorie free, fat filled does not mean off limits. Within nutritional reason, you should spend your calories on the foods you want to eat and enjoy eating. That includes cheese, chips, and ice cream, all of which can be balanced into a good diet and into your fat and calorie budget in diet portions. If you deny yourself your favorite foods, you will be more likely to end up bingeing on those items.

Myth: Food eaten after 8:00 P.M. readily turns into body fat while you sleep.

Truth: If you are hungry at night, you should honor hunger and eat, particularly if you have calories left in your calorie budget for the day. Many active people, because of their hectic work or training schedule, enjoy most of their calories at night. Other people, however, undereat by day only to blow the diet at night. They eat more than what their bodies require and consume excess calories.

The verdict is unclear about whether night eating is inherently fattening. One survey of 1,800 women found no connection between weight and big evening meals (Kant et al. 1995). But the night eaters did consume more fat, protein, and alcohol, and less carbohydrate, vitamin C, B-6, and folic acid, indicative of a fast-food diet low in fruits and vegetables. At night, people tend to eat fewer carrots and more cakes.

My clients' experiences suggest that cultivating an enormous evening appetite easily ends up with overeating and weight gain. This overeating is easy to rationalize. After all, as one working mother commented, "I feel as though I deserve to eat whatever I want. I've starved myself all day, I've worked hard, I'm tired, and I need a reward."

Gymnasts and runners who eat skimpily during the day tend to have more body fat than those who keep themselves better fueled. By minimizing the time they are in calorie deficit, they are less likely to conserve energy (Deutz et al. 2000). Hence, the bottom line for dieters is that you should fuel appropriately during the day and then eat less at night. You'll not only have more energy for training but also prevent yourself from becoming too hungry and overeating. Remember that when you get too hungry, you may no longer have the energy to care about how much you eat. You simply want to eat. That drive to eat is physiological and has little to do with willpower.

Myth: Exercise kills your appetite.
Truth: Exercise may temporarily kill your appetite, but hunger will catch up with you within one to two hours. Temperature control regulates appetite to some extent. Therefore, if you feel hot after a hard workout, you may experience a temporary drop in appetite. But if you are chilled, such as after swimming, you may feel ravenous.

The effect of exercise on appetite varies according to gender. Regularly exercising male rats tend to lose their appetite and drop weight, whereas female rats get a bigger appetite, eat more, and maintain weight. Limited human research supports those findings (Staten 1991). Postexercise appetite also varies according to body fatness. Studies with obese women who added moderate exercise to their sedentary lifestyle indicate that they did not eat more, and hence they lost weight. Diet and exercise studies with men suggest that the fatter they were, the more weight they lost (in comparison with their thinner peers) because their meals didn't compensate for the calories burned during exercise (Westerterp et al. 1992).

Myth: The more you exercise, the more weight you'll lose.
Truth: Often, the more you exercise, the hungrier you get and the more you eat. For example, you may spend an hour on the stair stepper burning off 500 calories and then devour 12 Oreos (600 calories) in less than six minutes. After a hard workout, your body is hungry. Your soul may also be hungry for a reward. You now deserve a treat for having survived the workout, right?

The effects of exercise on weight loss are complex and unclear. Nature seems to replenish fat stores of lean athletes efficiently to prevent them from wasting away. Lean female athletes, in particular, struggle harder than do males to lose body fat and maintain an even leaner physique. This makes sense in terms of evolution. Nature wants women to be able to reproduce; men are supposed to be lean hunters.

Managing Obesity

My obese clients repeatedly report that they don't have time for breakfast and commonly have to work through lunch. The fact is that they choose to skip those meals. They believe that they don't deserve to eat. They skip meals (in an effort to diet), eat meagerly during the day, but then succumb to excessive amounts of food at night. Even obese people deserve to eat. As one of my obese clients said, "Nancy, you are the only person who has ever told me it's OK to eat."

The unspoken rule is that the fatter you are, the fewer the calories you should eat. Wrong. Just as 18-wheel trailer trucks need more fuel than do compact cars, large bodies need more calories than do smaller bodies. Contrary to popular belief, obese people rarely have slow metabolism. Rather, they require significant amounts of food. For example, a 250-pound (114-kilogram) person may need 3,000 to 4,000 calories per day to maintain weight. An appropriate reducing plan would be 2,400 to 3,200 calories. That's far more than the 800 to 1,000 calories offered by many quick weight-loss programs (that fail in the long run).

If you have a spouse or a child who is obese, do not malign him or her and try to assist weight loss by restricting food. Rather, help your spouse or child become healthier by encouraging him or her to be more active. For you, this may mean accompanying your relative on walks or bike rides, and planning active family outings that everyone enjoys. You should also have more fruits and vegetables in the house rather than cookies and chips. As a society, we need to create community walking groups, fitness centers that welcome overweight clients, and swimming pools that allow people to wear T-shirts and shorts instead of embarrassing bathing suits.

If your child is overweight, note that children commonly grow out before they grow up. That is, they often gain body fat before embarking on a growth spurt. Instead of putting your child on a diet (which can damage self-esteem and imprint the message that they aren't good enough the way they are), get them involved in sports and other activities. Turn off the TV and be active with them.

You can delicately ask if your child is comfortable with his or her body. If he or she is not and expresses a desire to learn how to eat better, arrange a consultation with a registered dietitian who specializes in pediatric weight control. (Call the American Dietetic Association's referral network at 800-366-1655 or visit www.eatright.org.) You can also read books such as Ellen Sattyr's *How to Feed Your Child, But Not Too Much.* Clearly, preventing childhood obesity is preferable to treating adult obesity. Raising healthy kids invests in healthy adults.

Wrestling With Weight:
Athletes and Weight Limits

If you are a wrestler, boxer, jockey, or rower, you are probably not overweight. But you may have to cut weight to achieve a lower weight standard for your sport or else be denied permission to compete. Use the following tips, as well as the other information in this chapter, to help you lose weight healthfully. Despite popular belief, you do not need to starve yourself!

- First of all, get a realistic picture of how much weight you have to lose by getting your body fat measured (see chapter 9). The absolute minimal weight includes 5 percent fat for men and 12 percent fat for women. The minimum weight recommended for wrestlers commonly includes about 7 percent body fat. Trying to achieve a weight that will result in your having to starve yourself to lose muscle or dehydrate yourself to lose water weight is difficult and can hurt rather than enhance your health and performance.

    If you don't have access to calipers or another means to measure your percent body fat, give yourself the less professional pinch test. If you can pinch more than half an inch of thickness over your shoulder blade or hips, you can safely lose a little more weight.

- Start to lose weight early in the season or, better yet, before the start of the season. That way you'll have the time to lose weight slowly (0.5 to 1.0 pounds per week, or 0.23 to 0.45 kilograms) and more enjoyably. Your goal is to achieve and stay at your lowest healthy body-fat level.

- Remember that it is counterproductive to lose weight rapidly before an event. If you do, depleted muscle glycogen and dehydration will take their toll. In a study with wrestlers who quickly lost about 8 pounds (4.5 percent of their body weight), the wrestlers performed 3.5 percent worse on a six-minute arm-crank test designed to be similar to a wrestling competition. These results suggest that rapid weight loss by athletes before competition may be a detriment rather than a competitive advantage (Hickner et al. 1991).

    Athletes who struggle and starve to reach a low weight tend to fool only themselves. Remember, the odds are against the starved wrestler who crash diets to make weight as compared with the well-fueled wrestler who routinely maintains or stays within a few pounds of his fighting weight during training.

- To lose weight, follow the calorie guidelines outlined on pages 221-222. No matter how much weight you have to lose, do not eat less than that required to sustain your resting metabolic rate. Most athletes need to eat at least 1,500 calories of a variety of wholesome foods every day to prevent vitamin, mineral, and protein deficiencies. Do not eliminate any food group.

- Water is not extra weight. Your body stores the precious water in a delicate balance. If you disrupt this balance, you will decrease your ability to exercise at your best. Using diuretics, rubber suits, saunas, whirlpools, or steam rooms to dehydrate yourself is dangerous.

- When replacing sweat loss after workouts, note that juices, sports drinks, and soft drinks all have calories. Ration them wisely! The fluid replacer with the fewest calories is water.

- If you are worried that strict dieting as a teenager will stunt your growth, note that you will catch up after the competitive season. Many wrestlers are short in stature not because of malnutrition but because of genetics. They tend to have short parents. Small people often select a low-weight sport because they are more suited for that than they are for football or basketball.

Bottom Line

As the debate continues regarding the best way to lose weight, here's what I think you need to know and account for in your weight-loss plans.

- **Diets don't work.** Dieting and denial lead to overeating, if not binge eating.
- **Your body has a set point,** a predetermined weight that is appropriate for your genetics. You may not like this number, but you can't easily change it (Leibel, Rosenbaum, and Hirsch 1995).
- **Calories count,** but the mathematics of weight loss is not consistent. Just as your body can rev up its engines to burn off a few excess calories if you overeat, it can also lower the throttle when energy is scarce. This is how the body tries to maintain a set weight (Leibel, Rosenbaum, and Hirsch 1995).

Losing Weight After Your Pregnancy

If you are a new mother who worries that you'll never lose the weight gained during pregnancy, be patient. New mothers need to remember that life has seasons. The first year after pregnancy may not be the season to be as lean or as athletic as desired. Pregnancy lasts for 9 months, and many women need an additional 9 to 12 months to return to their prepregnancy physiques. Don't try to crash diet now.

Your better bet is to focus on eating healthfully and trust that healthy eating will contribute to the return of your appropriate weight. But this process often gets confounded because motherhood brings its own set of nutritional challenges and frustrations. When your baby cries, your life stops, and so do many healthful eating habits! Fatigue, stressful life changes, family adjustments, and lack of energy to food shop and cook can also take their toll on the quality of your diet. You may also lack the mental energy you need to reduce your weight.

The stresses and frustrations that accompany motherhood can interfere with your desired weight-loss plans and may even contribute to weight gain. If you are now home all day with readily available food, you may comfort yourself with soothing "drugs" such as candy, cookies, and other special treats. Physical exhaustion, lack of time, and child-care responsibilities may thwart your intentions to exercise. If this is the case, you might want to pay a babysitter so that you can have some time to exercise. This may help you feel better, and feel better about yourself.

If you fear that you'll end up overweight for the rest of your life, take note of a survey of new moms. The women, who were all runners, reported that most returned to running five weeks after delivery and were at their prepregnancy weight in five months (Lutter and Cushman 1982). Yes, there can be a lean life after pregnancy, as verified by the many mothers you see around you who are lean. For now, love yourself from the inside out, enjoy your baby, and be gentle on yourself.

12

Eating Disorders and Food Obsessions

For most active people, the *e* in *eating* stands for enjoyment. But for some, the *e* stands for evil, and food is the enemy. These food- and weight-obsessed exercisers spend their days trying not to eat. They worry constantly about what they'll eat, when and where they'll eat, how much weight they'll gain if they eat a normal meal with their friends, how many hours they will have to exercise to burn off those calories, how many meals they should skip if they overeat by a few morsels, and so on. The endless frets revolving around food, weight, exercise, and dieting consume them. But many of them fail to understand that their anxiety is abnormal. After all, doesn't everyone talk about food and diets all the time?

Eating Disorders and Active People

Eating disorders among active people seem to be on the rise. The staff at health clubs commonly express concerns about some of their clients, as do coaches about their athletes, especially athletes in sports that emphasize weight, such as running, gymnastics, and wrestling. Research indicates that eating disorders are widespread among athletes in all sports. An estimated 15 to 30 percent of collegiate female athletes have some type of disordered eating pattern, be it anorexia (self-induced starvation), bulimia (binge eating, followed by self-induced vomiting), laxative abuse, excessive exercise, crash diets, or other unhealthy weight-loss practices that place them at risk of developing a full-blown eating disorder (Beals and Manore 2002). Most people with eating disorders exercise compulsively, be it to create a calorie deficit and be thinner or to burn off the calories consumed during a binge.

Approximately half of all dieters report abnormal eating binges. Many of these dieters abuse exercise as a means to help control their weight. Some call themselves athletes, when in reality they can be better named compulsive exercisers. Many live in fear of becoming fat, and they constantly restrict their food in hopes of losing weight. They live with chaotic eating patterns and body hatred.

If you are among the lucky few who effortlessly maintain their desired weight, you probably think that all this talk about food and weight is ridiculous. But if you are a runner, dancer, gymnast, wrestler, or other weight-conscious athlete who constantly strives to be thinner, you may experience some degree of obsession with food. If you believe that you spend more time thinking about food than the average person does, keep reading.

I estimate that at least 40 to 50 percent of my clients at Sports-Medicine Associates are obsessed with food, and they represent only a minority of people who seek professional nutrition guidance. Most people who are obsessed with food struggle on their own for years before asking for help. They are embarrassed that they can't seem to resolve their food imbalances. One 65-year-old woman, a regular at the health club, confided that I was the first person in 50 years to whom she had talked about her bulimia.

Food, for these people, is not fuel. It is the fattening enemy that thwarts their desire to be perfectly thin. Their goal is thinness at any price, and that price is often mental anguish, physical fatigue, injuries that fail to heal, weakened bones, stress fractures, and impaired athletic performance. These athletes perform suboptimally because they eat poorly. One high school runner failed to connect her inability to finish track workouts with her one-banana-a-day diet. She thought that she fell asleep in classes because she had stayed up too late, not because she was underfed!

If you struggle with anorexia or bulimia, I recommend that you seek help from a professional counselor experienced with eating disorders and obtain nutritional guidance from a registered dietitian. (See appendix B for Web sites that offer referral networks.) Extreme eating disorders usually reflect an inability to cope with the day-to-day stresses of life. For example, a woman in charge of fund-raising for a charitable organization smothered her stress with homemade chocolate-chip cookies, warm from the oven. This treat certainly diverted her attention from her problems, but it didn't resolve any of them. Afraid of gaining weight, she'd burn off the calories with a long workout that was pure punishment. She became injured from the excessive exercise, panicked at her inability to exercise, tried to eat next to nothing, became ravenous, binged, and then resorted to self-induced vomiting as a means to purge the calories because she could no longer exercise the way she desired. She came to me looking for help with food. I insisted that she also get psychological counseling to help her deal with stress and her feelings of being out of control.

Eating disorders plague all types of casual exercisers and competitive athletes, males and females alike, and perhaps even you or one of your friends. About 4 percent of female athletes struggle with anorexia, 39 percent with bulimia. Among male athletes, an estimated 1.5 percent struggle with anorexia, 14 percent with bulimia. These numbers, if anything, are conservative because people who feel ashamed about their eating habits commonly give inaccurate self-reports.

These numbers exclude the large group of people with subclinical eating disorders who do not fit the diagnosis of anorexia (because they have a seemingly normal weight) but have an abnormal relationship with food and spend too much time thinking about food and weight. They fritter away each day, trying to get thinner.

In-depth interviews of women with subclinical eating disorders delineate these characteristic eating behaviors:

1. They restrict their calorie intake to lose weight and eat a repetitive diet, with little or no variety in the types and amounts of foods they consume.
2. They follow strict dietary rules and experience guilt and self-anger if they break one of their rules.
3. They limit their intake of "bad foods" and usually choose low- or non-fat foods.
4. Almost all these women perceive themselves as being slightly to very overfat and are preoccupied with weight (Beals and Manore 2000).

Surprisingly, women with subclinical eating disorders tend to have higher body fat than normal eaters do, despite exercising more and eating less than their normal-eating counterparts do. They also tend to consume less dietary fat than the normal eaters do. These findings challenge the two commonly held nutrition beliefs: (1) the more you exercise, the thinner you'll be, and (2) avoiding dietary fat helps you lose body fat.

The women seemingly adapt to the combination of intense exercise with high calorie expenditure and restricted calorie intake. The big deficit causes the body to shut down and conserve energy (similar to hibernation). As mentioned in chapter 9, this seems to be nature's survival technique to prevent women from becoming too thin to reproduce.

If you believe that your body is hibernating and you feel that you eat less than you "deserve" to eat given your exercise level, the solution is to increase your daytime calorie intake gradually to an appropriate level and stop living in calorie deficit. You can do this by adding about 100 calories to your daily intake for four days, then adding another 100 calories for the next four days, and so on until you approach your calorie requirements as outlined in chapter 11. A registered dietitian can be helpful with this process.

Hunger: A Simple Request for Fuel

Being hungry all the time is not a personality quirk. Rather, hunger is the body's request for fuel. Hunger is a powerful physiological force that creates a strong desire to eat. Unfortunately, in our thin-is-in society, many active people fail to honor this simple request because they fear food as being fattening. The thought of eating elicits a sense of panic: "Oh no, if I eat, I'll get fat. But if I stay hungry, I know I am not gaining weight." This is a sick mind-set.

Most athletes eat without getting fat. Food, after all, is fuel. But problems arise when a person denies himself or herself food (as happens with a strict reducing diet), when hunger becomes the norm. The result is an abnormal physiological state known as starvation.

Starvation has been inflicted on many people, including people in developing countries suffering from famines, poverty-stricken people at the end of the month when they have no money for food, and victims of World War II concentration camps. Starvation is also common among exercisers who are intent on losing weight. These include dieters who simply believe that thinner is better as well as people who participate in sports with weight limits (wrestlers, lightweight rowers, jockeys, dancers).

A question arises: What is the cost of starvation? What happens to the body and the mind when food is restricted and body weight is abnormally low? In 1950 Ancel Keys and his colleagues at the University of Minnesota studied the physiology of starvation (Keys et al. 1950; Garner 1998). They carefully monitored 36 young, healthy, psychologically normal men who for six months were allowed to eat only half their normal intake (an amount similar to that consumed on a strict reducing diet or with anorectic eating). For three months before this semistarvation diet, the researchers carefully studied each man's behaviors, personality, and eating patterns. The men were then observed for three to nine months of refeeding.

As their body weight fell to 25 percent below baseline, the researchers learned that many of the symptoms that might have been thought to be specific to anorexia or bulimia were actually the result of starvation. The most striking change was a dramatic increase in preoccupation with food. The subjects thought about food all the time, just as people with anorexia do. They talked about it, read about it, dreamed about it. They even collected recipes. They dramatically increased their consumption of coffee and tea, and they chewed gum excessively. They became depressed, had severe mood swings, and experienced irritability, anger, and anxiety. They became withdrawn, had little interest in sex, and lost their sense of humor. They had cold hands and feet, felt weak and dizzy, and their hair fell out. Their basal metabolic rate (the amount of food needed to exist) dropped by 40 percent as their bodies adapted to conserve energy. Perhaps these changes sound familiar.

During the study, some of the men were unable to maintain control over food; they would binge eat if the opportunity presented itself. During the refeeding period, many of the men ate continuously—large meals followed by snacking. Several ate until they were uncomfortably full, became nauseous, and then vomited. These abnormal eating behaviors lasted for about five months. By eight months most of them regained their standard eating behaviors. On average they initially regained 10 percent more than their original weight but then gradually lost that excess and returned close to their baseline weight.

So what can we learn from this starvation study?

1. Preoccupation with food is a sign that your body is too hungry. Hunger creates a strong physiological drive to eat.

2. Binge eating stems from starvation. If you worry about being unable to stop eating once you start, you have likely become too hungry.

3. Weight is more than a matter of willpower. That is, if you lose weight, your body will fight to return to a genetically normal level.

4. Dieters who restrict to the point of semistarvation are likely to regain the weight they lost, plus more. If you have weight to lose, lose it slowly, not by starvation.

To prevent hunger, you might find it helpful to know how many calories your body requires to maintain or to lose weight (see chapter 11). Then, the next time you get into a food tizzy, overeat, and wonder if you are borderline bulimic, you can compare your intake to your requirements. You'll likely see a huge discrepancy between what you have eaten and what your body deserves. Hunger is powerful. Avoid becoming too hungry!

Thin at Any Cost

The restriction of food that accompanies the struggle to be perfectly thin creates health problems for casual exercisers and competitors alike. The restrictive intake can greatly reduce the intake of vitamins, minerals, and protein, placing the athlete at risk of poor nutritional status. The restrictiveness can also lead to health problems such as chronic fatigue, compromised immune function, poor or delayed healing, anemia, electrolyte imbalance, menstrual dysfunction, reduced bone density, and a four times higher risk of stress fracture.

At SportsMedicine Associates, I counsel many people with eating disorders and disordered eating; they fill the majority of my counseling hours. They come believing that if only they were thinner, they'd be better athletes. I disagree. Their efforts to achieve their desired thinness reduce their energy and performance. They would be better athletes if they fed themselves better. Such was the case with Gretchen, an avid cyclist. She came to me complaining about her inability to lose five pounds (2.3 kilograms): "If only I could shed this extra fat I'd be so much faster climbing hills." She was severely restricting her food intake. I pointed out how few calories she was eating compared with what her body deserved. Once she started to eat adequately, she discovered she could keep up with the other cyclists. Food works!

Why Eating Disorders Happen

Eating disorders commonly occur in people with low self-esteem. They believe that thinness will make them into better and almost perfect people. The truth is that a smaller body does not make a person better, just smaller. There is simply less of the person to love. The individual is the same person, just obsessed, withdrawn, and tired. And when someone severely restricts food, he or she loses muscle, strength, and stamina. This is not the way to become a star athlete.

When an athlete with low self-esteem is physically beautiful, has traits of perfectionism, and tends to be hypercritical and anxious, the risk of developing an eating disorder increases dramatically. Add to the scenario a mother who may have had (or still has) food and weight issues, and her daughter becomes a prime target for developing a full-blown eating disorder.

Athletes with eating disorders are less available to their friends. After all, when that person is constantly exercising and counting calories (calories eaten at meals, calories burned during exercise, calories saved by skipping lunch, calories about to be eaten at dinner, and so on) as well as counting fat grams and sit-ups, his or her brain has little energy left to manage bigger issues like life's problems and relationships. The eating disorder creates a smokescreen that masks the underlying issues.

Eating Isn't Cheating

The following case studies are typical of the clients I treat. They may sound familiar and might help those of you who constantly struggle with food and exercise.

The Stair-Stepper Mistress

Alicia, a 41-year-old teacher, had never been concerned about her weight and had never dieted until her 39th birthday. But in the past two years, she had gained a few pounds because of the stress of a new job. Not liking the extra weight, she decided to join a health club. She forced herself through 60 minutes of stair stepping every morning before school, ate very little during the day, but would then devour any food in sight on arriving home from work. "I feel so guilty about the boxes of crackers, pretzels, and cookies I devour. After a binge, I won't eat dinner. Instead, I'll go back to the health club to burn off the excess calories. I'm exhausted all the time. I'm doing a poor job of teaching. I get easily irritated and feel like yelling at the students. I'm frustrated that I'm unable to do something as simple as lose a few pounds. I can't even eat normally now. I either starve or binge. I don't know if I should be seeing you or a therapist."

To help Alicia balance her food and exercise goals and to normalize her disordered eating patterns, I measured her percent body fat (a very lean 18 percent) and calculated how many calories her body required each day. She needed 1,200 calories for her resting metabolic rate, 600 calories for moderate daily activity, and 500 calories for purposeful exercise, adding up to 2,300 total calories per day. Then I devised a meal plan to stabilize her eating.

Like many of my clients, she dieted too hard and unrealistically restricted her calories. She would burn off 500 calories at the health club but would not eat anything until lunch, when she limited herself to 250 calories of a frozen diet dinner. No wonder she felt starved and stuffed herself with food the minute she arrived home after school. I advised her to stop dieting, start eating breakfast and lunch, and eat reasonably at night. She changed her habits and stopped binge eating after school.

Alicia followed my recommendations to eat 2,300 calories, divided into four even meals: breakfast, first lunch, second lunch (after school), and dinner. When she returned two weeks later she reported with a big smile, "When I get home after school, I no longer act like a maniac in the kitchen, eating whatever I can get my hands on. I feel so much better and am even losing a little weight because I'm not binge eating. Having a substantial breakfast and lunch helps me feel better and have enough energy to have fun with my students. I'm less irritable—back to my old happy self. And, most importantly, I'm back in control of my food."

Alicia normalized her eating by stopping her dieting and starting to eat appropriate meals at breakfast and lunch. She simply needed a better food plan to correct her food binges that stemmed from extreme hunger, not from an eating disorder. She'd thought that dieting would help her lose weight, but instead she learned that normal, healthful eating is really the better path to weight management.

The Exercise Addict

Bill, a regional sales manager for a computer company, was addicted to exercise. He'd get up at 5:15 A.M. and arrive at the front door of the health club when it opened at 6:00. There he'd do the morning spin class from 6:00 to 7:00 and then lift weights from 7:00 to 8:00. At lunchtime, he'd do a step-aerobics class at his company's fitness facility. After work he'd swim laps for an hour at the Y. Because he exercised at three different locations, few people knew how much time he spent exercising, except his wife and family. They constantly complained that he was never home.

Holidays brought even more complaints. "Why do you have to exercise on Christmas morning?" his eight-year-old daughter complained when Bill announced that he was going for his two-hour Merry Christmas run, his present to himself. His family knew he would be incredibly irritable if he didn't run, so they waited patiently for his return before opening gifts.

Without question, Bill was addicted to exercise. He'd feel irritable, anxious, guilty, and depressed if he was unable to do at least four hours of exercise a day. He needed to do increasingly more exercise to achieve the same physical and emotional highs. He'd exercise even when injured or sick. He had little energy for the rest of his life and was fearful that he would lose his job because of a steady decline in his work performance.

Bill's ability to exercise came to a halt when he experienced debilitating back pain. He could barely walk without severe anguish. While seeing the back doctor at SportsMedicine Associates, he noticed information on the bulletin board about my nutrition checkup and asked to speak to me.

"I need help," he admitted. "I can no longer exercise the way I'd like to and I'm petrified of getting fat. I'm trying not to eat because I cannot exercise, but I end up sneaking food—and stealing my daughter's M&Ms."

To my eyes, Bill had a long way to go before anyone would consider him fat. He was five feet, 10 inches (178 centimeters) and weighed 130 pounds (59 kilograms), but I listened to his fears. I reminded him that people in the hospital still eat and that they do little or no exercise but fail to get fat.

I worked with Bill on normalizing his eating and exercise practices, suggested readings (such as *Hooked on Exercise* by Rebecca Prussin), and convinced him that meeting with a counselor would help keep his life from falling apart. With a doctor, therapist, and nutritionist on his medical team, as well as a family therapist and the love of his wife and children, he evolved to become a happier person. He learned to communicate his wants and needs so that he no longer felt the desire to run away from his problems. He came to understand that his underlying belief that he wasn't good enough was a misperception. He came to like and accept himself as being the truly loving person he wanted to be.

The Marathon Runner With Bulimia

Carol, a 29-year-old graduate student, had gained 12 pounds (5 kilograms) in the two years since she had started studying for her MBA. She tended to overeat when schoolwork became overwhelming, and she felt like she couldn't do all that was expected of her. "I binge at night and then vomit and go for a long run. I'm exhausted all the time and think of little else other than what, when, and how I'll binge. I've stopped socializing with my friends at mealtimes because I'm afraid

I'll overeat and be unable to purge. Instead, I spend my time studying and training for a marathon. I'm hoping the added exercise will contribute to weight loss. But I'm a foodaholic. When I finish my run, I inevitably end up at the corner store, where I buy at least two big muffins and heaven only knows what else. I just can't seem to control my food intake."

After listening to Carol's story, I recognized that she seemed addicted not only to food but also to schoolwork and exercise. She constantly pushed herself to meet self-imposed deadlines, weight goals, and exercise demands. She always felt stressed and overextended. She lacked healthy balance in her life.

I asked if anyone in Carol's family had trouble with alcohol. She quietly admitted that her mother was an alcoholic. She seemed ashamed of this family secret. At least one-third of my clients with eating disorders grew up in families with some type of dysfunction, most commonly related to alcohol. The clients themselves may not be addicted to alcohol, but some are recovering alcoholics or drug abusers (Varner 1995). Alternatively, they express other addictive behaviors through overworking, overeating, overachieving, and overexercising. The traits and attitudes outlined in table 12.1 are characteristic of people who grew up in an alcoholic or otherwise dysfunctional family.

TABLE 12.1

Red-Flag Traits

Athletes who have disordered eating tend to have similar personality traits that affect their attitudes toward food, exercise, and weight. The traits may be the result of growing up in a family in which a parent had alcoholism or in an otherwise dysfunctional family in which a parent may have been unavailable for the child. If you find yourself struggling with food and fitting the following description, you should understand that food is not a problem; it's likely a symptom of problems with life.

Characteristic trait	How commonly expressed
Drive for perfection	"I've exercised for an hour every day for the past two years."
Desire for control	"I never eat after 7:00 p.m."
Compulsive behavior	"I work out for two hours every day, regardless of injuries, illness, or travel."
Feelings of inadequacy	"I could have biked even faster if I'd lost more weight."
Difficulty having fun	"Thanks for inviting me to the movie. I'll pass—I have to do my workout at the gym."
Trouble with intimate relationships	"My husband gets angry with me for spending two hours every night exercising and absent from my family."

Carol displayed all these traits. She had a strong drive to be perfect and a desire for control. Since childhood she had tried to be perfect to compensate for her family's problems. Now, she was trying to eat the perfect diet, achieve the perfect weight, develop the perfect career, and maintain the perfect training schedule. She ran 10 miles (16 kilometers) every day, despite blizzards, illness, or fatigue. She lived on calorie-free coffee, diet soda, and fat-free foods, until ravenous hunger overwhelmed her good intentions. After a binge, she'd vomit (to bring control back to her life and compensate for her imperfect eating).

I helped Carol get a better perspective on an appropriate weight by measuring her percent body fat. By designing a meal plan, I helped her eat an appropriate diet. A referral to a coach at the local running club allowed her to train with an appropriate program. I also advised her to read some books about adult children of alcoholics, seek guidance from a suitable counselor, and perhaps join a support group such as Al-Anon or ACoA (Adult Children of Alcoholics). For additional readings, see appendix A.

"For the past two years, I have tried to avoid food, thinking it was fattening," she wrote in a follow-up letter. "I've come to learn food wasn't the problem. My inability to handle stress was the problem. I'm now gentler on myself. I no longer strive to be the perfect student. For example, I took three days off from both school and running when I went on a ski weekend with my friends! I'm eating well and exercising healthfully rather than punishing myself with megamiles to burn off calories. I feel better and am at peace with myself and my body."

Hunger Scale

If you have you spent years dieting and not eating when you are hungry, then blowing your diet and stuffing yourself until you have to loosen your belt, you may feel troubled by the struggle to regulate your food intake. The hunger scale can help you get back in touch with normal eating, that is, eating like a child. Children eat when they are hungry and stop when they are content— and they never run out of energy!

1	5	10
Starved	Content	Stuffed
Lightheaded	Pleasantly fed	Uncomfortable
Unable to concentrate	Satiated	Painfully full

Your job is to listen to your body and eat until you are satisfied and feel pleasantly fed—not stuffed, not hankering for more because you are still hungry. The trick to feeding yourself appropriately is to eat slowly and mindfully, paying attention to the pleasant feeling of satiety that is midway between starved and stuffed.

The Figure Skater With Anorexia

Emily, a 16-year-old student at a highly competitive figure-skating school, was sent to me by her coach. Emily's mother made the appointment for her. Because she was chronically tired, Emily was compromising her ability to jump high and skate hard. Emily's first words to me were, "My coach and mother made me come here. They think I don't eat enough."

Emily weighed 92 pounds (42 kilograms). A year ago, she had weighed 110 pounds (50 kilograms), and at 63 inches (160 centimeters), she could have appropriately weighed 115 pounds (53 kilograms). She was limiting herself to 1,000 calories per day but deserved to eat about 1,800 calories, if not more. Because she was eating so little food, she was consuming inadequate amounts of protein, calcium, iron, zinc, and numerous other vitamins and minerals that her body needed to be healthy.

Emily was so afraid that she'd get fat if she were to eat more, I had to constantly remind her that food is fuel and health. She was currently unhealthy. She had stopped menstruating (one sign of poor health), and her complexion was splotchy and grayish (a second sign). Emily needed to eat a wider variety of food than cottage cheese, egg whites, and apples to balance her diet and provide the nutrients in which she was deficient. She also needed to include more dietary fat.

I reminded Emily that she deserved to eat, even if she was not exercising. I asked her to take notice of all her friends who were nonexercisers. All ate, and most were lean! Eating more would not provide excess calories but fundamental fuel. We established the following goals:

- Follow a food plan that would optimize her health.
- Fuel her body appropriately by gradually increasing calories at meals and snacks.
- Rebuild her body to an appropriate weight to optimize her strength and health.
- Reduce the risk of stress fractures and future osteoporosis by achieving regular menstrual periods.
- Attain peace with food and weight.

Emily agreed to increase her intake gradually, by 100 calories per week, adding more food at breakfast and lunch until she had three 500-calorie meals that included at least three or four kinds of foods (such as cereal, milk, and fruit; pita bread, turkey, and yogurt; fish, rice, broccoli, and milk). These dietary improvements would help her have more energy to concentrate better at school and skate with enthusiasm. I suggested that she *practice* eating more healthfully, just as she practiced her skating, and that she focus on how much better she felt when she fueled herself better.

Over the course of weeks, Emily stopped rigidly controlling her food and started to eat more appropriately. My nutrition advice had provided helpful guidelines, but a key factor in her recovery was counseling. A psychologist skilled with eating disorders counseled her, as did a family therapist who met with her and her parents and sister. By communicating and resolving many of the family's issues, Emily was able to express her needs rather than withhold words and use food restriction to starve her feelings and be her silent cry for help.

Within three months, Emily started to menstruate, a good sign that she was adequately nourishing her body. She was feeling physically stronger, was happier with her family, and felt at peace with food and her body. She no longer felt that she had to be perfect to earn her parents' love, nor did she need to be perfectly thin, eat the perfect diet, and be the perfect student and figure skater. She learned to enjoy being human, like the rest of her family and friends. She let go of her fantasy that a perfect body would bring a perfect life. "I thought I'd be happier once I was thinner, but I was wrong. I've learned that happiness comes from loving myself from the inside out, not from the outside in."

What Is Anorexia?

People with anorexia nervosa tend to either consistently restrict food or restrict and then binge and purge. The American Psychiatric Association (1994) uses the following definition:

- Intense fear of gaining weight or becoming fat, even though underweight
- Disturbance in the way a person experiences his or her body (that is, claiming to feel fat even when emaciated), with an undue influence of body weight or shape on self-perception
- Weight loss to less than 85 percent of normal body weight or, if during a period of growth, failure to make expected weight gain leading to 85 percent of that expected
- Refusal to maintain body weight over a minimal normal weight for age and height
- Denial of the seriousness of the current weight loss
- Absence of at least three consecutive menstrual cycles

Data from *Diagnostic and Statistical Manual of Mental Disorders,* 4th ed., revised, 2000. Copyright 2000 American Psychiatric Association.

What Is Bulimia?

The person with bulimia nervosa may purge by self-induced vomiting, by misusing laxatives, diuretics, or enemas (purging type), or by using other inappropriate compensatory mechanisms to prevent weight gain, such as fasting or exercising excessively (nonpurging type). The definition used by the American Psychiatric Association (1994) includes these aspects:

- Recurrent episodes of binge eating, characterized by
    1. eating an unusually large amount of food in a discrete period of time (the amount eaten is larger than most people would eat during a similar time period and under similar circumstances) and
    2. feeling out of control during the eating episode and unable to stop eating or control what and how much is eaten
- Compensating for the food binge to prevent weight gain, such as inducing vomiting; misusing laxatives, enemas, or other medications; fasting; or exercising excessively
- Binge eating and purging, on average, at least twice a week for three months
- Evaluating self-worth according to body shape and weight

Data from *Diagnostic and Statistical Manual of Mental Disorders*, 4th ed., revised, 2000. Copyright 2000 American Psychiatric Association.

Athletes and Amenorrhea

Athletes with eating disorders commonly stop menstruating. If you are an athlete who previously had regular menstrual periods but have stopped menstruating (amenorrhea), don't ignore it! Although you may think amenorrhea is desirable because you no longer have to deal with the hassles of monthly menstrual periods, amenorrhea can lead to problems that interfere with your health and ability to perform at your best. These problems include

- almost a three-times-higher incidence of stress fractures that put you on the sideline,
- premature osteoporosis that can affect your bone health in the not-too-distant future, and
- an inability to conceive easily should you want to start a family.

Amenorrhea Is Complex

If you believe you lack periods only because you are too thin and are exercising too much, you are wrong. Studies have shown no body-fat differences between athletic women who menstruate regularly and those who don't (Sanborn et al. 2000). Many very thin athletes do have regular menses. Clearly, leanness and intense exercise are not the simple explanation to the complexities of amenorrhea.

But the question remains unanswered: Why are you amenorrheic when your peers, who have similar exercise programs and the same low percent body fat, are not? Are you

- striving to maintain a weight lower than your natural set point,
- struggling harder to maintain your desired leanness, or
- eating inadequately to achieve your desired leanness?

If so, you are probably experiencing nutritional amenorrhea.

Resolving the Problem

To resume menses, you need to eat enough calories to support not only your exercise program but also your body's ability to reproduce. Current research suggests that amenorrhea is not due to exercising too much, but to eating too little food (Loucks 2001). A registered dietitian or sports nutritionist can help you reverse your patterns of skimpy eating—a task that for some women is easier said than done. The following tips may also be of help.

1. Throw away the bathroom scale. Rather than strive to achieve a certain number on the scale, let your body weigh what it weighs. Rather than exert willpower to achieve a desired weight, let your body acquire its genetic weight. The information in chapters 9 and 11 can help you to estimate a weight you can comfortably maintain without constantly dieting. Your physician or dietitian can also give unbiased professional advice.

2. If you have weight to lose, don't restrict calories by more than 20 percent or eat less than 1,200 calories (Woolsey 2001). By following a healthy reducing program, you'll not only have greater success with long-term weight loss but also be able to enjoy enough energy to participate in your sports program.

3. If you are at an appropriate weight, practice eating as you did when you were a child. That is, eat when you are hungry and stop when you are content. If you are always hungry and constantly obsessing about food, you are undoubtedly trying to eat too few calories. Your body is complaining and requesting more food; hunger is simply a request for fuel. The information in chapter 11, plus advice from your doctor and dietitian, can help you determine an appropriate calorie intake.

Amenorrheic women commonly eat in nontraditional ways with chaotic eating patterns (Wilmore et al. 1992). For example, they may eat little at breakfast and lunch only to overeat at night, or they restrict themselves on Monday through Thursday and then overeat on the weekends. If your weight is stable, you are somehow consuming the number of calories you need, so you might as well eat them on a regular schedule of wholesome, well-balanced meals. A registered dietitian can help you develop an appropriate food plan if you are struggling on your own.

4. Eat adequate protein. In one study, 82 percent of the women with amenorrhea ate less than the recommended intake for protein (Nelson et al. 1986). Vegetarians, in particular, need to be sure to get adequate protein. Vegetarian women who consume adequate protein and calories tend to have regular menstrual periods (Barr 1999).

5. Eat at least 20 percent of your calories from fat. Amenorrheic athletes tend to avoid meat and other protein-rich foods because they are afraid of eating fat. For most active women, eating 40 to 60 grams of fat per day would be an appropriate low-fat diet. This plan clearly allows salmon, peanut butter, nuts, olive oil, and other health-promoting fats, as well as smaller amounts of saturated fat as in lean beef, low-fat cheese, and other nourishing foods that provide balance to a sports diet.

6. Include small portions of red meat two to four times per week, if you are not opposed to doing so. Surveys of runners show that those with amenorrhea tend to eat less red meat and are more likely to follow a vegetarian diet than their regularly menstruating counterparts are (Kaiserauer et al. 1989). Although lean red meats can have a slightly higher fat content than chicken or fish, an overall low-fat sports diet can accommodate some fat, and eating lean meats may help achieve regular menses.

7. Maintain a calcium-rich diet. If you are amenorrheic, you should regularly consume three to four eight-ounce (240-milliliter) servings of low-fat milk or yogurt (or other calcium-rich foods) daily to protect your bones. Your bones benefit from the protective effect of exercise, but exercise does not compensate for lack of calcium or lack of estrogen. Although you may cringe at the thought of spending so many calories on dairy foods, remember that milk is a wholesome food that contains many important nutrients (see chapters 1 and 2) and contributes to fat loss, not gain. Women who consume three or more glasses of milk or yogurt tend to be leaner than those who do not (Pereira, Jacobs,

Van Horn et al. 2002). If you are eating a diet that includes lots of bran cereal, fruits, and vegetables, you may have an even higher need for calcium because the fiber may interfere with calcium absorption.

Many amenorrheic women worry about their bone health and wonder if there is long-term damage. That is likely the case. Women who resume menses do restore some of the bone density lost during the months of amenorrhea, but they do not restore all of it. Hence, your goal should be to minimize the damages of amenorrhea by eating appropriately and taking the proper steps to resolve the problem.

Although female athletes fear that eating more and exercising less will hurt their performance, this is not the case. A 19-year-old amenorrheic runner reduced her training by one day per week, increased her daily food intake with one can of a 360-calorie liquid meal supplement, gained 6 pounds (2.7 kilograms) over about four months (from 106 to 112, or from 48 to 51 kilograms), and resumed menstruation. She set more personal records than she did during any prior season, broke two school records, and qualified for a national track meet (Dueck et al. 1996). Food works!

How to Help

Perhaps you have friends, family, or teammates who struggle with food, and you wonder what you can do to help resolve the problem. Seeing a loved one seemingly waste away can be sad and scary. Often it's hard to tell if the person is really struggling or just being a dedicated athlete. Even health professionals can have trouble distinguishing between the person who is lean and mean and the one who is suffering with anorexia.

The athlete with anorexia is generally a compulsive exerciser who trains frantically out of fear of gaining weight and never takes rest days. In comparison, the dedicated athlete trains hard with hopes of improving performance but also enjoys days with no exercise. Both push themselves to perfection—to be perfectly thin or to be the perfect athlete. Sometimes the two intertwine.

Approximately half of those with anorexia become bulimic. Some purge by vomiting, others by excessive exercise. For example, some triathletes who train two or three times per day may be bulimic, and they purge themselves of excess calories under the guise of building endurance.

This constant battle with food endangers an athlete's physical and mental health and overall well-being. Unfortunately, too many coaches, parents, friends, and teammates fail to confront the devastating stressfulness of this struggle for ultimate thinness. After all, how can anyone who is training hard and seems happy be sick?

If you suspect that your friend, training partner, child, or teammate has a problem with food, don't wait until medical problems prove you right. Speak up in an appropriate manner. Anorexia and bulimia are life-threatening conditions that shouldn't be overlooked. Here are 10 tips for approaching this delicate subject.

1. **Heed the signs.** You may notice that people with anorexia wear bulky clothes to hide their abnormal thinness or that their food consumption is abnormally restrictive and spartan in comparison to the energy they expend. Anorexic runners, for example, may eat only a yogurt for dinner after having completed a strenuous 10-mile (16-kilometer) workout. Perhaps you'll never see them eating in public, at home, or with friends. They find some excuse for not joining others at meals. Or if they do, they may push the food around on the plate to fool you into thinking that they're eating. You may also notice other compulsive behaviors, such as excessive studying or working.

Signs and Symptoms of Anorexia

- Significant weight loss
- Wearing layers of baggy clothing to hide thinness
- Loss of menstrual periods
- Loss of hair
- Growth of fine body hair, noticeable on the face and arms
- Cold hands and feet and extreme sensitivity to cold temperatures
- Wearing sweaters in summer heat because of feeling cold all the time
- Lightheadedness
- Inability to concentrate
- Low pulse rate
- Hyperactivity, compulsive exercise beyond normal training
- Recurrent overuse injuries and stress fractures
- Comments about how fat they are, distorted body image
- Expression of intense fear of becoming fat
- Nervousness at mealtime, avoidance of eating in public
- Food rituals, such as cutting food into small pieces and playing with it
- Antisocial behavior, isolation from family and friends
- Excessive working or studying, compulsiveness, and rigidity
- Extreme emotions: tearful, uptight, oversensitive, restless

Bulimic behavior can be subtler. The athlete may eat a great deal of food and then rush to the bathroom. You may hear water running to cover up the sound of vomiting. The person may hide laxatives or even speak about a magic method of eating without gaining weight. She or he may have bloodshot eyes, swollen glands, and bruised fingers (from inducing vomiting). The following list describes other symptoms of bulimia.

Signs and Symptoms of Bulimia

- Weakness, headaches, dizziness
- Frequent weight fluctuations because of alternating binges and fasts
- Swollen glands that give a chipmunklike appearance
- Difficulty swallowing and retaining food, damage to throat
- Frequent vomiting
- Damaged tooth enamel from exposure to gastric acid when vomiting
- Petty stealing of food or stealing of money to buy food for binges
- Strange behavior that surrounds secretive eating
- Disappearance after meals, often to the bathroom to "take a shower"
- Running water in the bathroom after meals to hide the sound of vomiting
- Extreme concern with body weight, shape, and physical appearance
- Ability to eat enormous meals without weight gain
- Compulsive exercise beyond normal training
- Depression
- Bloodshot eyes

2. **Express your concern carefully.** Approach these individuals gently but persistently, saying that you are worried about their health: "I'm concerned that your injuries are taking so long to heal." Talk about what you see: "I've noticed that you seem tired and your race times are getting slower and slower." Give evidence for why you believe they are struggling to balance food and exercise and ask if they want to talk about it.

Individuals who are truly anorexic or bulimic commonly deny the problem, insisting that they're perfectly fine. Continue to share your concerns about their lack of concentration, lightheadedness, or chronic fatigue. These health issues are more likely to be stepping-stones for the athlete to accept help, given that she or he undoubtedly clings to food and exercise as attempts to gain control and stability.

3. **Do not discuss weight or eating habits.** The athlete takes great pride in being perfectly thin and may dismiss your concern as

jealousy. Avoid any mention of starving and bingeing as the issue. Focus on life issues, not food issues.

4. **Suggest unhappiness as the reason for seeking help.** Point out how anxious, tired, or irritable the athlete has been lately. Emphasize that he or she doesn't have to be that way.

5. **Be supportive and listen sympathetically.** Don't expect someone to admit right away that there's a problem. Give it time and constantly remind your friend that you believe in him or her. Your support will make a difference in recovery.

6. **Offer a list of professional resources.** If someone you know is suffering from a full-blown or subclinical eating disorder, you may feel frustrated with your unsuccessful efforts to resolve the problem. You may think, "If only my friend would eat normally, everything would be OK." Likely not. Food is just the symptom. The problem is this person is unhappy. To help you understand more about these underlying issues, you might want to read *Surviving an Eating Disorder: A Survival Guide for Parents and Friends* by J. Siegal and J. Brisman. This helpful resource can teach you what to say to your friend. (This book and many other helpful books on the topic of eating disorders are available at www.bulimia.com.)

   Your job is to help your friend or loved one by taking her or him to get professional guidance. This might mean finding a registered dietitian in your area who specializes in sports nutrition and eating disorders. (Use the American Dietetic Association's referral network at www.eatright.org or call 800-366-1655.)

   Remind your friend that no weight will ever be good enough to create happiness. Happiness comes from within, not from a number on the scale. And although the athlete may deny the problem to your face, she or he may admit despair at another moment. If you don't know of a mental-health counselor skilled with eating disorders, ask the national organizations for the closest resource. Here's a list of organizations that may be able to provide more information and help for someone with anorexia or bulimia.

National Eating Disorders Association
603 Stewart St., Suite 803
Seattle, WA 98101
206-382-3587
www.NationalEatingDisorders.org
Offers educational materials, referrals, reports on new research.

American Dietetic Association
120 S. Riverside Plaza, Suite 2000
Chicago, IL 60606
800-877-1600
www.eatright.org
Referral service for sports nutritionists skilled with handling eating disorders and knowledgeable about local counseling services.

Something Fishy Web Site on Eating Disorders
www.something-fishy.org
Extensive online information and recovery support for individuals and loved ones; referral network.

Gurze Books
P.O. Box 2238
Carlsbad, CA 92018
800-756-7533
www.bulimia.com
An eating disorders self-help library with online bookstore.

You can also call your local sports-medicine clinic and ask to speak to their physician or nutritionist, your university health center or eating-disorders program, or your local medical center and ask to have an eating disorders assessment.

7. **Limit your expectations.** You alone can't solve the problem. It's more complex than food and exercise; it's a life problem. Share your concerns with others. Seek help from a trusted family member, medical professional, or health service. Don't try to deal with the problem alone, especially if you are making no headway and the athlete is becoming more self-destructive.

8. **Recognize that you may be overreacting.** Maybe there is no eating disorder. Maybe the athlete is appropriately thin for enhanced sports performance. But how can you decide? To clarify the situation, insist that the athlete have a mental-health evaluation. If necessary, make the appointment and take the athlete there yourself. Only then will you get an unbiased opinion of the degree of danger, if any. The therapist may tell you to go home and stop worrying, or might detect misery and suicidal tendencies in the athlete and encourage immediate care.

9. **Seek advice from health-care professionals about your concerns.** You may need to discuss your feelings with someone. Remember that you are not responsible for the other person's health. You can only try to help. Your power comes from using guidance counselors, registered dietitians, medical professionals, or eating-disorder clinics.

10. **Be patient.** Recognize that the healing process can be long and arduous with many relapses and setbacks, but your reward will be that you can make a critical difference in that person's life. People die from anorexia and bulimia.

Preventing Eating Disorders

Many people think, or feel pressured to believe, that by restricting their food intake to lose weight they will exercise better, look better, and enhance their overall performances. Ironically, restricting food in an attempt to improve performance can result in depleted fuel stores, muscle depletion, amenorrhea, stress fractures, fainting, weakness, fatigue, and eventually impaired performance. Some athletes may manage to do well for a while without an obvious decline in performance, but then injuries and lack of energy will catch up with them.

Eating disorders would fade if people could learn to love their bodies. As a society, we must

- dispel the myth that thinness equals happiness and success,
- discourage the notion that the thinnest athlete is the best athlete,
- love our bodies for what they are rather than hate them for what they are not,
- emphasize being fit and healthy as more appropriate goals than being skinny, and
- be careful about how we acknowledge weight loss.

When Your Friends Lose Weight, What Should You Say?

When someone has lost weight, the knee-jerk response is to exclaim, "Wow! Don't you look great!" This praise is intended to be positive, but it implies that

1. the person looked horrible before,
2. physical size is more important than health, and
3. she is a better person if she is lighter.

Be it 2 pounds or 20 (1 kilogram or 10), the better way to acknowledge weight loss is to shift the focus away from physical weight change and focus instead on the praiseworthy aspect: the person's improved health status. Here are some recommended phrases to share with people who are losing or have lost weight:

- "You look like you've been working hard at losing weight." The dieter will be ever ready to talk about how proud she or he is of the hard work it took to lose weight. Listen to the story and be sure that the person is healthy.

- "You look smaller. . . . Is there less of you to love?" The message is that your friend is not a better person for having lost weight; she or he is just smaller.

- "You look pleased with your weight loss. How do you feel about it?" The person may feel healthier and more energetic, but you may also hear her or him express frustration in not being quite thin enough yet.

- "You are looking more fit. How are your workouts going? How is your energy level? How do you feel?" If your friend is losing weight appropriately, she or he will feel great.

- "You appear to be trading some of your excess fat for muscle." Acknowledge what you see but don't suggest that your friend is a better person.

Regardless of the dieter's response, the goal is to help the person hold a solid appreciation of her or his value as a person. The beauty of a person is in the smile, in friendship and caring, not in being size 2 instead of size 12. People need to know they are loved from the inside out, not judged from the outside in. If dieters lose weight, they need to realize that there is simply less of them to love. They are not better or more likable. They are just smaller. With appropriate dieting, they are healthier, more energetic, stronger, and happy with those benefits. But sometimes dieting goes awry.

PART III

Winning Recipes

RECIPE CONTRIBUTORS

Gloria Averbush   *Sesame Pasta With Broccoli*
Helen Baker   *Shrimp Fettuccine*
Annie and David Bastille   *Thick and Frosty Milk Shake*
Janice Clark   *Apple Crisp*
Cook's Illustrated   *Oven-Fried Chicken*
Candace Crowell   *Mediterranean Shrimp and Scallops With Pasta*

Molly Curran   *Sautéed Chicken With Mushrooms and Onions*

Karin Daisy   *Turkey Teriyaki*
Barbara Day   *Chicken Salad With Almonds and Mandarin Oranges*

Diana Dyer   *Diana's Soy Shake*
Anne Fletcher   *Peanut Butter Banana Roll-Up*
Paul Friedman   *Cereal-to-Go*
Jenny Hegmann   *Carrot Cake, Jenny's Favorite Oatmeal*
Peter Hermann   *Chicken Black Bean Soup*
Anne LeBarron   *Oven French Fries*
Sue Luke   *Ground Turkey Mix for Spaghetti or Chili*
John McGrath   *Quick and Easy Chili*
Brenda Ponichtera   *Brenda's Greek Salad*
National Peanut Board   *Peanutty Energy Bars*
Linda Press Wolfe   *Gourmet Lasagna*
Diane Sinski   *Chicken and Oriental Noodles in Peanut Sauce*

Jean Smith   *Spinach Salad*
Terri Smith   *Pasta and White Bean Soup With Sun-Dried Tomatoes*

Evelyn Tribole   *Carrot Raisin Muffins*
Natalie Updegrove Partridge   *Oatmeal Cookies*
Shannon Weirlot   *Sugar and Spice Trail Mix*
Sue Westin   *Chocolate Lush*

Introduction to Recipes

Active people generally prefer to spend their time exercising rather than preparing meals. These recipes will enable you to spend minimal time preparing food for maximal nutrition. With them, you can produce meals that taste good and invest in health and top sports performance. All of the recipes are quick and easy to fix and use commonly available ingredients. Some have moderate amounts of sodium; athletes on a salt-restricted diet should eliminate or reduce the salt or salty foods in the recipes.

Many of the recipes are low-fat favorites contributed by athletes or food lovers. I've also adapted favorite higher-fat recipes to the more appropriate versions here. I've compiled a collection of foods that will be popular with all members of the family—athletes and support crew alike. My primary criterion for selection was whether the taste-testers requested a second helping.

Using Nutrition Information

The calorie and nutrition information provided with each recipe represent approximate values, not including optional ingredients. If two ingredients are listed (i.e., 2 to 4 tablespoons oil), the nutrition analysis is based on the lower amount. Remember that your total daily calorie intake should be about 55 to 65 percent carbohydrates, 20 to 30 percent fat, and 10 to 15 percent protein. To convert these targets into grams, multiply your daily calorie needs (see chapter 11) by the targets, and then divide the carbohydrate and protein products by 4 and the fat product by 9. For example, the calculations for an active woman who needs about 2,000 calories per day follow:

60% carb × 2,000 calories = 1,200 carb calories
Divided by 4 = 300 grams carb

25% fat × 2,000 calories = 500 fat calories
Divided by 9 = 55 grams fat

15% protein × 2,000 calories = 300 protein calories
Divided by 4 = 75 grams protein

If you feel ambitious, you can add up the grams of carbohydrates, proteins, and fats you consume daily to be sure that you balance your intake. Or, you can simply follow the Food Guide Pyramid (see chapter 1) and you'll end up with the right balance of carbs, protein, and fat. That is, if the foundation of each meal is a grain food, and it's accompanied by a fruit, vegetable, and protein-rich food, your diet will likely be close to the recommended 60% carbohydrate, 10-15% protein, and 20-30% fat.

Cooking Efficiently

Following are a few tips on how to prepare and cook efficiently:

1. Read a recipe completely before you start making it to be sure you understand the entire process clearly.

2. Be sure you have adequate amounts of all the ingredients on hand. Make a double recipe to freeze or to use later in the week.

3. Hang a grocery list on the refrigerator door or in another convenient place so you and your family can easily add items when your supply of a particular item begins to dwindle.

4. You can make cooking easier by using frozen or precut vegetables, prechopped garlic (in a jar in the produce section of the market), dried onions instead of fresh, etc.

5. For continental cooking, remember these approximate metric conversions:

1 teaspoon (tsp) = 5 ml

1 tablespoon (Tbsp) = 15 ml

1 cup (8 oz) = 250 ml

350°F = 180°C

1 quart (4 cups) = 1 liter

1 pound (16 oz) = 450 grams

2.2 pounds = 1 kilo

Spicing Up Your Diet

Many busy people eat the same foods all the time. If that sounds like you, you can easily add variety to your limited repertoire by adding herbs, spices, and other seasonings. Use about 1/4 teaspoon of dry herbs (or 3/4 teaspoon fresh) for a dish that serves four people. Be conservative at first. It's better to use too little seasoning and have to add more than it is to have to double the recipe to dilute the flavor of too much seasoning. To enhance their flavor, crumble herbs between your fingers and heat them in oil. Add herbs during the last hour of cooking soups and stews. Store herbs in a cool place to retain their flavor; do not keep them near the stove. The following list are examples of a few harmonious combinations:

- **Basil**   Tomato dishes, fish, salads
- **Cinnamon**   Cooked fruits, winter squash, baked goods
- **Cloves**   Hot cider or tea, cooked fruits, tomatoes, winter squash
- **Ginger**   Cooked fruits, curry, chicken, stir-fry
- **Marjoram**   Fish, meat, poultry, stuffing
- **Nutmeg**   Apple desserts, puddings, winter squash
- **Oregano**   Tomato dishes, fish, salads
- **Parsley**   Soups, salads, vegetables, or as garnish for almost any plate
- **Poppy seeds**   Cottage cheese, noodles, cole slaw, baked goods
- **Rosemary**   Fish, meat, poultry, stuffing, vegetables
- **Sage**   Soups, stews, stuffing
- **Thyme**   Tomato dishes, stews, salads, vegetables

These additional flavor boosters are also worth stocking:

- **Sesame oil** in chicken, fish, vegetables, soups
- **Dijon mustard** in chicken, fish

- **Sun-dried tomatoes** in pasta, tomato sauces
- **Salsa** in fish, chicken, cheese, beans
- **Tabasco or hot chili oil** in stir-fry, soups, vegetables, pasta
- **Balsamic vinegar** in salads, vegetables
- **Canned green chiles** in eggs, tomato, cheese
- **Chicken broth** in rice, vegetables

Microwave Cooking

Microwave ovens have revolutionized the way many people eat. They can help you eat well yet spend minimal time cooking and cleaning. On weekends, you might want to make a big pot of chili or curry or a chicken-rice casserole. You can then freeze some and leave the rest in the refrigerator, creating a ready supply of microwaveable entrées. Following are tips to use when cooking with the microwave:

- When cooking separate items such as pieces of meat or whole potatoes, arrange food with the thickest parts toward the outer edge of the dish. Leave a space in the center, allowing the microwaves to penetrate from all sides.
- Fish cooks well in microwave ovens. Sprinkle with seasonings as desired (pepper, lemon, oregano, basil, etc.), cover with waxed paper, and "zap."
- Cover vegetables loosely with waxed paper or plastic wrap to retain moisture. Veggies will continue to cook after the oven is off, so prevent overcooking by planning this into the preparation time. Since microwave cookery is quick and waterless, it retains a high percentage of a food's nutrients.
- Prick potatoes several times with a fork before baking them to reduce the risk of explosion due to steam buildup. Allow baked potatoes to stand for 5 minutes to finish cooking and improve their texture.

Freezing Foods Properly

When you cook, you can easily make a double batch and freeze the leftovers. Here are five tips for proper freezing:

1. Do not let food sit in the refrigerator for a few days and then freeze it. You might be freezing lots of bacteria, too.

2. Cool foods before freezing them. Hot food causes your freezer to work too hard.

3. Use the proper size container with a tight cover. Allow one-half to one inch of space above the food for expansion.

4. Label the container with the name of the food and the date you freeze it.

5. Use the food within 6 to 8 weeks.

Keeping Food Safe

When you are planning for any event that involves packing food, here are some tips to keep meals safe so they won't spoil—nor spoil your event.

- Keep cold foods below 40°F and hot foods above 140°F. Bacteria multiply most rapidly in foods kept between these temperatures.

- Use insulated bags and coolers with reusable freezer packs to keep food safe longer. Make sure foods are very cold or frozen before you place them in the cooler. You can freeze sandwiches (without mayonnaise, lettuce, and tomatoes), individual containers of yogurt, or juice boxes in advance. They will be thawed but still cool several hours later.

- Pack the cooler so the foods you plan to eat first are located near the top. Store meat items near the bottom, where it's coolest. Allow space between items so cool air can circulate properly.

- Bring a separate cooler for beverages. Otherwise, every time someone opens the cooler for a beverage, the temperature inside will rise and warm the food items.

- Place your cooler or lunch bag in the coolest location possible. In the summer, do not put it in the trunk. Wrap it with a blanket or towels to keep out the heat. At the beach, you can make a cool spot by digging a large hole in the sand, placing the cooler inside, and then covering it with a folded towel to shade the top from the sunlight.

- After the event, throw away any food that has been outside of the cooler for more than 2 hours. Throw out leftover food that's inside the cooler, unless the cooler still has chunks of ice remaining in it. The safest rule is this: When in doubt, throw it out!

13

Breads and Breakfasts

Fresh from the oven, breads are one of the favorite carbohydrates for active people. Here are some baking tips to help you prepare the yummiest of breads.

- The secret for light and fluffy quick breads, muffins, and scones is to stir the flour lightly and for only 20 seconds. Ignore the lumps! If you beat the batter too much, the gluten (protein) in the flour will toughen the dough.

- Breads made entirely with whole-wheat flour tend to be heavy. In general, half whole-wheat and half white flour is an appropriate combination. Many of these recipes have been developed using this ratio. You can alter the ratio as you like. When substituting whole-wheat for white flour in other recipes, use 3/4 cup whole-wheat for 1 cup white flour.

  Breads made with 100-percent whole-wheat flour do offer slightly more nutritional value than those made with white flour. However, if you or your family dislike whole-wheat products, compensate by consistently eating other whole grains, such as oatmeal and brown rice.

- Most of these recipes have reduced sugar content. To reduce the sugar content of your own recipes, use one-third to one-half less sugar than indicated; the finished product will be just fine. If you want to exchange white sugar with honey, brown sugar, or molasses, use only 1/2 teaspoon baking powder per 2 cups flour, and add 1/2 teaspoon baking soda. This prevents an "off" taste.

- Most quick-bread recipes instruct you to sift together the baking powder and flour. This method produces the lightest breads and best results. In some of these recipes, I direct you to mix the baking powder in with the wet ingredients and gently add the flour last. My method is easier, produces an acceptable product, and saves time and energy.

- To prevent breads from sticking, use nonstick baking pans or cooking spray or place a piece of waxed paper in the baking pan before pouring the batter. I've found that using waxed paper is foolproof. After the bread has baked, I let it cool for 5 minutes, tip it out of the pan, then peel off the paper.

- To hasten cooking time, bake quick breads in a 8" × 8" square pan instead of a loaf pan. They bake in half the time. You can also bake muffins in a loaf or square pan, eliminating the hard-to-wash muffin tins!

Oatmeal can be not only a healthful addition to your sports diet (it helps lower cholesterol) but also an easy-to-digest pre-exercise breakfast. Many people like oatmeal before long runs, hard workouts at the gym, swim practices or whatever the sport might be. The following additions to oatmeal might add some variety to your breakfasts:

- Dried apricot pieces + honey + dash nutmeg
- Raisins + cinnamon
- Sliced banana (cooked in with the oatmeal) + brown sugar + peanut butter
- Dried cranberries + honey + chopped pecans
- Diced apple (cooked in with the oatmeal) + maple syrup

Instead of adding sweetener to the oatmeal, some people choose to just add a little salt then eat the oatmeal as a grain (as opposed to a sweetened cereal). Because active people need some salt to replace that which they lose in sweat, eating salted oatmeal is certainly an acceptable practice—plus most athletes find the oatmeal tastes a lot better. See chapter 2 for more information on salt and high blood pressure.

BANANA BREAD. 276
BLUEBERRY OATMEAL MUFFINS. 277
CARROT RAISIN MUFFINS 278
MOLASSES MUFFINS WITH FLAX AND DATES 279
COLD CEREAL WITH HOT FRUIT 280
CEREAL-TO-GO 281
JENNY'S FAVORITE OATMEAL. 282
SWISS MUESLI 283
HONEY NUT GRANOLA 284
OATMEAL PANCAKES 285
WHEAT GERM AND COTTAGE CHEESE PANCAKES 286

See also: Tofu Burritos, Oatmeal Cookies, Peanutty Energy Bars, Peanut Butter Banana Roll-Up, Diana's Soy Shake, Fruit Smoothie, Protein Shake

For additional suggestions, visit www.quakeroatmeal.com.

BANANA BREAD

This is the all-time favorite banana bread recipe. Its key to success is using well-ripened bananas that are covered with brown speckles.

Banana bread is a favorite for premarathon carbohydrate loading and for snacking during long-distance bike rides and hikes. Add some peanut butter and you'll have a delicious sandwich that'll keep you energized for a long time!

3 large well-ripened bananas
1 egg or 2 egg whites
2 tablespoons oil, preferably canola
1/3 cup milk
1/3 to 1/2 cup sugar
1 teaspoon salt
1 teaspoon baking soda
1/2 teaspoon baking powder
1 1/2 cups flour, preferably half whole-wheat and half white

1. Preheat the oven to 350°F.

2. Mash bananas with a fork.

3. Add egg, oil, milk, sugar, salt, baking soda, and baking powder. Beat well.

4. Gently blend the flour into the banana mixture and stir for 20 seconds or until moistened.

5. Pour into a 4" × 8" loaf pan that has been lightly oiled, treated with cooking spray, or lined with wax paper.

6. Bake for 45 minutes, or until a toothpick inserted near the middle comes out clean.

7. Let cool for 5 minutes before removing from the pan.

Yield: 12 slices

Nutrition Information :   Total calories: 1,600
Calories per slice: 135

Nutrients	Grams
Carbohydrate	24
Protein	3
Fat	3

BLUEBERRY OATMEAL MUFFINS

Blueberries and oatmeal are a tasty combination. Enjoy these muffins for breakfast or snacks. With any baked product, buttermilk offers a nice flaky texture. If you don't have any on hand, you can substitute 1 cup milk mixed with 1 teaspoon vinegar (let stand for a few minutes).

1 cup uncooked oatmeal, instant or regular
1 cup buttermilk (or 1 cup milk + 1 teaspoon white vinegar)
1 egg or 2 egg whites
1/4 to 1/3 cup sugar, as desired
1/4 to 1/3 cup oil, as desired, preferably canola
1 cup flour
1 teaspoon baking powder
1/2 teaspoon baking soda
1 teaspoon salt
1 to 1 1/2 cups blueberries, fresh or frozen

Optional: 1/4 teaspoon nutmeg or cinnamon

1. Preheat oven to 400°F. Prepare 12 muffin cups with cooking spray or paper liners.
2. In a medium bowl, combine oatmeal, buttermilk, egg, oil, and sugar. Beat well; if time allows, let the batter stand for 5 to 10 minutes for the oatmeal to soften.
3. In a small bowl, combine the flour, baking powder, baking soda, and salt (and nutmeg or cinnamon). Mix well, then combine with the wet ingredients. Stir just until moistened.
4. Gently add the blueberries.
5. Fill the muffin cups. Bake for 15 to 20 minutes or until a toothpick inserted in the middle comes out dry. Cool for five minutes, then remove from the pan.

Yield: 12 muffins

Nutrition Information: Total calories: 1,600
Calories per muffin: 135

Nutrients	Grams
Carbohydrate	18
Protein	4
Fat	5

CARROT RAISIN MUFFINS

These muffins are a favorite of Evelyn Tribole, RD, sports nutritionist and author of *Healthy Homestyle Cooking*. I can understand why she enjoys these muffins . . . they're tasty warm from the oven, and even tastier on the second day, when the flavors have blended. If you prefer a fat-free muffin, replace the canola oil with 1/3 cup of applesauce and use 6 egg whites instead of the whole eggs.

1 cup whole-wheat flour
1 cup white flour
3/4 cup sugar
2 teaspoons baking powder
2 teaspoons cinnamon
1/2 teaspoon baking soda
3 eggs or substitute
1/2 cup buttermilk (or 1/2 cup milk mixed with 1/2 teaspoon
   vinegar and left to stand for 5 minutes)
1/3 cup oil, preferably canola
2 teaspoons vanilla extract
1 teaspoon salt
2 cups finely shredded carrots
1 medium apple, peeled and shredded
1/2 cup raisins
1/2 cup chopped nuts

1. Preheat the oven to 350°F. Prepare 12 muffin tins with papers or cooking spray.
2. In a large bowl, stir together the flours, sugar, baking powder, salt, cinnamon, and baking soda.
3. In a separate bowl, stir together the eggs, buttermilk, oil, and vanilla, then the carrots, apple, raisins, and nuts. Add to the flour mixture and stir just until blended.
4. Spoon the batter into the muffin cups. Bake about 30 minutes or until a toothpick inserted near the center comes out clean.

Yield: 12 muffins

Nutrition Information: Total calories: 2,750
Calories per muffin: 230

Nutrients	Grams
Carbohydrate	37 grams
Protein	5 grams
Fat	7 grams

MOLASSES MUFFINS
WITH FLAX AND DATES

Flax is rich in substances that have been shown to lower the risk of heart disease and cancer. It has a very mild taste, and is good mixed into muffins and breads, as well as sprinkled on cereal. This flax muffin recipe is one way to add the recommended daily one tablespoon of flaxseed to your breakfast and snacks.

These muffins are remarkably sweet and moist, despite having no added fat. (The 3 grams of fat per muffin are from the health-protective fats in the ground flaxseed meal.)

1 cup chopped dates
1 egg or 2 egg whites
1/3 cup molasses
1 cup buttermilk (or 1 cup milk mixed with 1 teaspoon vinegar)
3/4 cup ground flaxseed meal
1/2 teaspoon salt
1 teaspoon baking soda
1 1/2 cups flour, preferably half while, half whole-wheat

Optional: 1/2 teaspoon cinnamon; 1 teaspoon grated orange rind; 1 teaspoon vanilla extract

1. Preheat the oven to 350°F, and prepare the muffin cups with papers or cooking spray.
2. In a large bowl, mix together the egg, molasses, buttermilk, flax, and salt and add the dates to the batter.
3. In a separate bowl, mix together the flour and baking soda (and cinnamon).
4. Gently stir in the flour mixture (and cinnamon, orange rind, and vanilla) into the egg mixture.
5. Fill the muffin cups 2/3 full. Bake for 18 to 20 minutes, or until a toothpick inserted near the center comes out clean.

Yield: 12 muffins

Nutrition Information: Total calories: 2,000
Calories per muffin: 165

Nutrients	Grams
Carbohydrate	30
Protein	4
Fat	3

COLD CEREAL WITH HOT FRUIT

This recipe is one of my favorites. I love the combination of hot fruit with cereal and cold milk—reminds me of dessert, similar to a fruit crisp a la mode. Bananas, pears, apples, berries . . . any and all fruits work well. Be creative!

In the winter, having warm fruit takes the cold chill away from the quick-and-easy cereal breakfast. Sometimes I even heat the milk along with the fruit, then add the crunchy cereal. It's easier than making hot oatmeal, and has the same warming effect.

This recipe also works well with frozen fruits. For example, I generally stock blueberries in the freezer, so they are ready and waiting to be enjoyed for breakfast. Then any day I can make "blueberry crisp" for breakfast by simply shaking a handful on to the cold cereal and heating them up.

1 cup Life cereal
1/2 cup All-Bran
1/4 cup low-fat granola
1/2 cup blueberries or other fruit
1 cup low-fat milk

1. In a microwaveable bowl, combine the cereals.
2. Sprinkle with blueberries or other fruit of your choice.
3. Heat in the microwave oven for 20 to 40 seconds, until the blueberries are warm.
4. Pour the cold milk over the top. Dig in!

Yield: 1 serving

Nutrition Information: Total calories: 500

Nutrients	Grams
Carbohydrate	85
Protein	20
Fat	7

CEREAL-TO-GO

This is a favorite of Paul Friedman, a runner and soccer-dad who often travels to events. He combines the ingredients in a container that doubles as a bowl, then adds water and shakes: an instant breakfast! Just be sure to pack a spoon.

This recipe can be especially handy for traveling athletes who are on a budget. The cereal, dried milk, and dried fruit won't spoil, and they travel well not only to sports events but also on business trips. You can save yourself great expense (as well as time and hassle) by packing this simple preevent meal. The trick is to plan ahead and organize your menu so you'll have this breakfast available for a tried-and-true meal.

1/2 cup raw rolled oats
1/4 cup Grape-Nuts (or 1/2 cup of your favorite cereal)
1/4 to 1/3 cup raisins or other dried fruit
1/3 to 1/2 cup milk powder

Optional: Brown sugar; diced fresh apple, banana, or other
   fruit added just before eating

Yield: 1 serving

Nutrition Information: Total calories: 520

Nutrients	Grams
Carbohydrate	104
Protein	15
Fat	5

JENNY'S FAVORITE OATMEAL

This recipe is a favorite of Jenny Hegmann, a sports nutritionist, cyclist, and outdoor sports enthusiast. She claims it's a handy way to get a jump-start on your day's vegetable intake! This recipe can also be made with applesauce in place of the pumpkin.

1/2 cup rolled oats
1 cup milk or water
1/4 cup cooked (canned) pumpkin or winter squash (frozen)
Dash cinnamon
Salt to taste
1 tablespoon brown sugar or molasses, as desired

Optional: Chopped pecans; sunflower seeds; dried fruit

1. In a small saucepan, cook the oats in the milk or water according to the package directions.
2. When the oatmeal is done, add the pumpkin, cinnamon, salt, and brown sugar, stirring constantly for about a minute or until hot.
3. Pour into a serving bowl and if desired, top with more brown sugar, milk, dried fruit, and chopped nuts.

Yield: 1 serving

Nutrition Information: Total calories: 325

Nutrient	Grams
Carbohydrate	60
Protein	14
Fat	3

SWISS MUESLI

This a standard breakfast in Switzerland, and can also be eaten for lunch or a light supper. It's a tasty, cook-free way to add fruit and whole grains into your daily diet.

1/2 cup oats (regular or quick-cooking)
1/2 cup plain yogurt, preferably low-fat
1 tablespoon lemon juice
1 small apple, grated
1 small banana, sliced
3 tablespoons raisins
Honey or sugar to taste

Optional: 1/2 cup chopped nuts (walnuts, almonds, hazelnuts); 1 cup berries (strawberries, blueberries, blackberries, raspberries); 1 cup sliced peaches, apricots, or pears

1. In a large bowl, combine the oats and yogurt. Add the lemon juice and the grated apples. Mix immediately to avoid discoloration of the apples.
2. Add the bananas and raisins, and any of the optional ingredients.
3. Sweeten to taste with sugar or honey.

Yield: 1 serving

Nutrition Information: Total calories: 450

Nutrients	Grams
Carbohydrate	95
Protein	11
Fat	3

HONEY NUT GRANOLA

The nice thing about making your own granola is you can avoid the unhealthful trans-fats that are in most commercially made granolas. Instead, this recipe offers healthful fats from nuts and canola oil, with a nice blend of carbohydrate-rich whole oats, dried fruits, and other add-ins of your choice to add crunch and goodness.

Mixed with fresh fruit and yogurt, this recipe offers a delicious and healthful way to start the morning or to recover after a tiring workout. The milk powder and nuts add a protein boost.

3 cups rolled oats (not instant oatmeal!)
1 cup chopped almonds
2 teaspoons cinnamon
1/3 cup honey
1/3 cup canola oil
1 cup powdered milk
1 cup dried fruit bits, raisins, dried cranberries, chopped dates, etc.

Optional: 1 teaspoon salt; 1/2 cup sesame seeds (untoasted); 1/2 cup sunflower seeds (unsalted, untoasted); 1/2 cup wheat germ; 1/2 cup ground flaxseed meal

1. In a large bowl, combine the oats, almonds, cinnamon, and powdered milk (and salt, sesame seeds, and sunflower seeds, as desired).
2. In a saucepan or microwaveable bowl, combine the honey and oil. Heat until almost boiling. Pour the honey mixture over the oat mixture and stir well.
3. Spread the mixture onto two large baking sheets.
4. Bake at 300°F for 20 to 25 minutes, stirring every 5 minutes.
5. After the granola has cooled, add the dried fruit (and wheat germ and flaxseed meal, as desired). Store in an airtight container.

Yield: 10 1/2-cup servings

Nutrition Information: Total calories: 3,300
Calories per 1/2 cup: 330

Nutrients	Grams
Carbohydrate	40
Protein	10
Fat	14

OATMEAL PANCAKES

The pancakes are light and fluffy prizewinners, perfect for carbo-loading or recovering from a hard workout. For best results, let the batter stand for 5 minutes before cooking.

1/2 cup uncooked oats (quick or old fashioned)
1/2 cup plain yogurt, buttermilk, or milk mixed with
   1/2 teaspoon vinegar
1/2 to 3/4 cup milk
1 egg or 2 egg whites, beaten
1 tablespoon oil, preferably canola
2 tablespoons packed brown sugar
1/2 teaspoon salt, as desired
1 teaspoon baking powder
1 cup flour, preferably half whole-wheat and half white

Optional: dash cinnamon

1. In a medium bowl, combine the oats, yogurt, and milk. Set aside for 15 to 20 minutes to let the oatmeal soften.
2. When the oatmeal is through soaking, beat in the egg and oil and mix well. Add the sugar, salt, and cinnamon, then the baking powder and flour. Stir until just moistened.
3. Heat a lightly oiled or nonstick griddle over medium-high heat (375°F for electric frying pan).
4. For each pancake, pour about 1/4 cup batter onto the griddle.
5. Turn when the tops are covered with bubbles and the edges look cooked. Turn only once.
6. Serve with syrup, honey, applesauce, yogurt, or other topping of your choice.

Yield: 6 6-inch pancakes

Nutrition Information: Total calories: 1,000
Calories per serving (2 pancakes): 330

Nutrients	Grams
Carbohydrate	57
Protein	10
Fat	7

WHEAT GERM AND COTTAGE CHEESE PANCAKES

These pancakes are a tasty way to add protein and satiety to a carbohydrate-rich sports breakfast. Although cottage cheese may sound like an unusual addition to pancakes, you won't even notice it. The wheat germ adds vitamin E, B-vitamins, and fiber.

1/2 cup cottage cheese, preferably low-fat
1/2 cup wheat germ
2 to 4 tablespoons firmly packed brown sugar or honey
1 egg or 2 egg whites
1 to 2 tablespoons oil, preferably canola
1 cup milk, preferably low-fat
1 teaspoon vanilla extract
1 teaspoon baking powder
1/2 teaspoon baking soda
1 cup flour, preferably half while, half whole-wheat

Optional: 1/2 teaspoon cinnamon or 1/4 teaspoon nutmeg

1. In a medium bowl, beat together the cottage cheese, wheat germ, brown sugar, egg, and oil.
2. Beat in the milk and vanilla, then the baking powder and soda (and cinnamon or nutmeg). Gently stir in the flour.
3. For each pancake, pour about 1/4 cup of batter onto a hot griddle. Cook pancakes until the edges are done and bubbles form on the top. Turn and cook until golden.
4. Serve plain or with maple syrup, applesauce with cinnamon, or yogurt.

Yield: 3 servings

Nutrition Information: Total calories: 1,200
Calories per serving: 400

Nutrients	Grams
Carbohydrate	54
Protein	19
Fat	12

14

Pasta, Rice, and Potatoes

Although some weight-conscious people mistakenly try to stay away from dinner starches such as pasta, rice, and potatoes, these carbohydrate-rich foods are actually important for a high-energy sports diet. (See chapters 7 and 11 for information about why these foods are important, not fattening.)

Pasta

When trying to decide which shape of pasta to use for a meal, the rule of thumb is to use twisted and curved shapes (such as twists and shells) with meaty, beany, and chunky sauces. The shape will trap more sauce than the straight strands of spaghetti or linguini.

Perfectly cooked pasta is tender yet firm when bitten with the teeth—"al dente," as the Italians say. The quickest cooking pastas include angel hair, alphabets, and little stars (stelline). Here are some tips for cooking pasta perfectly.

- Allow 4 quarts (4 liters) of water per pound of dry pasta. Plan to cook no more than 2 pounds of pasta at a time; otherwise, you may end up with a gummy mess.

- Use a big pot filled with water so the individual pieces of pasta can float freely. Allow 10 minutes for the water to reach a rolling boil. (If you are rushed for time, you can cook the pasta in half the amount of water, and it will cook OK—in less time.)
- To keep the water from boiling over, add 1 tablespoon of oil to the cooking water. You can also add 1 to 2 tablespoons of salt, as desired, to heighten the flavor of the pasta.
- Bring the water to a vigorous, rolling boil before you add the pasta. Then add the pasta in small amounts that will not cool the water too much and cause the pieces to clump. When cooking spaghetti or lasagna, push down the stiff strands as they soften, using a long-handled spoon.
- If the water stops boiling, cover the pan, turn up the heat, and bring the water to a boil again as soon as possible.
- Cooking time will depend on the shape of the pasta. Pasta is done when it starts to look opaque. To tell if it is done, lift a piece of pasta (with a fork) from the boiling water, let it cool briefly, then carefully pinch or bite it (being sure not to burn yourself). The pasta should feel flexible but still firm inside.
- When the pasta is done, drain it into a colander set in the sink, using potholders to protect your hands from the steam. Shake the pasta briefly to remove excess water, then return it to the cooking pot or to a warmed serving bowl.
- To prevent the pasta from sticking together as it cools, toss the pasta with a little oil or sauce.

The following quick and easy pasta toppings are a change of pace from the standard tomato sauce straight from the jar.

- Steamed, chopped broccoli
- Salsa
- Salsa heated in the microwave, then mixed with cottage cheese
- Red pepper flakes
- Low-fat Italian salad dressing mixed with a little Dijon mustard
- Low- or no-fat salad dressings of your choice
- Low- or no-fat Italian salad dressing with tamari, chopped garlic, steamed vegetables
- Nonfat sour cream and Italian seasonings
- Cottage cheese, parmesan, and Italian seasonings

- Parmesan cheese and a sprinkling of herbs (basil, oregano, Italian seasonings)
- Chicken breast sautéed with oil, garlic, onion, and basil
- Chili with kidney beans (and cheese)
- Lentil soup (thick)
- Spaghetti sauce with a spoonful of grape jelly (adds a sweet and sour taste)
- Spaghetti sauce with added protein: canned chicken or tuna, tofu cubes, canned beans, cottage cheese, ground beef or turkey
- Spaghetti sauce with added fresh diced tomato and parsley

Rice

Rice is the world's third leading grain, after wheat and corn. Brown rice is made into white rice when the fiber-rich bran is removed during the refining process. This also removes some of the nutrients, but you can compensate for this loss (if you prefer white to brown rice) by eating other whole grains such as bran cereals and whole-wheat breads at your other meals. Here are some tips for cooking rice:

- Because of its tough bran coat and germ, brown rice needs about 45 to 50 minutes to cook; white rice needs only about 20 to 30 minutes.
- Consider cooking rice in the morning while you are getting ready for work, so that it will only need to be reheated when you get home.
- When cooking rice, cook double amounts to have leftovers that you can freeze or refrigerate.
- Portion size:
  1 cup raw white rice = 3 cups cooked = 700 calories
  1 cup raw brown rice = 3 to 4 cups cooked = 700 calories
- Rice is popularly cooked in two ways. Bring a saucepan of water to a full boil, stir in 1/3 to 1/2 cup rice per person plus 1 to 2 teaspoons of salt, as desired. Simmer about 20 minutes, or until a grain of rice is tender when you bite into it. Drain into a colander, rinse it under hot tap water to remove the sticky starch, and put it back into the saucepan. Keep the rice warm over low heat, fluffing it with a fork. Or, for each 1 cup of rice, put 2 cups of water into a saucepan, and 1 teaspoon salt, as desired. Bring to a boil, then

cover and turn the heat down low. Let the rice cook undisturbed until it is tender and all the water has been absorbed. Then, stir gently with a fork. (Stirring too much may result in a sticky mess.) This method retains more of the vitamins that otherwise get lost into the cooking water.

Here are a few rice suggestions for hungry athletes.

Cook rice in these liquids:
- Chicken or beef broth
- Mixture of orange or apple juice and water
- Water with seasonings: cinnamon, soy sauce, oregano, curry, chili powder, or whatever might nicely blend with the menu.

Combine rice with these foods:
- Leftover chili
- Low- or no-fat Italian dressing and mustard
- Toasted sesame seeds, chopped nuts
- Steamed vegetables
- Chopped mushrooms and green peppers, either raw or sautéed
- Nonfat sour cream, raisins, tuna, and curry powder
- Raisins, cinnamon, and applesauce
- Soy sauce and diced scallions
- Honey, raisins, and toasted sliced almonds

Potatoes

The potato is a carbohydrate-rich vegetable that actually offers more vitamins and minerals than plain rice or pasta. To help you include more potatoes in your sports diet, here are some tips.

- Potatoes come in different varieties. Some varieties are best suited for baking (russets), others for boiling (red or white rounds). Ask the produce manager at your grocery store for guidance.
- Potatoes are best stored in a cool, humid (but not wet) place that is well ventilated, such as your cellar. Do not refrigerate potatoes because they will become sweet and off-colored.
- Rather than peel the skin (under which is stored most of the vitamin C), scrub the skin well and cook the potato skin and all. Yes, even mashed potatoes can be made with unpeeled potatoes!

- One pound of potatoes equals three medium or two large potatoes. The large, "restaurant size" potato has about 200 calories.
- To bake a potato in the oven, allow about 40 minutes at 400°F for a medium potato, closer to an hour for a large potato. Because potatoes can be baked at any temperature, you can adjust the cooking time to whatever else is in the oven.
- You can tell that the potato is done when you can easily pierce it with a fork.
- To cook a potato in the microwave oven, prick its skin in several places with a fork, place it on some paper toweling on the bottom of the microwave, and cook it for about 4 minutes if it is medium-sized, or 6 to 10 minutes if it's large. Cooking time will vary according to the size of the potato, the power of your oven, and the number of potatoes being cooked. Turn the potato over halfway through cooking. Remove the potato from the oven, wrap it in a towel, and allow it to finish cooking outside the oven for about 3 to 5 minutes.

To spice up your potato, try the following toppings.

- Plain yogurt
- Imitation butter granules (such as Molly McButter) and milk
- Mustard
- Mustard and Worcestershire sauce
- White and flavored vinegars
- Soy sauce
- Pesto
- Chopped chives and green onion
- Herbs such as dill and parsley
- Steamed broccoli or other cooked vegetables
- Chopped jalapeño peppers
- Low- or no-fat salad dressing
- Nonfat sour cream, chopped onion, and grated low-fat cheddar cheese
- Cottage cheese and garlic powder
- Cottage cheese and salsa
- Chili and grated low-fat cheddar cheese
- Cooked chopped spinach and crumbled feta cheese
- Soup broth

- Milk mashed into the potato
- Lentils or lentil soup
- Baked beans or refried beans
- Applesauce

COLORFUL PASTA SALAD 293
EASY LASAGNA 294
GOURMET LASAGNA. 295
SESAME PASTA WITH BROCCOLI 296
SOUTHWESTERN RICE AND BEAN SALAD 297
OVEN FRENCH FRIES 298
EGG-STUFFED BAKED POTATO 299

See also: Pasta and White Bean Soup With Sun-Dried Tomatoes, Chicken With Pasta and Spinach, Chicken and Oriental Noodles in Peanut Sauce, Country Pasta With Turkey Sausage and White Beans, Ground Turkey Mix for Spaghetti or Chili, Shrimp Fettuccine, Mediterranean Shrimp and Scallops With Pasta, Salmon Pasta Salad, Tofu Lo Mein, Sweet and Spicy Orange Beef, Minestrone Soup

For additional recipes, see www.ilovepasta.org, www.usarice.com, or www.potatohelp.com.

COLORFUL PASTA SALAD

The colorful vegetables make this pasta salad pretty to look at—and tasty to eat. You can be creative and use other pasta shapes (rotini, bow ties), toss in other ingredients (tofu, diced chicken, beans, grated cheese), and simply use a bottled lowfat dressing of your choice.

8 ounces dry pasta shells
1 cup cherry tomato halves
1 cup zucchini slices
1 cup yellow pepper strips
1 cup broccoli florets
1 cup carrot slices
1/2 cup onion slices

Dressing:
2 tablespoons oil, preferably olive or canola
1/4 cup cider vinegar
1/4 cup honey
1 tablespoon dijon mustard
1 teaspoon ground ginger
Salt and pepper, as desired

1. Cook the pasta according to the package directions. Drain and rinse with cold water.
2. In a large bowl, toss together the pasta and all the vegetables.
3. In a small bowl, whisk together the oil, vinegar, honey, mustard, ginger, salt, and pepper.
4. Pour the dressing over the pasta mixture. Stir gently, cover, and refrigerate until ready to serve.

Yield: 4 servings

Nutrition Information: Total calories: 1,500
Calories per serving: 375

Nutrients	Grams
Carbohydrate	70
Protein	8
Fat	7

EASY LASAGNA

This recipe is "easy" because it eliminates the step of cooking the lasagna noodles before assembly.

When eating this lasagna pre-event, be aware that half the calories come from protein and fat. (Most lasagnas are even higher in protein and fat!) Be sure to boost your carb intake with (whole-grain) bread, fruit salad, juice, and other carbohydrate-rich foods.

1 pound (2 cups) part-skim ricotta or cottage cheese or a mixture
1 egg or 2 egg whites
1 teaspoon dried oregano
1 teaspoon salt, as desired
1 48-ounce jar spaghetti sauce
2 cups water
20 lasagna noodles
4 to 6 ounces (1 to 1 1/2 cups) mozzarella cheese, shredded

Optional: 10-ounce package frozen chopped spinach, thawed and drained; 4 cups diced vegetables (onions, mushrooms, carrots, zucchini, summer squash, etc.) steamed or sautéed in a little oil; 1 pound extralean hamburger or ground turkey, browned and drained; 1 pound tofu, crumbled

1. In a bowl, mix the ricotta cheese with the egg, spinach, oregano, salt (and vegetables and meat).
2. Set aside 2 cups of spaghetti sauce for the topping, then mix 2 cups of water into the remaining sauce.
3. In a 9" × 13" pan, place four uncooked lasagna noodles, then add a layer of cheese/vegetable mixture, then spaghetti sauce. Repeat three times, ending with noodles. Sprinkle shredded mozzarella over the top.
4. Pour the 2 cups of reserved spaghetti sauce on the top layer. Sprinkle shredded mozzarella over the top.
5. Cover with foil and bake at 350°F for 1 hour and 15 minutes, uncovering for the last 10 minutes. (Try to prevent the foil from sticking to the top cheese by covering it carefully.)

Yield: 8 servings

Nutrition Information: Total calories: 3,700
Calories per serving: 460

Nutrients	Grams
Carbohydrate	64
Protein	22
Fat	13

GOURMET LASAGNA

This "company is coming" lasagna has a wonderful flavor and is a nice variation from standard lasagnas. The sun-dried tomatoes and pine nuts make the difference—well worth the effort of buying them if you have none stocked!

15 lasagna noodles
8 to 9 sun-dried tomatoes
1/2 cup pine nuts (pignoli nuts)
1 to 3 cloves garlic, peeled and finely chopped
1 teaspoon oil, preferably olive or canola
1 pound ricotta cheese, part-skim or nonfat
4 to 8 ounces shredded lowfat mozzarella cheese
1 to 2 dashes nutmeg
1/4 teaspoon oregano
1 10-ounce package frozen spinach, thawed and drained
1 28-ounce jar spaghetti sauce
Optional: 1/4 cup grated parmesan cheese

1. Cook the lasagna noodles according to the package directions.
2. Put the sun-dried tomatoes in a small bowl. Cover with boiling water and set aside for 5 minutes if oil-packed, 10 to 15 minutes if dried. Drain, cool, and chop finely. Set aside.
3. Toast the pine nuts in the oven at 350°F for five minutes or on the stovetop in a nonstick skillet over medium-high heat for 2 to 3 minutes.
4. In a separate skillet, sauté the garlic in oil for 2 minutes. Do not brown. Set the pan aside.
5. In a large mixing bowl, combine the ricotta, mozzarella, nutmeg, oregano, spinach, sun-dried tomatoes, pine nuts, and garlic.
6. In a 9" × 13" pan, pour enough tomato sauce to coat the bottom. Cover with lasagna noodles, then add a layer of ricotta mixture, then spaghetti sauce. Repeat, making three layers of ricotta, and ending with noodles and tomato sauce. Sprinkle with parmesan, as desired.
7. Cover with foil. Bake at 350°F for 30 to 40 minutes or until hot.

Yield: 8 servings

Nutrition Information: Total calories: 3,600
Calories per serving: 450

Nutrients	Grams
Carbohydrate	53
Protein	21
Fat	17

SESAME PASTA WITH BROCCOLI

Sesame paste (tahini) is the secret ingredient in this recipe. Not only does it have a wonderful flavor but it's also a good source of vitamin E. Look for tahini in the ethnic food section of the supermarket or at the health food store. You can also use it in the recipe for hummus on page 352. If you can't find tahini, substitute peanut butter diluted with 1 or 2 tablespoons of boiling water.

8 ounces dry pasta
2 cups fresh or frozen broccoli, chopped
1/4 cup tahini (sesame butter) or peanut butter

Optional: cayenne pepper; garlic powder; vegetables such as diced carrot, celery, red peppers, and scallions

1. Cook pasta according to directions on the package. Drain.
2. While pasta is cooking, steam broccoli (and other vegetables, as desired) until tender-crisp.
3. Add tahini to drained pasta, mix well. Add cooked broccoli and the water in which it was cooked if the pasta is "dry."
4. Add a dash of cayenne or garlic powder, as desired.

Yield: 4 side servings; 2 main dish servings

Nutrition Information: Total calories: 1,300
Calories per side serving: 325

Nutrients	Grams
Carbohydrate	50
Protein	11
Fat	9

SOUTHWESTERN
RICE AND BEAN SALAD

This makes a nice side dish with barbequed chicken. If you do not have lime juice on hand, you can use lemon juice, rice vinegar, or white vinegar.

2 cups cooked rice, cooled (about 2/3 cup when uncooked)
1 15-ounce can black beans, drained and rinsed
1 large tomato, chopped
3 ounces low-fat cheddar cheese, diced into small 1/4" cubes

Dressing:
1 tablespoon oil, preferably olive or canola
2 tablespoons lime juice, lemon juice, or vinegar
1 tablespoon taco seasoning mix (or 1 teaspoon cumin and
   1/8 teaspoon cayenne pepper)

Optional: 2 tablespoons chopped cilantro; 1/4 cup diced onion;
   salt and pepper

1. In a large bowl, combine the cooked rice, beans, tomato, and cheese (and cilantro and onion).

2. In a small bowl, whisk together the oil, lime juice, and taco seasonings. Pour over the rice mixture and mix well. Adjust the seasonings to the desired taste. Refrigerate until ready to serve.

Yield: 4 servings (as a side dish)

Nutrition Information: Total calories: 960
Calories per serving: 240

Nutrients	Grams
Carbohydrate	27
Protein	15
Fat	8

OVEN FRENCH FRIES

This healthful french fry recipe is a popular family favorite—and no one will realize it is low in fat! For a flavor boost, dip the fries in salsa, nonfat yogurt mixed with fresh herbs, or ketchup.

1 large baking potato, cleaned, unpeeled
1 teaspoon oil, preferably canola or olive
Salt and pepper to taste

Optional: red pepper flakes; dried basil; oregano; minced garlic; parmesan cheese

1. Cut each potato lengthwise into 10 or 12 pieces. Place in a large bowl; cover with cold water and let stand for 15 to 20 minutes. (This soaking can be eliminated, but it shortens the cooking time and improves the final product.)

2. Drain the potatoes, dry them on a towel, then put them in a bowl or ziplock bag. Drizzle them with the oil and sprinkle with the salt and pepper, as desired. Toss to coat evenly.

3. Place the potatoes evenly on a nonstick shallow baking pan.

4. Bake at 425°F for 15 minutes. Turn the potatoes over, sprinkle with the optional seasonings, as desired, and continue baking for another 10 to 15 minutes. Serve immediately. Be careful; the potatoes will be very hot!

Yield: 1 serving

Nutrition Information: Calories per potato: 260

Nutrients	Grams
Carbohydrate	52
Protein	4
Fat	4

EGG-STUFFED BAKED POTATO

If you let the potato bake while you are exercising, dinner will be ready when you are! Or, prepare it in the microwave oven. One of these potatoes alone may not provide adequate calories for a dinner. Plan to supplement this meal with soup and salad, or eat two potatoes.

1 large baking potato (1/2 pound)
1 egg
1 ounce shredded cheese, preferably low-fat
Salt and pepper as desired

Optional: 1 to 2 tablespoons milk

1. Prick the potato in several places with a fork. Bake in a 400°F oven for an hour or until done; the potato should be tender if pierced with a fork. Or cook the potato for about 8 minutes in a microwave oven, letting it rest for an additional 3 minutes.
2. Cut an X on top of the baked potato. Fluff up the insides and make a well.
3. Optional: For moistness add 1 to 2 tablespoons of milk.
4. Break the egg into the well. Top with cheese and salt and pepper as desired.
5. Return to the oven until the egg is cooked, about 10 minutes. Or microwave at medium power for 1 to 2 minutes, being sure to pierce the yolk (otherwise it will explode).

Yield: 1 serving

Nutrition Information: Calories per potato: 270

Nutrients	Grams
Carbohydrate	35
Protein	15
Fat	8

15

Vegetables and Salads

Vegetables are perfectly delicious when served plain, without added flavorings. That's why you won't find many vegetable recipes in this section. When cooking vegetables, carefully cook them just until they are tender-crisp and still flavorful. Limp, overcooked veggies lose their appeal as well as some of their nutrients.

Most vegetables contain negligible amounts of protein and fat but offer carbohydrates, fiber, and abundant vitamins and minerals. Eating vegetables is the best way to boost your vitamin intake—preferable to taking vitamin pills.

The first four recipes offer basic advice about cooking methods. Nutrition information is provided only for the final four recipes. Tables 1.2 on page 12 and 4.1 on page 73 provide more nutrition information.

STEAMED VEGETABLES 303
STIR-FRIED VEGETABLES 304
BAKED VEGETABLES 305
MICROWAVED VEGETABLES 306
SPINACH SALAD WITH SWEET AND SPICY DRESSING 307
SPINACH SALAD WITH ORIENTAL DRESSING 308
BRENDA'S GREEK SALAD 309
CARROT-RAISIN SALAD 310

See also: Minestrone Soup, Easy Lasagna, Gourmet Lasagna, Tofu Lo Mein, Jenny's Favorite Oatmeal, Fish and Spinach Bake, Carrot Cake, Carrot Raisin Muffins

For abundant recipes with vegetables, visit www.aboutproduce.com.

STEAMED VEGETABLES

Vegetable of your choice. Examples of good choices include:

- Broccoli
- Spinach
- Carrots
- Green beans
- Brussel sprouts

Optional: Sprinkle vegetables with herbs before or after cooking. Add basil and oregano to zucchini squash, ginger to carrots, and garlic powder to green beans. With carrots, add a teaspoon of honey afterward. Be creative!

1. Wash the vegetables thoroughly to remove soil. Cut into the desired size.

2. Put 1/2 inch of water in the bottom of a pan with a tight lid. Bring to a boil, then add the vegetables. Cover tightly, or put the vegetables in a steamer basket and put the basket into a saucepan with 1 inch of water (or enough to prevent the water from boiling away). Cover tightly and bring to a boil.

3. Cook over medium heat until tender-crisp, about 3 to 10 minutes, depending on the type and size of vegetable.

4. Drain the vegetables, reserving the cooking liquid for soup, sauces, or even for drinking as vegetable broth.

STIR-FRIED VEGETABLES

A large nonstick skillet is useful for stir-frying vegetables. The goal is to end up with vegetables that are cooked until tender-crisp and flavorful. By combining only two or three vegetables, you'll get more distinguished flavors. Plus, this makes it easier to time the cooking so they are all done at the right time.

Olive and canola oils are among the heart-healthiest choices for stir-frying. For a wonderful flavor, add a little sesame oil (available in the Chinese food section of larger supermarkets or health food stores). If you are watching your weight, be sure to add only a little oil.

Vegetables of your choice (popular combinations are: carrots, broccoli, and mushrooms; onions, zucchini, and tomatoes; Chinese cabbage and water chestnuts; sugar snap peas, Chinese pea pods, and green peas)
Cooking oil of your choice: canola, olive, sesame

Optional: toasted sesame seeds; nuts; mandarin orange sections; pineapple chunks

1. Wash, drain well (to prevent oil from spattering when the vegetables are added), and cut the vegetables into bite-sized pieces or 1/8-inch slices. When possible, slice the vegetables diagonally to increase the surface area; this allows faster cooking. Try to make the pieces uniform so they will cook evenly.

2. Heat the nonstick skillet, wok, or large frying pan over high heat until very hot, then add 1 to 3 teaspoons of canola, olive, or sesame oil—just enough to coat the bottom of the pan. For interesting flavor, try adding a slice of ginger root or minced garlic to the oil. Stir-fry for a minute to flavor the oil.

3. First add vegetables that take the longest to cook (carrots, cauliflower, broccoli); a few minutes later, add the remaining veggies (mushrooms, bean sprouts, cabbage, spinach). Rather than stir constantly (as the name would imply), wait about 30 seconds between each stirring so the pan can regain its heat. Adjust the heat to prevent scorching.

4. Don't overcrowd the pan. Cook small batches at a time. The goal is to cook the vegetables until they are tender but still crunchy, about 2 to 5 minutes.

5. Optional: Garnish the vegetables with toasted sesame seeds or toasted nuts (almonds, cashews, peanuts), or mandarin orange sections or pineapple chunks.

BAKED VEGETABLES

If the oven is already hot because you are baking potatoes, chicken, or a casserole, you might as well make good use of the heat and bake the vegetables, too. Roasting vegetables evaporates much of their water, concentrates their natural sugars, and yields a rich, sweet taste and meaty texture.

Vegetables of your choice. Popular combinations are:

- Eggplant halves sprinkled with garlic powder
- Zucchini or summer squash halves covered with onion slices
- Carrot chunks
- Sweet potato slices and apples

1. Cut vegetables into equal-sized chunks, rub with a little canola or olive oil, and spread them on a nonstick baking sheet, uncovered.
2. Bake at 350°F for 30 to 45 minutes, until tender.

Alternatively:

1. Wrap the vegetables in foil or put them in a covered baking dish with a small amount of water. (This actually steams them, rather than roasts them.)
2. Bake at 350°F for 20 to 30 minutes (depending on the size of the chunks) until tender-crisp.
3. When you open the foil, be careful of escaping steam so that you don't get burned.

MICROWAVED VEGETABLES

Microwave cookery is ideal for vegetables because it cooks them quickly and without water, retaining a greater percentage of nutrients than with conventional methods.

Vegetables of your choice. All cook fine in the microwave oven, but some nice options are:

- Green beans
- Peas
- Broccoli
- Cauliflower
- Carrots

Optional: Sprinkle vegetables with herbs (basil, parsley, oregano, garlic powder), soy sauce, or whatever suits your taste

1. Wash the vegetables and cut them into bite-sized pieces.
2. Put them in a microwaveable dish and cover with plastic wrap. If the vegetables vary in thickness (like stalks of broccoli do), arrange them in a ring with the thicker portions toward the outside of the dish.
3. Microwave until tender-crisp. The amount of time will vary according to your particular oven and the amount of vegetables you are cooking. You'll learn by trial and error! Start off with 3 minutes for a single serving; larger quantities take longer. The vegetables will continue cooking after they are removed from the microwave, so plan that into the time allotment.

SPINACH SALAD WITH
SWEET AND SPICY DRESSING

Spinach is a powerhouse vegetable, rich in vitamin C, folate, beta-carotene and many other nutrients. You can easily incorporate more spinach into your diet with tasty spinach salads. Here is one version.

1 10 oz. package or large bunch fresh spinach, rinsed well and cut up

Optional: 1 cup sliced mushrooms; 2 fresh tomatoes, cut into wedges; 2 hard-boiled eggs, sliced; 1/2 cup broken walnuts

Sweet and Spicy Dressing:
3 tablespoons olive oil
2 tablespoons red wine vinegar
1 tablespoon sugar
1 teaspoon salt as desired
1 tablespoon ketchup

1. In a salad bowl combine the spinach (and mushrooms and tomatoes, as desired).
2. In a jar combine the olive oil, vinegar, sugar, salt, and ketchup. Cover and shake until well blended.
3. Pour the dressing over the salad; toss well then garnish with eggs and walnuts, as desired.

Yield: 4 large salads

Nutrition Information: Total calories: 480
Calories per serving: 120

Nutrients	Grams
Carbohydrate	7
Protein	2
Fat	9

SPINACH SALAD
WITH ORIENTAL DRESSING

This goes nicely with a simple baked fish or chicken meal and some fresh whole-grain bread.

1 10-ounce bag or large bunch fresh spinach, rinsed well and cut up

Optional: 4 ounces water chestnuts, sliced; 1/2 pound mushrooms, sliced; 1/2 pound bean sprouts; 1/2 teaspoon toasted sesame seeds; 1 11-ounce can mandarin oranges

Dressing:
1 tablespoon soy sauce, light or regular
1/4 cup vinegar, preferably rice vinegar
2 teaspoons fresh lemon juice (or 2 teaspoons more vinegar)
1 teaspoon sugar
1/2 teaspoon grated ginger
1/4 teaspoon garlic powder
2 tablespoons sesame oil

1. In a salad bowl combine the spinach (and water chestnuts, mushrooms, bean sprouts, and mandarin oranges, as desired).
2. In a jar combine the soy sauce, vinegar, lemon juice, sugar, ginger, garlic powder, and sesame oil. Cover and shake until well blended.
3. Pour the dressing over the salad and toss well.
4. Garnish with sesame seeds, as desired.

Yield: 4 large salads

Nutrition Information: Total calories: 320
Calories per serving: 80

Nutrients	Grams
Carbohydrate	4
Protein	2
Fat	6

BRENDA'S GREEK SALAD

This recipe is a favorite of Brenda Ponichtera, RD, cookbook author of *Quick and Healthy Recipes and Ideas: For People Who Say They Don't Have Time to Cook Healthy Meals* (www.quickandhealthy.net). Brenda says the combination of red and yellow peppers give the salad an especially good flavor. If time allows, let it marinate for several hours—and make enough for leftovers because it'll be great the next day. (I like to make it into a wrap for lunch!)

The salad can be made with only green peppers; it'll taste just fine. For a richer flavor, you can add a drizzle of olive oil.

1 green pepper, sliced
1 red pepper, sliced
1 yellow pepper, sliced
1 unpeeled cucumber, sliced
2 tablespoons lemon juice
3 tablespoons red wine vinegar
1/4 teaspoon dried oregano
4 ounces feta cheese, crumbled

1. Mix peppers and cucumber in a bowl.
2. Add lemon juice, vinegar, and oregano. Mix well.
3. Top with crumbled feta cheese.

Yield: 4 servings

Nutrition Information: Total calories: 400
Calories per serving (about 1 cup):
 100 calories

Nutrients	Grams
Carbohydrate	8
Protein	5
Fat	6

Reprinted, by permission, from Brenda J. Ponichtera, 1991, *Quick and healthy recipes and ideas: for people who say they don't have time to cook healthy meals* (The Dalles, Oregon: ScaleDown Publishing, Inc.).

CARROT-RAISIN SALAD

Carrots are an excellent source of beta-carotene, the plant form of vitamin A. This vitamin helps your eyes adjust to the dark, as they do when you come indoors after exercising outside on a sunny day.

4 medium carrots, grated
1/2 cup raisins
3 tablespoons orange juice

Optional: 1/2 cup lowfat yogurt or mayonnaise, or mixture;
   1 tablespoon honey; 1/2 cup chopped walnuts

1. In a salad bowl, combine the carrots, raisins, and orange juice.
2. Add the yogurt or mayonnaise, honey, and nuts, as desired.

Yield: 4 servings

Nutrition Information: Total calories: 440
Calories per serving: 110

Nutrients	Grams
Carbohydrate	26
Protein	1
Fat	0

16

Chicken and Turkey

The white and dark meat of chicken and turkey are excellent examples of muscle physiology. They represent two types of muscle fibers.

- The white breast meat is primarily fast-twitch muscle fibers. These are used for bursts of energy. Athletes such as elite gymnasts, basketball players, and others who do sprint types of exercise tend to have a high percentage of fast-twitch fibers.

- The dark meat in the legs and wings is primarily slow-twitch muscle fibers that function best for endurance exercise. Elite marathoners, long-distance cyclists, and other successful endurance athletes tend to have a high percentage of slow-twitch fibers.

   The dark meat (endurance muscle fibers) of poultry contains more fat than the white meat (sprint fibers) because the fat provides energy for greater endurance; the dark meat also has slightly more fat calories than light meat:

   3 oz chicken breast (white meat) = 120 calories

   3 oz chicken thigh (dark meat) = 150 calories

The dark meat also has more iron, zinc, B vitamins, and other nutrients. I recommend that athletes who don't eat beef select skinless dark meat poultry to boost their intake of these important nutrients. Because the highest source of fat in chicken is in the skin, be sure to remove the skin prior to cooking. This eliminates the temptation to eat it!

- For a basic chicken meal, put 1/2 inch of water in a saucepan, add the chicken, cover tightly, and bring just to a boil. Turn down heat; gently simmer over medium-low heat for 20 to 25 minutes, or until the juices run clear when the chicken is poked with a fork. You may also choose to remove the skin from the chicken; place the skinless chicken on a rack in a baking pan. Bake uncovered at 350°F for 20 to 30 minutes or until the juices run clear when it is poked with a fork.

- For easy cleanup when baking chicken, use a nonstick pan or a regular baking pan treated with cooking spray, or line the pan with aluminum foil.

Some of my clients eat so much chicken, they claim they'll turn into a chicken! If that sounds familiar, here are some ways to add variety to your chicken meals.

- Replace cooking water with orange juice, white wine, or a can of stewed tomatoes.
- Add seasonings to the cooking water: a chicken bouillon cube, soy sauce, curry, basil, or thyme.
- Cook rice along with the chicken (add extra water).
- Make stuffing with the chicken broth and stuffing mix.
- Add vegetables in the last 5 minutes.
- Dice the cooked chicken and wrap it in a tortilla with salsa, shredded lettuce, and grated lowfat cheese.
- Smear the chicken with a teaspoon of dijon mustard, then add a generous sprinkling of parmesan cheese.
- Smear the chicken with a teaspoon of honey, then sprinkle on curry powder.
- Wrap a chicken breast around a piece of string cheese sliced in half lengthwise; secure with toothpicks, then bake.
- Marinate the chicken for 10 to 60 minutes in a ziplock bag with soy sauce, a shake of ground ginger, mustard, and garlic powder, then bake (or sauté in a little oil in a frying pan).
- Dip in sesame seeds, cracker crumbs, or corn flake crumbs, then bake (or sauté in a little oil in a frying pan).

- Place chicken breast on a piece of foil, cover with vegetables (your choice of onion, mushrooms, carrots, potato, tomato) and seasonings (your choice of garlic, rosemary, thyme, basil). Wrap well by folding the edges of the foil together, then bake at 375°F for about 20 minutes. (Be careful to not get burned by the steam that escapes when you open the foil packet!)

OVEN-FRIED CHICKEN 314
SAUTÉED CHICKEN WITH MUSHROOMS AND ONIONS 315
CHICKEN WITH PASTA AND SPINACH. 316
CHICKEN AND ORIENTAL NOODLES IN PEANUT SAUCE 317
CHICKEN SALAD WITH ALMONDS AND MANDARIN ORANGES. 318
CHICKEN BLACK BEAN SOUP. 319
TURKEY TERIYAKI. 320
TURKEY PICCATA 321
COUNTRY PASTA WITH TURKEY SAUSAGE AND WHITE BEANS. 322
TURKEY MEATBALLS OR TURKEY BURGERS 323
GROUND TURKEY MIX FOR SPAGHETTI OR CHILI 324
MEXICAN BAKED CHICKEN WITH PINTO BEANS 325

See also: Stir-Fried Vegetables, Easy Lasagna, Pasta and White Bean Soup With Sun-Dried Tomatoes, Tofu Lo Mein, Fish in Foil Mexican Style, Quick and Easy Chili, Mexican Tortilla Lasagna, Warm Taco Salad

For more recipes, visit www.eatchicken.com and www.eatturkey.com.

OVEN-FRIED CHICKEN

Deep fat fried chicken is popular with many athletes, but fails to be the healthiest of sports foods. This recipe offers a lower-fat alternative that will get "thumbs up" from even fussy eaters. The recipe is reprinted with permission from the May/June 1999 issue of *Cook's Illustrated*, a cooking magazine that I highly recommend if you want to learn more about the what's, how's, and why's of cooking (www.cooksillustrated.com).

1 box (5 ounces) Melba toast
2 to 4 tablespoons olive or canola oil
2 egg whites or 1 egg
4 boneless, skinless chicken breasts

Optional: 1 tablespoon dijon mustard; salt and pepper

1. Heat oven to 400°F. Set a wire rack in a shallow baking pan. If desired, line the pan with foil for ease with clean-up. Cooking the chicken on a rack allows air to circulate on all sides, resulting in a crisper chicken without turning.

2. Put the Melba toast into a heavy-duty plastic bag, seal, and pound with a rolling pin or other hard object (wine bottle, can, fist). Leave some crumbs the size of small pebbles to add crunchiness.

3. Put the crumbs in a shallow dish and drizzle the oil over them, tossing well to distribute the oil evenly.

4. Beat the egg in a medium bowl. Add optional seasonings as desired.

5. One piece of chicken at a time, coat the chicken with the egg mixture, then place in the crumbs. Sprinkle the crumbs over the flesh and press them in.

6. Gently shake off excess crumbs and place the chicken on the rack.

7. Bake about 40 minutes, or until the coating is a deep brown and the juices run clear when the meat is slit with a knife.

Yield: 4 servings

Nutrition Information: Total calories: 1,200
Calories per serving: 300

Nutrients	Grams
Carbohydrate	12
Protein	40
Fat	10

Reprinted, by permission, from *Cooks Magazine*, May/June 1999. www.cooksillustrated.com

SAUTÉED CHICKEN
WITH MUSHROOMS AND ONIONS

This simple recipe is tasty enough for an impromptu gourmet dinner. It includes common ingredients that are easy to keep stocked: (frozen) chicken breasts, (canned) mushrooms, onions, low-fat cheese, and wine. Enjoy it with rice, crusty whole-grain rolls, and a green vegetable.

1 to 2 tablespoons oil, preferably olive or canola
4 chicken breasts, boneless and skinless
1 medium onion, diced
1 cup dry white wine
2 cans (6 ounces each) sliced mushrooms, drained
2 ounces low-fat swiss cheese

Optional: 1 to 2 cloves garlic, minced or 1 teaspoon ground thyme

1. In a large nonstick skillet, heat the oil and add the chicken breasts and onions (and garlic). Cook for about 5 minutes per side.
2. Add the wine and drained mushrooms (and thyme).
3. Cover and simmer for about 10 minutes, or until the chicken is done and the juices run clear when the meat is slit with a knife.
4. Place a half-ounce of cheese on top of each cooked chicken breast. Cover the pan and simmer for another three minutes, or until the cheese is melted.
5. Serve by placing the chicken on top of a bed of mushrooms.

Yield: 4 servings

Nutrition Information: Total calories: 1,200
Calories per serving: 300

Nutrients	Grams
Carbohydrate	10
Protein	42
Fat	10

CHICKEN WITH PASTA AND SPINACH

This recipe is not only quick and easy, but also includes three different food groups (grain, protein, and vegetable), creating a well balanced meal. Food variety can help you be strong to the finish—as can the spinach itself!

1 pound pasta, such as fettuccine
1 pound boneless, skinless chicken breasts, thinly sliced
2 tablespoons oil, preferably olive or canola
1 to 4 cloves garlic, finely chopped or 1/4 to 1 teaspoon garlic powder
1 pound fresh spinach, washed, drained, and roughly chopped
1 10-ounce can chicken broth
Salt and pepper to taste

Optional: 10 ounces mushrooms, sliced; 1/4 cup parmesan cheese

1. Cook the pasta according to the package directions.
2. While the pasta is cooking, in a large skillet heat the oil and sauté the sliced chicken breasts for 30 seconds.
3. Toss in the garlic (and mushrooms) and stir well. Cook for about 5 minutes.
4. Pour in the chicken broth and bring it to a simmer. Add the spinach, stirring until it wilts.
5. Drain the pasta and return it to the cooking pot. Pour in the chicken and spinach mixture and toss well. Heat for 2 minutes.
6. Season to taste with salt and pepper (and parmesan cheese, as desired).

Yield: 5 servings

Nutrition Information: Total calories: 2,800
Calories per serving: 560

Nutrients	Grams
Carbohydrate	75
Protein	40
Fat	11

CHICKEN AND ORIENTAL NOODLES IN PEANUT SAUCE

You can serve this satiating meal either hot or chilled; it will be sure to please your palate. Hoisin sauce, rice vinegar, and sesame oil, which are found in the Asian food section of large grocery stores, are worth buying so you'll have them on hand for other meals. (For example, you can use the hoisin sauce in the recipe on page 318 for Chicken Salad with Almonds and Mandarin Oranges.) Note: If the noodle mixture becomes too dry, simply add a little warm water for moisture.

This recipe also works well with beef, shrimp, scallops, and tofu, as well as an assortment of vegetables—broccoli, celery, green beans, and so on.

9 ounces uncooked Japanese udon (or any oriental noodle)
1/2 cup chicken broth, canned, homemade, or from bouillion
1/4 cup hoisin sauce
1/4 cup peanut butter, creamy-style
2 tablespoons vinegar, preferably rice vinegar or white
2 tablespoons ketchup
1/4 teaspoon crushed red pepper
2 teaspoons oil, canola or sesame
1 pound chicken breast, sliced thinly
1 large green or red pepper, sliced into strips

Optional: 1/2 teaspoon ground ginger; 1/4 teaspoon garlic powder or 1 clove fresh garlic, finely diced

1. Cook the noodles according to the package directions; drain.
2. Heat the chicken broth in a small microwaveable bowl, then add the hoisin sauce, peanut butter, vinegar, ketchup, and crushed red pepper (and ginger and garlic). Stir to blend.
3. Heat the oil in a large nonstick skillet over medium-high heat. Add the chicken and green pepper slices, and stir-fry for 3 to 5 minutes.
4. Pour the hoisin sauce mixture into the chicken-pepper mixture and heat for a minute, then add the noodles. Toss well and serve.

Yield: 4 servings

Nutrition Information: Total calories: 2,200
Calories per serving: 550

Nutrients	Grams
Carbohydrate	55
Protein	48
Fat	15

CHICKEN SALAD WITH ALMONDS AND MANDARIN ORANGES

This is nice served on a bed of salad greens with whole-grain bread.

1 pound boneless, skinless chicken breasts
1/4 to 1/2 cup slivered almonds
1 can (11 ounces) mandarin oranges, drained
Optional: 1 can (8 ounces) pineapple chunks; 1 can (6 ounces) sliced water chestnuts; 1/2 cup raisins or chopped dates

Lemon Dressing:
1/2 to 1 cup (8 ounces) low-fat lemon yogurt, or mixture of half yogurt, half low-fat mayonnaise

Oriental Dressing:
2 tablespoons hoisin sauce
2 tablespoons juice from the mandarin oranges
4 tablespoons low-fat mayonnaise
Optional: 1/2 teaspoon dry mustard; 1/4 teaspoon garlic powder

1. Simmer the chicken in 1 cup water in a covered pan for about 20 minutes, or until the juices run clear when pricked with a fork. Cool, then dice and place in a large bowl along with the almonds and oranges (and pineapple, water chestnuts, and raisins).
2. For the lemon dressing: Add the lemon yogurt and mix well. For the oriental dressing: In a small bowl, mix the hoisin sauce, mandarin orange juice, and low-fat mayonnaise (and mustard and garlic).
3. If time allows, chill. Serve on a bed of salad greens.

Yield: 4 servings

Nutrition Information: Total calories, with lemon dressing: 1,100; calories per serving: 270

Nutrients	Grams
Carbohydrate	12
Protein	40
Fat	7

Total calories with oriental dressing: 1,200; calories per serving: 300

Nutrients	Grams
Carbohydrate	17
Protein	40
Fat	8

CHICKEN BLACK BEAN SOUP

Fitness enthusiast and chef Peter Hermann gave me this simple yet delicious and nutritious recipe. It's a tasty way to add more fiber-rich beans into your diet. You can make it a heartier meal by adding cooked pasta.

4 chicken breasts, skinned and boned
5 cups chicken broth or water
2 carrots, peeled and sliced
2 tomatoes, chopped
1/2 onion, chopped
3 to 5 cloves garlic, crushed
2 16-ounce cans black beans, rinsed and drained
1 tablespoon fresh oregano leaves or 1 teaspoon dried

Optional: 2 to 4 cups cooked pasta, shells or bow-ties; 2 ounces grated cheddar cheese; hot red pepper flakes; 1/2 cup marsala wine

1. In a large stock pot, place the chicken breasts, broth, carrots, tomatoes, garlic, beans, and seasonings (and wine) in the water or broth. Cover and bring to a boil, reduce the heat, and simmer for about 20 minutes or until done.

2. Remove the chicken pieces from the broth and set them aside to cool. Keep the broth warm over low heat. (Optional: Add the cooked pasta.)

3. Dice the chicken into small pieces. Return it to the soup and heat it through.

4. Garnish with grated cheese and red pepper flakes, if desired.

Yield: 4 servings

Nutrition Information: Total calories 1,200
Calories per serving: 300

Nutrients	Grams
Carbohydrate	33
Protein	35
Fat	3

TURKEY TERIYAKI

Although the recipe calls for the turkey to marinate for several hours, you can coat it in the marinade and then sauté or grill it right away—and it'll taste just fine!

This recipe also works equally well with chicken and shrimp, and goes nicely with rice and broccoli. If desired, you can skewer it on a stick for easier grilling.

1 pound turkey or chicken cutlets

Marinade:
2 tablespoons soy sauce, regular or low sodium
2 tablespoons cooking sherry or apple juice
1 teaspoon ground ginger
1 tablespoon oil, preferably canola
1 teaspoon brown sugar

Optional: 1/2 teaspoon pepper; 1/4 teaspoon garlic powder or
     1 clove garlic, minced

1. In a medium bowl, combine the soy sauce, cooking sherry, ginger, oil, and brown sugar (and pepper and garlic, as desired).
2. Add the turkey and mix well.
3. If time allows, cover and refrigerate for several hours or overnight.
4. Sauté in a nonstick skillet or grill until the meat is no longer pink on the inside.

Yield: 4 servings

Nutrition Information: Total calories: 840
                             Calories per serving: 210

Nutrients	Grams
Carbohydrate	2
Protein	35
Fat	7

TURKEY PICCATA

This goes well with pasta, roasted potato, or rice. The recipe can also be made with chicken breasts.

2 tablespoons oil, olive or canola
1 pound mushrooms, sliced
1 1/2 pounds turkey breast, flattened to 1/4-inch thickness
3 tablespoons dry madeira wine
1 to 3 tablespoons lemon juice
1/4 cup chicken broth

Optional: 1/4 cup fresh diced parsley or lemon slices for garnish

1. In a nonstick skillet, add 1 tablespoon oil and the sliced mushrooms. Sauté over medium-high heat for about 5 minutes. Remove the mushrooms from the pan and set aside.
2. Heat the second tablespoon oil in the skillet and add 1 or 2 pieces of turkey breast, sautéing for 2 to 3 minutes per side. Transfer the turkey to a plate and keep it in a warm oven while sautéing the remaining pieces.
3. Drain any excess oil from the pan and stir in the wine, lemon juice, and chicken broth, scraping off any browned bits. Boil the sauce for a few minutes until it is slightly thickened.
4. Pour the sauce over the turkey, top with the mushrooms, and garnish with fresh parsley and lemon slices, if desired.

Yield: 4 servings

Nutrition Information: Total calories: 1,000
Calories per serving: 250

Nutrients	Grams
Carbohydrate	4
Protein	36
Fat	10

COUNTRY PASTA WITH TURKEY SAUSAGE AND WHITE BEANS

This recipe is versatile and allows for being creative: you can make it without the turkey sausage, without the beans, or with different protein sources, such as ground beef, diced chicken, tofu, or seafood.

When I make this, I like to remove the casing from the sausage by cutting it with a sharp knife and then scrambling the sausage meat. The alternative is to cook the sausage whole, then cut it into coins.

1 pound turkey sausage, casing removed
12 ounces uncooked pasta, such as shells, ziti, or rotini.
1 14-ounce can diced tomatoes, drained
1 15-ounce can white canellini beans, drained
1 1/2 tablespoons cornstarch mixed into
1 1/2 cups milk, low-fat
1/4 cup grated parmesan or romano cheese

Optional: 1 small onion, diced; 1-2 cloves garlic, minced;
1/8 teaspoon crushed red pepper flakes; salt and pepper

1. Heat a large nonstick skillet and add the turkey sausage (and onion, garlic, and red pepper flakes) and cook over medium heat for about 10 minutes or until done.
2. While the sausage is cooking, cook the pasta according to package directions; drain.
3. To the scrambled sausage, add the drained diced tomatoes and canellini beans. Heat through, then add the cornstarch-milk mixture. Stir until thickened, then add the parmesan cheese.
4. Add the cooked pasta; toss well and let set for a few minutes for the flavors to blend. Adjust the seasonings with salt and pepper.

Yield: 5 large servings

Nutrition Information: Total calories: 2,500
Calories per serving: 500

Nutrients	Grams
Carbohydrate	75
Protein	25
Fat	11

TURKEY MEATBALLS
OR TURKEY BURGERS

This recipe works well for either meatballs or burgers. Adding oatmeal makes the burgers juicier than when they're made with plain ground turkey. It also works well with extralean ground beef, but when feeding people who don't eat red meat, these turkey burgers or meatballs will appeal to everyone.

1/3 cup oatmeal, uncooked
1/2 cup chicken broth, canned, homemade, or from bouillon cubes
1 pound ground turkey
1 egg or 2 egg whites
2 tablespoons grated onion
Salt and pepper as desired

Optional: 1/8 teaspoon nutmeg or 1/4 teaspoon allspice

1. In a medium bowl, combine the oatmeal, broth, turkey, egg, onion, and seasonings.
2. For meatballs: Shape into 1 1/2 inch meatballs, place on a nonstick cooking sheet, and bake at 350°F for 20 to 25 minutes. (Or, cook them in a nonstick skillet on the stovetop.)

   For burgers: Shape into 4 patties. Cook over medium-high heat in a nonstick skillet for about 5 minutes per side.

Yield: 4 servings

Nutrition Information: Total calories: 760
Calories per serving: 190

Nutrients	Grams
Carbohydrate	5
Protein	26
Fat	7

GROUND TURKEY MIX
FOR SPAGHETTI SAUCE OR CHILI

This recipe is popular with Sue Luke, RD, sports nutritionist in Charlotte, North Carolina. She makes double or triple this recipe and stores the extra in the freezer to use as needed. For example, it's a simple way to add protein to spaghetti sauce or soups. It also works well for sloppy joes and tacos.

1 1/2 pounds ground turkey
1 tablespoon oil, preferably olive or canola
1 small onion, chopped
1 small green pepper, chopped
8 ounces fresh mushrooms, chopped

1. In a large nonstick skillet, sauté the ground turkey until cooked. Transfer the turkey to a colander and let any excess fat drip away. Wipe the skillet.
2. In the same skillet, heat the oil and sauté the onions and green pepper until tender-crisp.
3. Add the mushrooms and continue cooking until the mushrooms are softened.
4. Return the turkey to the pan and mix well.
5. Either use immediately for spaghetti sauce or chili, or divide the mixture into the desired portion size, place in resealable plastic bags, and freeze for future use.

Yield: 4 servings

Nutrition Information: Total calories: 900
Calories per serving: 225

Nutrients	Grams
Carbohydrate	5
Protein	35
Fat	7

MEXICAN BAKED CHICKEN WITH PINTO BEANS

A spicy favorite! When cooking for myself, I wrap one piece of chicken, a quarter of a can of beans, and 1/4 cup of salsa in a piece of foil, bake it in the oven, and have no dishes to wash!

2 16-ounce cans pinto beans
4 pieces chicken, skinned
1 cup salsa

1. Drain the beans and put in the bottom of a baking dish.
2. Put the skinless chicken on top; pour salsa over beans and chicken.
3. Cover and bake in a 350°F oven for 25 to 30 minutes. If desired, bake uncovered the last 10 minutes to thicken the pan juices.

Yield: 4 servings

Nutrition Information: Total calories: 1,350
Calories per serving: 340

Nutrients	Grams
Carbohydrate	31
Protein	45
Fat	4

17

Fish and Seafood

Fish meals tend to be more popular in restaurants than at home, because many people don't know how to buy or prepare fish. The following tips will take the mystique out of fish cookery; fish is one of the easiest foods to prepare!

Fresh fish, when properly handled, has no fishy odor whether it is raw or cooked. The odor comes with aging and bacterial contamination. Whenever possible, ask to smell the fish you want to buy. Signs of freshness to look for are bulging eyes, reddish gills, and shiny scales that adhere firmly to the skin. After buying fresh fish, use it quickly, preferably within a day. Keep it in the coldest part of the refrigerator.

When buying commercially frozen fish, be sure the box is firm and square, showing no sign of thawing and refreezing. To thaw, defrost the fish in the refrigerator or microwave oven. Do not refreeze.

For each serving, allow one pound of uncooked whole fish (such as trout or mackerel) or 1/3 to 1/2 pound uncooked fish fillets or steaks (such as salmon, swordfish, halibut, or sole). To rid your hands of any fishy smell, rub them with lemon juice or vinegar. Wash cooking utensils with 1 teaspoon of baking soda per quart of water.

Here are a few tips to help you prepare your "catch."

- If possible, cook fish in its serving dish; fish is fragile, and the less it is handled the more attractive it is.
- Seasonings that go well with fish include lemon, dill, basil, rosemary, and parsley (and paprika for color).

- To test for doneness, gently pull the flesh apart with a fork. It should flake easily and not be translucent.
- Use leftover fish, warm or cold, in sandwiches as a change from chicken or turkey.

Here are four different ways to cook fish.

Broiling. Place fish on a broiling pan that has been lightly oiled or treated with cooking spray to prevent sticking, sprinkle with a little olive oil and seasonings (if desired), and place 4 to 6 inches from the heat source. Thin fillets (such as sole or bluefish) can be cooked in 5 minutes (without turning); thicker fillets (such as salmon or swordfish) may require about 5 or 6 minutes per side. Before broiling, spread with a mixture of equal parts low-fat mayonnaise and dijon mustard.

Baking. Set the fish in a baking dish that has been lightly oiled or treated with cooking spray, season as desired, cover, and bake at 400°F for 15 to 20 minutes, depending on thickness.

Poaching. Set the fish in a nonstick skillet, cover the fillets with water, white wine, or milk; season as desired, cover, and gently simmer on the stove top for about 10 minutes. For an Asian twist, add scallions and a little soy sauce.

Microwaving. If possible, place the thickest part of the fillet toward the outside of the dish, overlapping thin portions to prevent overcooking. Season as desired, cover with waxed paper, and microwave for the minimum amount of time to prevent the fish from turning tough and dry. Remove from the oven before the fish is totally cooked and allow it to stand for 5 minutes to finish cooking before serving. Whitefish fillets may need 4 minutes, salmon steaks 6 to 7 minutes.

CRUNCHY OVEN-BAKED FISH STICKS. 329
FISH AND SPINACH BAKE 330
SHRIMP FETTUCCINE 331
GREEK SHRIMP WITH FETA AND TOMATOES. 332
MEDITERRANEAN SHRIMP AND SCALLOPS WITH PASTA 333
FISH IN FOIL MEXICAN STYLE 334
SALMON PASTA SALAD. 335

See also: Chicken and Oriental Noodles in Peanut Sauce, Country Pasta With Turkey Sausage and White Beans, Turkey Teriyaki, Tofu Lo Mein

For additional recipes, see www.aboutseafood.com.

CRUNCHY OVEN-BAKED FISH STICKS

Most fried fish is cooked in fat that does not contribute to a heart-healthy diet. This recipe offers a low-fat alternative for fans of fried fish.

Many cereals make a nice topping for this fish dish, such as bran flakes or crushed shredded wheat. You can also use plain bread crumbs seasoned with grated parmesan cheese, garlic powder and oregano, or crushed Melba toast (see Oven-Fried Chicken on page 314).

1 pound fish fillets, cut into sticks
Salt and pepper as desired
2 to 4 teaspoons oil, preferably olive or canola
1/3 cup crispy rice cereal or cornflake crumbs

Optional: parsley flakes; parmesan cheese

1. Preheat the oven to 450°F.
2. Wash and dry the fish fillets. Cut into sticks.
3. Season with salt and pepper as desired; coat with the oil.
4. Dip the fish fillets into the cereal crumbs.
5. Arrange the fillets on shallow nonstick pan and bake for 12 minutes; don't turn.
6. Optional: Sprinkle with parsley flakes and/or parmesan cheese.

Yield: 2 servings

Nutrition Information: Total calories (made with cod): 480
Calories per serving: 240

Nutrients	Grams
Carbohydrate	8
Protein	40
Fat	5

FISH AND SPINACH BAKE

This recipe goes nicely with rice and a loaf of crusty whole-grain bread. If you want a fancier recipe, sauté 1/2 teaspoon of minced garlic, 1/2 pound of sliced mushrooms, and 1/4 teaspoon oregano in a little olive oil, then add that to the spinach before placing it in the baking dish.

1 10-ounce box frozen chopped spinach
1/2 cup (2 ounces) shredded mozzarella cheese
1 pound fish fillets
Salt, pepper, and lemon juice as desired

1. Preheat the oven to 400°F.
2. Thaw the spinach and squeeze out excess moisture. Spread on the bottom of a small baking dish.
3. Sprinkle with the cheese and top with the fish. Season as desired.
4. Cover with foil. Bake for 20 minutes, or until the fish flakes easily.

Yield: 2 servings

Nutrition Information: Total calories (made with cod): 560
Calories per serving: 280

Nutrients	Grams
Carbohydrate	6
Protein	50
Fat	6

SHRIMP FETTUCCINE

Yum! This is quick and easy, yet tasty enough to be a special company meal. Serve it with green vegetables (such as peas, green beans, or broccoli) that you steam while the pasta is cooking.

6 ounces pasta, preferably fettuccine
1 tablespoon margarine or olive oil
1 8-ounce package frozen, peeled, and deveined shrimp
1/2 teaspoon instant chicken bouillon granules or 1 cube
1 tablespoon cornstarch mixed into
1 cup milk, preferably low-fat
2 tablespoons grated parmesan cheese

Optional: 1 clove garlic, minced or 1/8 teaspoon garlic powder; 2 tablespoons white wine; tomatoes and parsley for garnish

1. In a large pot, cook the pasta according to package directions.
2. While the pasta is cooking, heat a large nonstick skillet, add the margarine, then the shrimp and chicken boullion (and garlic). Stir-fry for 3 to 4 minutes or until the shrimp turn pink.
3. Stir the cornstarch into the milk, then pour the mixture into the cooked shrimp. Cook, stirring constantly, until thick and bubbly. Stir in the cheese (and wine, as desired).
4. Add the cooked, drained pasta; toss to combine. Garnish with more parmesan, tomatoes, and parsley as desired.

Yield: 2 large servings

Nutrition Information: Total calories: 1,100
Calories per serving: 550

Nutrients	Grams
Carbohydrate	70 grams
Protein	40 grams
Fat	12 grams

GREEK SHRIMP
WITH FETA AND TOMATOES

Quick and easy, this goes nicely served over rice. Start the rice before you start makng the salad.

1 tablespoon oil
2 to 4 cloves garlic, chopped (or 1/4 teaspoon garlic powder)
1 pound cleaned, deveined shrimp
1 28-ounce can crushed or diced tomatoes
4 ounces feta cheese, crumbled

Optional: 1/2 cup chopped fresh parsley; 1/2 teaspoon dried oregano

1. In a nonstick skillet, heat the oil and sauté the garlic and shrimp until the shrimp turns pink, about 1 minute.
2. Add the tomatoes (and oregano) and simmer for 2 to 5 minutes.
3. Add the crumbled feta. Add the parsley just before serving.

Yield: 4 servings

Nutrition Information: Total calories: 1,000
One serving: 250 calories

Nutrients	Grams
Carbohydrate	9
Protein	28
Fat	11
With one cup of rice: 450 calories	
Carbohydrate	53
Protein	30
Fat	13

MEDITERRANEAN SHRIMP AND SCALLOPS WITH PASTA

This recipes uses pasta, but you could also serve it over (brown) rice. Feel free to be creative with the ingredients. You can use different types of seafood (clams, mussels, fish) as well as an assortment of vegetables (diced celery, green beans, etc.).

3/4 pound pasta, such as shells
0-1 tablespoons oil, as desired
1 28-ounce can diced tomatoes, drained
1 small green and/or red bell pepper, diced
1 cup white wine
2 teaspoons dried basil
1 bay leaf
Salt to taste
1 to 2 tablespoons corn starch
2 tablespoons water
1 pound scallops and/or shrimp

Optional: 1 small onion, chopped; 1 to 2 cloves garlic, minced or 1/4 teaspoon garlic powder

1. Cook the pasta according to the package directions.
2. If garlic and onions are desired, in a large skillet heat the oil and sauté the onions and garlic until tender, about 3 to 5 minutes.
3. In the skillet, add the tomatoes, bell pepper, wine, basil, bay leaf, and salt. Simmer uncovered for 10 minutes.
4. In a small bowl, dissolve the cornstarch in the water. Add the mixture to the skillet, stirring quickly until the broth thickens.
5. Add the scallops and/or shrimp. Cover and simmer for 3 to 5 minutes, or until the seafood is done. Serve over pasta.

Yield: 4 servings

Nutrition Information: Total calories: 2,100
Calories per serving: 525

Nutrients	Grams
Carbohydrate	83
Protein	30
Fat	8

FISH IN FOIL MEXICAN STYLE

Fish always comes out moist and flavorful when cooked in foil. For variety, you can bake the fish oriental style (with soy sauce, sesame oil, and scallions) or Italian style (with tomatoes, onions, and oregano). The recipe also works well with boneless, skinless chicken breasts.

The amount below is for two servings. Be sure to double it if you're feeding the family!

2 18-inch-long pieces of heavy duty foil
1 pound white fish fillets
1/2 cup salsa

Optional: 1 diced green pepper and 1 diced small onion, sautéed in 1 teaspoon olive oil; 1/8 teaspoon garlic powder; salt and pepper; low-fat grated cheddar cheese

1. If desired, sauté the onion and pepper in olive oil.
2. In the middle of the foil, place 1/2 pound of fish. Cover with 1/4 cup salsa (add peppers, onions, and other ingredients or seasonings, as desired).
3. Wrap by bringing together two edges of the foil, folding them over, then folding up the ends and crimping the edges.
4. Bake or grill the packets for 15 to 20 minutes. Lift with a spatula and open carefully, being sure to not burn yourself on escaping steam.

Yield: 2 servings

Nutrition Information: Total calories: 400
Calories per serving: 200

Nutrients	Grams
Carbohydrate	4
Protein	42
Fat	2

SALMON PASTA SALAD

Because the fat in oily fish such as salmon is health protective, the American Heart Association recommends two fish meals per week. This is a nice way to get one of them! The pasta is pretty to look at and tasty to eat; a nice light supper for two people.

1/2 pound salmon fillet
1 cup water
2 cups broccoli florets
2 medium carrots, thinly sliced diagonally
1 cup chicken broth, canned, homemade or from bouillon
1 tablespoon cornstarch mixed in 2 tablespoons broth or water
4 ounces (1 1/2 cups uncooked) pasta, spirals or shells

Optional: 1 to 2 teaspoons sesame oil

1. Cook the pasta according to the package directions.
2. Meanwhile place the salmon in a large nonstick skillet, add the water, cover, and bring to a boil. Reduce the heat and simmer for 10 to 12 minutes or until the fish flakes easily with a fork. Remove the salmon, let cool, then remove skin and flake the fish. Discard the water.
3. In a clean skillet, combine the broccoli, carrots, and chicken broth (and sesame oil). Cover, bring to a boil, reduce the heat, and simmer for 5 minutes or until the vegetables are just tender.
4. Combine the cornstarch with two tablespoons of broth or water. Stir into the vegetable mixture. Cook, stirring until the mixture thickens.
5. Add the cooked pasta and flaked salmon; combine gently.

Yield: 2 servings

Nutrition Information: Total calories: 920
Calories per serving: 460

Nutrients	Grams
Carbohydrate	60
Protein	26
Fat	13

18

Beef and Pork

Despite popular belief, lean beef and pork can be a part of a heart-healthy diet. They are excellent sources of protein, iron, and zinc—nutrients important for everyone, particularly athletes. The main health concern about red meat is its fat content. The solution is to choose lean cuts, trim the fat, and eat smaller portions.

These are the leanest cuts of beef:

- Top round roast and steak
- Bottom round roast
- Eye of the round
- Boneless rump roast
- Tip roast and steak
- Round, strip, and flank steak
- Lean stew beef

And here are the leanest cuts of pork:

- Sirloin roast and chops
- Loin chops
- Top loin roast
- Tenderloin
- Cutlets

Finally, the leanest cuts of ham:

- Lean and extralean cured ham (labeled 93- to 97-percent fat free)
- Center-cut ham
- Canadian bacon

For more information about iron and zinc, refer to the section on minerals in chapter 8.

ENCHILADA CASSEROLE 339
WARM TACO SALAD 340
SWEET AND SPICY ORANGE BEEF. 341
HONEY-GLAZED PORK CHOPS. 342
STIR-FRY PORK WITH FRUIT. 343

See also: Turkey Teriyaki, Chicken and Oriental Noodles in Peanut Sauce, Quick and Easy Chili, Ground Turkey Mix for Spaghetti or Chili, Mexican Tortilla Lasagna

For more beef and pork recipes, visit www.beef.org or www.otherwhitemeat.com.

ENCHILADA CASSEROLE

This particular recipe is made with beef, but you could just as easily make it with ground turkey, diced tofu, or kidney beans. For color, top the casserole with diced peppers.

1 pound extralean ground beef
28-ounce can diced tomatoes, drained (or fresh tomatoes, chopped)
10-ounce can enchilada sauce
16-ounce can refried beans, preferably low fat
6 ounces baked corn chips
4 ounces cheddar cheese, preferably reduced fat

Optional: 1 medium onion, chopped; 1 teaspoon chili powder; 1/2 teaspoon dried basil; 1 green pepper, diced

1. Brown the ground beef (and onion) in a large nonstick skillet.
2. Drain any fat, then add the diced tomatoes, enchilada sauce, and refried beans (and chili and basil, as desired). Heat until bubbly.
3. Preheat the oven to 350°F. Crumble the corn chips and spread all but 1 cup in the bottom of a 9″ × 13″ baking pan.
4. Pour the enchilada-beef sauce over the chips.
5. Grate the cheese and sprinkle it over the enchilada-beef sauce. Sprinkle with 1 cup corn chips (and diced green pepper, if desired).
6. Bake for 15 minutes or until the cheese is melted.

Yield: 6 servings

Nutrition Information: Total calories: 2,800
Calories per serving: 470

Nutrients	Grams
Carbohydrate	52
Protein	30
Fat	16

WARM TACO SALAD

This is a quick and easy Mexican dish that is popular after a busy day at work. You can also use leftover chili in place of the ground beef mixture. To boost the carbohydrate value, simply add an extra can of beans and a can of corn. If you prefer not to eat red meat, replace the beef with ground turkey—or eliminate it altogether.

1/2 to 1 pound extralean ground beef or turkey
1 packet taco seasoning mix
1 16-ounce can kidney beans, drained
6 ounces baked tortilla chips
4 ounces (1 cup) shredded low-fat cheddar cheese
4 cups shredded lettuce
2 medium tomatoes, diced

Optional: salsa; low-fat sour cream; guacamole

1. In a nonstick skillet brown the beef. Drain the fat.
2. Add the taco seasoning mix.
3. Add the beans and heat through.
4. In a 2-quart bowl or casserole dish, layer in order the tortilla chips, hot beef-bean mixture, cheese, lettuce, and tomatoes.
5. Top with a dollop of salsa, low-fat sour cream, or guacamole if desired. Serve warm.

Yield: 4 servings

Nutrition Information: Total calories: 1,700
Calories per serving: 425

Nutrients	Grams
Carbohydrate	47
Protein	30
Fat	13

SWEET AND SPICY ORANGE BEEF

Here's a welcome treat after a hard workout when you're hankering for something sweet but healthful. This goes nicely with cooked carrots and peas.

1 cup uncooked rice
1 pound extralean ground beef
1/4 cup orange marmalade
1/4 teaspoon red pepper flakes or dash cayenne pepper

Optional: cooked peas; diced celery; green peppers; pineapple chunks

1. Cook the rice according to package directions.
2. In a skillet, cook the beef until browned; drain fat.
3. To the beef, add the marmalade, red pepper flakes, and cooked rice. Mix well. Add optional ingredients as desired.

Yield: 3 servings

Nutrition Information: Total calories: 1,500
Calories per serving: 500

Nutrients	Grams
Carbohydrate	70
Protein	42
Fat	6

HONEY-GLAZED PORK CHOPS

The combination of honey, cinnamon, and applesauce makes a nice glaze for pork chops. Enjoy these with rice, using the pan juices as a gravy.

4 extralean pork chops or pork cutlets, well trimmed (about 5 ounces, raw)

For the glaze:
2 tablespoons honey
1/4 cup applesauce
1/4 teaspoon cinnamon
Salt and pepper, as desired

1. In a small bowl, combine the honey, applesauce, and cinnamon (and salt and pepper, as desired).

2. Heat a nonstick skillet, then brown the pork for 3 minutes on one side.

3. Turn the pork, then spoon the glaze on top. Cover and cook for 3 minutes.

4. Uncover and cook over medium-low heat for 10 minutes or until done, turning once.

5. Serve the pork with rice, spooning the glaze over both the rice and the pork.

Yield: 4 servings

Nutrition Information: Total calories: 1,000
Calories per serving: 250

Nutrients	Grams
Carbohydrate	10
Protein	30
Fat	10

STIR-FRY PORK WITH FRUIT

This is a popular family food that appeals to children and adults alike. Pineapple is a nice alternative or addition to the mandarin oranges.

1 pound boneless pork cutlets, trimmed and sliced into thin strips
1 teaspoon oil
1/2 cup water
1/4 cup vinegar
2 tablespoons molasses or honey
2 tablespoons soy sauce
1 11-ounce can mandarin oranges
1 tablespoon cornstarch mixed in 1 tablespoon water

Optional: pineapple chunks; green pepper chunks; 1 medium apple, diced; 1/4 cup raisins; 1/4 cup chopped toasted nuts

1. In a large nonstick skillet, heat the oil and add the sliced pork. Stir until browned.
2. Add the water, vinegar, molasses, soy sauce, and mandarin oranges (and pineapple, green pepper, apple, and raisins, as desired).
3. Bring to a boil; cover and simmer for 5 minutes.
4. Thicken the broth by slowly adding the cornstarch and water mixture and cooking until thickened to the desired consistency.
5. Sprinkle with chopped nuts, as desired.

Yield: 4 servings

Nutrition Information: Total calories: 1,200
Calories per serving: 300

Nutrients	Grams
Carbohydrate	30
Protein	25
Fat	8

19

Beans and Tofu

Beans—protein-rich foods with little fat and no cholesterol—are some of nature's greatest foods. They help lower blood cholesterol, control blood sugar, fight cancer, reduce problems with constipation, build muscles with their protein, fuel muscles with their carbohydrate, and nourish muscles with lots of B vitamins, iron, zinc, magnesium, copper, folic acid, and potassium.

Because beans are a healthful source of both protein and carbohydrate, vegetarian meals such as chili, hummus, bean and rice casseroles, and other bean meals are perfect for a sports diet. When beans are the only protein source, be sure to eat them in large quantities to consume adequate protein (see chapter 8). Or if you are a meat-eater who wants to become more of a vegetarian, replace part or all of the meat in recipes with more beans, such as replacing ground beef in chili or lasagna with kidney beans.

Canned beans or home-cooked dried beans are nutritionally similar. I generally use canned; they're quicker and more convenient. Dried beans (except for lentils) should be soaked overnight or for 6 to 8 hours in water at room temperature. This soak shortens the cooking time and improves the flavor, texture, and appearance of the beans. Soaking also reduces the beans' gas-causing qualities. If you want to speed the soaking process, add beans to a large pot of boiling water, boil them for 2 minutes, cover, then remove them from the heat and let stand for an hour. Drain and rinse them and then they'll be ready to cook.

Beans cook nicely in a crock-pot (5 to 10 hours, moderate heat) or pressure cooker (10 to 35 minutes), depending upon how much time you have to cook. Be sure to use a large enough kettle. Beans expand! You may also want to cook enough beans for more than one meal. They refrigerate and freeze well. For convenience, freeze them in individual portions.

Here are some suggestions on preparing and serving beans:

- In a blender, mix black or pinto beans, salsa, and cheese. Heat in the microwave and use as a dip or on top of tortillas or potatoes.
- Sauté garlic and onions in a little oil; add canned beans (whole or mashed), and heat together. Eat with rice or rolled in a tortilla.
- Add beans to salads, spaghetti sauce, soups, and stews for a protein booster.
- Make an easy burrito: top a tortilla with 1/2 can heated vegetarian refried beans, 1/2 cup cottage cheese, salsa, chopped lettuce, and tomato as desired. Roll into a burrito.
- Combine black beans, refried beans, and salsa to taste. Spoon onto a tortilla. Top with more salsa and cheese, as desired.

For more complete information about preparing homemade beans and creating bean dishes, read cookbooks that specialize in vegetarian cookery. Appendix A has some additional reading suggestions.

Tofu, also known as bean curd, is made from an extract of soybeans. It is a complete protein that contains all the essential amino acids. Tofu has no cholesterol and is relatively low in calories and sodium. Surprisingly, about half the calories in tofu come from fat—unsaturated fat, that is. Tofu is a popular alternative to meat, and can be a source of calcium for people who limit their intake of dairy foods. It is protective against heart disease and cancer and is a very healthful addition to your diet.

Tofu is found in most supermarkets in the refrigerated vegetable section. You can buy soft or firm tofu cakes that are packaged in water; be sure to check the "sell by" date, and buy the freshest brand. Soft or silken tofu is preferable for blending into a smooth cream; firm tofu is good to crumble or slice. To store tofu, drain off the water, place the tofu in a container with a tight lid, cover with fresh cold water, and keep it in the refrigerator. If you change the water every other day, it will keep up to a week without spoiling.

Tofu itself has very little flavor; it takes on the flavors of the foods with which it's prepared. For example, tofu mixed with soy sauce takes on a Chinese flavor; with chili, a Mexican flavor. Due to this versatility, tofu lends itself to many recipes: spaghetti, salads, chili, Chinese stir-fry, and even salad dressings. To achieve an interesting, spongy texture, freeze the tofu for at least two days. After it has thawed, squeeze out the water (as if it were a kitchen sponge), tear the tofu into chunks, and add them to spaghetti sauce, chili, soups, or other dishes.

MINESTRONE SOUP 348
PASTA AND WHITE BEAN SOUP WITH SUN-DRIED TOMATOES 349
QUICK AND EASY CHILI 350
MEXICAN TORTILLA LASAGNA 351
HUMMUS ROLL-UPS. 352
TOFU LO MEIN 353
TOFU BURRITOS 354

See also: Chicken Black Bean Soup, Country Pasta With Turkey Sausage and White Beans, Mexican Baked Chicken With Pinto Beans, Chicken and Oriental Noodles in Peanut Sauce, Diana's Soy Shake, Protein Shake, Quick and Easy Chili, Warm Taco Salad

For more recipes with beans and tofu, visit www.vegweb.com and www.vegancooking.com.

MINESTRONE SOUP

This soup offers an enjoyable way to boost your intake of not only beans but also vegetables. Feel free to vary the ingredients, depending on what's available. Serve with crusty whole-grain rolls.

2 to 4 tablespoons oil, preferably olive or canola
2 cloves garlic, minced or 1/2 teaspoon garlic powder
1 medium onion, diced
1 large carrot, diced
2 stalks celery, diced
2 large potatoes, diced
2 small zucchini, diced
4 to 6 mushrooms, diced
1 cup fresh or frozen green beans, cut into 1-inch pieces
1 28-ounce can diced tomatoes with liquid
6 cups broth (beef or vegetable) or water
1 19-ounce can cannellini beans (white kidney beans)

Optional: 2 teaspoons dried basil; 2 bay leaves; grated parmesan cheese

1. In a large pot, heat the oil and add the onions and garlic; sauté until the onions are softened.
2. Add the carrot, celery, potato, zucchini, mushrooms, green beans, tomatoes, broth (and basil and bay leaves). Bring to a boil, reduce the heat and simmer for about 30 minutes.
3. Add the cannellini beans and heat through. Adjust the seasonings.
4. Serve and sprinkle with parmesan cheese, as desired.

Yield: 6 large servings

Nutrition Information: Total calories: 1,300
Calories per serving: 220

Nutrients	Grams
Carbohydrate	36
Protein	10
Fat	4

PASTA AND WHITE BEAN SOUP WITH SUN-DRIED TOMATOES

This soup is delicious—worth the trip to the store to get the sundried tomatoes! If desired, add more beans and pasta—and even diced chicken—to the soup and you'll have a heartier meal.

1 tablespoon oil, preferably olive or canola
1 large onion, diced
1 medium carrot, diced
1/4 to 1/2 teaspoon red pepper flakes
1 12-ounce can cannellini beans, drained
5 cups chicken or vegetable broth, homemade, canned or from boullion
3 ounces (about 2/3 cup) dry bowtie or shell pasta
1/3 cup sun-dried tomatoes, diced
3 tablespoons fresh parsley

Optional: 1 clove garlic, minced or 1/4 teaspoon garlic powder; 1 bay leaf; grated parmesan cheese

1. In a large nonstick pot, heat the oil and sauté the onion, carrot, and red pepper flakes (and garlic). Cover and cook for 10 minutes, stirring occasionally.
2. Add the drained beans and broth (and bay leaf). Bring the soup to a boil.
3. Add the pasta and sun-dried tomatoes. Reduce the heat and simmer until the pasta is tender, about 10 minutes.
4. Season to taste with salt and pepper. Add the parsley. Serve with grated parmesan cheese.

Yield: 4 12-ounce servings

Nutrition Information: Total calories: 900
Calories per serving: 225

Nutrients	Grams
Carbohydrate	38
Protein	9
Fat	4

QUICK AND EASY CHILI

This is a simple family favorite. Although using packaged chili seasonings may seem like cheating, it actually simplifies the cooking process and perhaps enhances the likelihood you'll even make the recipe. Adding a second can of beans and halving the meat makes this a higher carbohydrate meal. You can also eliminate the beef and turkey and add tofu, if desired.

1 pound extralean ground beef or ground turkey
1 16-ounce can stewed tomatoes, preferably Cajun-style
1 16-ounce can beans, kidney or pinto
1 package chili seasonings, hot or mild
1 2/3 cup rice, uncooked

Optional: 1 11-ounce can corn, drained; 1 green pepper, diced

1. In a skillet with high sides, brown the beef or turkey. Drain the fat, if any.
2. Add the stewed tomatoes, beans, and chili seasonings (and corn and pepper). Bring the mixture to a boil, then reduce the heat.
3. Simmer for 5 to 50 minutes, depending on how much time you have.
4. While the chili is simmering, cook the rice according to package directions.
5. Serve the chili over rice.

Yield: 6 servings

Nutrition Information: Total calories without rice: 1,650
Calories per serving without rice: 275

Nutrients	Grams
Carbohydrate	20
Protein	24
Fat	11

Calories per serving with 1 cup rice: 480

Nutrients	Grams
Carbohydrate	64
Protein	27
Fat	13

MEXICAN TORTILLA LASAGNA

Tortillas are easy, precooked alternatives to lasagna noodles, and they taste great.

1 16-ounce container cottage cheese
1 16-ounce can kidney or pinto beans
1 tablespoon flour
1/4 teaspoon dried red pepper flakes or 1/8 teaspoon cayenne
Salt, pepper, and garlic powder, as desired
1 tablespoon chili powder, as desired
6 tortillas, flour or corn

Sauce:
1 32-ounce can crushed tomatoes
2 tablespoons chili powder
1/4 teaspoon red pepper flakes
1 tablespoon molasses

Optional: 1 10-ounce package frozen chopped spinach or broccoli, cooked; 1 cup chopped mushrooms, peppers, or other vegetables; 1 cup corn; 1 pound extralean ground beef or turkey, browned and drained

1. Mix together the cottage cheese, beans, flour, and seasonings (and vegetables and meat, as desired).
2. Make sauce by combining the tomatoes and seasonings.
3. Preheat the oven to 375°F.
4. In a 9" × 13" nonstick pan or casserole dish, alternate layers of sauce, tortillas, and cheese mixture. Top with sauce.
5. Bake, covered, for 30 minutes. Let stand about 5 minutes before cutting into squares.

Yield: 4 servings

Nutrition Information: Total calories: 1,800
Calories per serving: 450

Nutrients	Grams
Carbohydrate	70
Protein	27
Fat	7

HUMMUS ROLL-UPS

Traditional hummus, made with olive oil and tahini, can be a surprisingly high-fat meal. This recipe reduces the fat.

The secret ingredient in hummus is tahini, or sesame paste. You can buy tahini in the ethnic food section of larger supermarkets or health food stores. Store leftover tahini in the refrigerator and use it for other dishes, such as Sesame Pasta With Broccoli on page 296.

1 16-ounce can chickpeas
1 to 2 tablespoons lemon juice, bottled or fresh
1 clove garlic or 1/4 teaspoon garlic powder to taste
2 to 4 tablespoons tahini or peanut butter
Salt and pepper as desired
8-inch tortillas, preferably whole-wheat

Optional: dash of cayenne; 1 tablespoon parsley; 1/4 teaspoon cumin; diced or shredded vegetables for topping

1. Drain the chickpeas, saving 1/4 cup of the liquid.
2. In a blender or food processor, mix the chickpeas, 1/4 cup liquid, lemon juice, garlic, tahini, and seasonings.
3. Blend until smooth. If you don't have a blender, mash the chickpeas with the back of a fork.
4. Spread 1/3 cup hummus on a tortilla. Add 1/2 cup diced or shredded vegetables of your choice: tomato, pepper, scallion, beans, nuts, carrot, lettuce.

Yield: about 1 1/2 cups hummus

Nutrition Information:

Total calories: 625
Calories per serving (1/3 cup): 125

Nutrients	Grams
Carbohydrate	18
Protein	5
Fat	4

In tortilla roll-up (with 1/2 cup hummus):

Nutrients	Grams
Calories:	300
Carbohydrate:	49
Protein:	8
Fat:	8

TOFU LO MEIN

This versatile recipe can be made according to your tastes—with extra veggies, hot pepper, or garlic. You can also replace the tofu with chicken, shrimp, beef, or just vegetables. If the noodles seem dry, add a little water or broth.

9 ounces Chinese noodles (or 4 ounces dry spaghetti)
4 teaspoons oil, preferably half sesame, half canola
1/2 to 3/4 teaspoon ground ginger or 2 teaspoons fresh chopped ginger
1/4 to 1/2 teaspoon garlic powder or 1 to 2 cloves garlic, minced
2 to 4 cups shredded napa cabbage or bok choy
1 large carrot, grated
8 ounces extra-firm tofu, drained and cut into 1/2 inch cubes
2 tablespoons soy sauce or tamari sauce

Optional: 1/8 teaspoon of sugar (adds a nice hint of sweetness); dash hot pepper flakes; 4 scallions, chopped; 1 to 2 cups diced mushrooms, onions, pea pods, peppers, and/or other vegetables of your choice; sunflower seeds or sliced almonds for garnish

1. Cook the noodles according to the package directions. Drain, return to the pot, and using two knives as scissors, cut them into smaller, more manageable pieces.

2. While the noodles are cooking, in a large nonstick skillet heat the 4 teaspoons of oil, then add the ginger, garlic powder, cabbage, and carrots (and sugar, hot pepper, and vegetables). Stir-fry over medium-high heat for 1 to 2 minutes.

3. Add the soy sauce and cubed tofu. Stir-fry for another 1 to 2 minutes, or until the vegetables are tender-crisp.

4. Add the noodles, toss well, adjust the seasonings, then serve.

Yield: 5 servings as a side dish; 3 large servings as a main dish

Nutrition Information: Total calories: 1,500
Calories per serving: 300 (side dish)

Nutrients	Grams
Carbohydrate	35
Protein	10
Fat	13

TOFU BURRITOS

This is a simple lunch, dinner—or even breakfast. I like it with a dollop of hummus.

2 teaspoons margarine or olive oil
1 small onion, diced
1 green pepper, diced
1 cake (14 ounces) firm tofu, crumbled
4 tortillas, white, whole wheat, or corn, warmed
Salt and pepper, to taste

Optional: raisins, chopped walnuts, and curry powder; sesame seeds, sesame oil (instead of margarine), and soy sauce; garlic powder; hummus

1. In a nonstick skillet, melt the margarine, add the onion and green pepper. Sauté until tender.
2. Add the crumbled tofu and desired seasonings; heat thoroughly.
3. Place 1/4 of the mixture in the middle of a tortilla, fold over one end, fold in the sides, and roll up.

Yield: 4 small servings (or two large)

Nutrition Information: Total calories: 1,200
Calories per serving: 300

Nutrients	Grams
Carbohydrate	40
Protein	15
Fat	9

20

Beverages and Smoothies

Beverages are not only a way to quench your thirst and replace fluids lost through sweat, but also a way to refuel your muscles with carbohydrates. Some of the smoothies can even be a quick meal—to say nothing of boosting your fruit intake at the same time.

To spur your creativity, here are a few smoothie suggestions. If you don't have frozen fruit handy, you can add ice cubes to the smoothie for that cool and frosty feeling.

- Frozen strawberries + banana + milk powder + orange juice
- Vanilla yogurt + instant coffee powder (decaf or regular) + ice cubes
- Frozen raspberries + silken tofu + cranberry juice + honey
- Frozen banana chunks + orange juice + pineapple juice + protein powder
- Soy milk + peaches + vanilla low-fat frozen yogurt

HOMEMADE SPORTS DRINK 356
FRUIT SMOOTHIE 357
DIANA'S SOY SHAKE 358
PROTEIN SHAKE 359
THICK AND FROSTY MILKSHAKE 360

355

HOMEMADE SPORTS DRINK

The nutritional profile of commercial sports drinks is 50 to 70 calories per 8 ounces, with about 110 milligrams sodium. Below is a simple recipe that offers this profile, but at a much lower cost than the expensive store-bought brands. You can make it without the lemon juice, but the flavor will be weaker.

You can be creative when making your own sports drink. For example, you can dilute many combinations of juices (such as cranberry + lemonade) to 50 calories per 8 ounces and then add a pinch of salt. Some people use flavorings such as sugar-free lemonade to enhance the flavor yet leave the calories in the 50 to 70 calories per 8-ounce range. The trick is to always test the recipe during training, not during an important event. You want to be sure it tastes good when you are hot and sweaty and settles well when you're working hard.

1/4 cup sugar
1/4 teaspoon salt
1/4 cup hot water
1/4 cup orange juice (*not* concentrate) plus 2 tablespoons
  lemon juice
3 1/2 cups cold water

1. In the bottom of a pitcher, dissolve the sugar and salt in the hot water.
2. Add the juice and the remaining water; chill.
3. Quench that thirst!

Yield: 1 quart

Nutrition Information: Total calories: 200
Calories per 8 ounces: 50

Nutrients	Grams
Carbohydrate	12
Sodium	110 mg

FRUIT SMOOTHIE

Fruit smoothies are popular for breakfasts and snacks. The ingredients can vary according to individual tastes. Some tried-and-true combinations include banana and strawberries in orange juice and melon and pineapple in pineapple juice. Almost any combination works!

For a thick, frosty shake, use fruit that has been frozen. To have fruit ready for blending into a smoothie, simply slice a surplus of ripe fresh fruit (that might otherwise spoil) into chunks, then freeze the chunks on a flat sheet. When frozen, pack them into ziplock bags. (If you freeze them in the bag, you'll end up with one big chunk of frozen fruit that is hard to break apart.)

1/2 cup low-fat yogurt (plain or flavored) or milk
1 cup fruit juice
1/2 to 1 cup fruit, fresh, frozen, or canned

Optional: 1/4 cup milk powder; dash cinnamon or nutmeg; sweetener as desired

1. Place all ingredients in a blender, cover, and whip until smooth.

Yield: 1 serving

Nutrition Information: Calories per serving: 220-290

Nutrients	Grams
Carbohydrate	50-60
Protein	5
Fat	0-3

DIANA'S SOY SHAKE

Diana Dyer, RD, a nutritionist and three-time cancer survivor, swears by this smoothie! It's full of vitamins, minerals, fiber, calcium, and health-protective phytochemicals. Diana enjoys it for breakfast every day. She drinks about half the shake right away, often accompanying it with a whole-grain bagel. Then she puts the rest of the shake in an insulated coffee mug to carry with her "on the go," sipping it through a straw over the next hour or so. Many people have told her how tasty the shake is and additionally, how "energizing" it is. She invites you to drink to your health and enjoy it! Her book *A Dietitian's Cancer Story* and her Web site (www.CancerRD.com) offer more anti-cancer food suggestions.

3/4 cup soy milk, preferably calcium fortified
3/4 cup orange juice, preferably calcium fortified
1 to 2 tablespoons* wheat or oat bran
1 to 2 tablespoons* wheat germ
1 to 2 tablespoons* whole flaxseed or ground flaxseed meal
2 to 3 ounces soft tofu
6-8 baby carrots or one large raw carrot, chopped
3/4 cup fresh or frozen fruit

* Increase the fiber content gradually, starting with a scant tablespoon each of the wheat bran, wheat germ, and flaxseed. Take a few weeks to work up to 2 tablespoons of each.

1. In a blender, combine the milk and juice. Turn on the blender, and carefully add the bran, wheat germ, and flax. (This keeps the dry ingredients from sticking to the side of the blender.)
2. Stop the blender, then add the tofu, carrots, and fruit. Cover and blend on high until smooth.
3. If the shake is too thick, thin with a little juice, soy milk, milk, water, or even iced green tea.

Yield: about 3 cups

Nutrition Information: Approximate calories: 450

Nutrients	Grams
Carbohydrate	65
Protein	25
Fat	10

PROTEIN SHAKE

This shake is a simple way to boost not only protein and calcium but also your intake of health-protective tofu (see chapter 2). This recipe uses silken tofu, which has about 5 grams of protein per quarter-cake. Extra-firm tofu has more protein (10 grams per quarter-cake), but it blends poorly. Dry milk powder, with 8 grams of protein per quarter-cup, boosts protein as well.

1/4 cake silken tofu
1/3 cup dried milk powder
1 cup low-fat milk
2 tablespoons chocolate milk powder

1. Combine ingredients in a blender.
2. Cover and blend for 1 minute, or until smooth.

Yield: 1 serving

Nutrition Information: Total calories: 350

Nutrients	Grams
Carbohydrate	52
Protein	26
Fat	4

THICK AND FROSTY MILKSHAKE

This thick and tasty milkshake is a healthful alternative to ones made with ice cream. The instant pudding adds a nice thick texture and the ice cubes make it frosty and refreshing. I like to make these for my kids—an enjoyable way to boost their protein and calcium intake.

By varying the flavor of the pudding (vanilla, lemon, chocolate), you can create numerous variations. You can also add fruit (preferably frozen chunks) for extra nutritional value.

Note: The shake thickens upon standing; you can add more (or less) pudding mix, depending on how thick you like your shakes. If there are pieces of ice cubes remaining in the shake, worry not—they'll just keep the beverage cool.

1 cup low-fat milk
1/4 cup instant pudding
1/4 cup powdered milk mix
3 ice cubes

Optional: 1/2 to 1 cup (frozen) fruit chunks

Place all ingredients in a blender and blend until smooth.

Yield: 1 serving

Nutrition Information: Total Calories: 280

Nutrients	Grams
Carbohydrates	55
Protein	15
Fat	—

21

Snacks and Desserts

Snacks and desserts are major parts of Americans' meal style. Fresh fruits are ideal choices for either, yet there is a time and a place for other sweets. The trick is to choose snacks and desserts low in fat and high in carbohydrates. These recipes provide healthy alternatives to empty-calorie temptations.

Remember, peanut butter is a staple for hungry athletes who want a satisfying, wholesome snack. Although peanut butter is fat-laden, it can healthfully fit into the fat budget for most sports diets (see chapter 2 for more information about dietary fat goals). If you are a peanut butter lover, the following ideas might add some variety to your sports snacks.

Bread or tortillas with peanut butter and any of these ingredients make a nice snack.

- Jelly (of course!)
- Honey
- Cinnamon or cinnamon sugar
- Applesauce, raisins, and cinnamon
- Raisins
- Banana slices
- Apple slices

- Sprouts
- Granola or sunflower seeds
- Cottage cheese
- Dill pickle slices (no kidding!)

You can also make yourself a homemade milkshake by combining 1 cup milk, 1 banana, 1 tablespoon peanut butter, and sweetener as desired.

OATMEAL COOKIES 363
PEANUTTY ENERGY BARS 364
SUGAR AND SPICE TRAIL MIX 365
SPICED WALNUTS 366
PEANUT BUTTER BANANA ROLL-UP 367
APPLE CRISP 368
PEACH CRUMBLE 369
PEAR UPSIDE-DOWN GINGERBREAD CAKE 370
CARROT CAKE 371
CHOCOLATE LUSH 373

See also: Fruit Smoothie, Thick and Frosty Milkshake

For more recipes for desserts with fruit, see www.aboutproduce.com.

OATMEAL COOKIES

These cakey, low-fat cookies digest easily and are good for a pre-exercise snack or recovery food. The recipe makes about 5 dozen cookies—enough to feed the whole team! If you are cooking for yourself, you might want to cut the recipe in half.

1 1/4 cup milk
1 cup oil, preferably canola
2 eggs or 4 egg whites
2 teaspoons vanilla
3/4 cup white sugar
1 cup packed brown sugar
4 cups uncooked oatmeal
2 teaspoons baking soda
2 teaspoons salt
2 teaspoons cinnamon
3 cups flour, half whole-wheat, half white, as desired
1 cup raisins

1. Preheat the oven to 350°F.
2. In a large bowl, mix together the milk, oil, sugar, oatmeal, eggs, and vanilla. Beat well.
3. Add the soda, salt, and cinnamon and mix well, then gently stir in the flour, then raisins.
4. Drop by rounded tablespoons onto an ungreased baking sheet.
5. Bake for 15 to 18 minutes or until firm when lightly tapped with a finger.

Yield: 5 dozen cookies

Nutrition Information: Total calories: 6,500
Calories per cookie: 110

Nutrients	Grams
Carbohydrate	16
Protein	2
Fat	4

PEANUTTY ENERGY BARS

This prizewinning recipe offers a yummy alternative to commercial energy bars. They are perfect for when you are hiking or biking, as well as for a satisfying afternoon snack. They are relatively high in fat—but it's healthful fat from peanuts and sunflower seeds.

For variety, you can make this recipe with cashews and cashew butter, and/or add a variety of dried fruits (cranberries, cherries, and dates).

1/2 cup salted dry-roasted peanuts
1/2 cup roasted sunflower seed kernels or use more peanuts or other nuts
1/2 cup raisins or other dried fruit
2 cups uncooked oatmeal, old-fashioned or instant
2 cups toasted rice cereal, such as Rice Krispies
1/2 cup peanut butter, crunchy or creamy
1/2 cup packed brown sugar
1/2 cup light corn syrup
1 teaspoon vanilla

Optional: 1/4 cup toasted wheat germ

1. In a large bowl, mix together the peanuts, sunflower seeds, raisins, oatmeal, and toasted rice cereal (and wheat germ). Set aside.

2. In a medium microwaveable bowl, combine the peanut butter, brown sugar, and corn syrup. Microwave on high for 2 minutes. Add vanilla and stir until blended.

3. Pour the peanut butter mixture over the dry ingredients and stir until coated.

4. For squares, spoon the mixture into an 8" × 8" pan coated with cooking spray; for bars spoon it into a 9" × 13" pan. Press down firmly. (It helps to coat your fingers with margarine, oil, or cooking spray.)

5. Let stand for about an hour, then cut into squares or bars.

Yield: 16 squares or bars

Nutrition Information: Total calories: 3,600
Calories per serving: 225

Nutrients	Grams
Carbohydrate	30
Protein	6
Fat	9

Courtesy of the National Peanut Board, Atlanta, GA

SUGAR AND SPICE TRAIL MIX

Shannon Weiderholt, RD, found this recipe on the American Heart Association's Web site, www.deliciousdecisions.com. She says it's a perfect snack for calming the afternoon munchies, be you on the trail, at home, or at work. Keep this in a resealable plastic bag in your desk drawer or gym bag and you'll have energy to enjoy your day! It's sweet, but not too sweet.

3 cups oat squares cereal
3 cups mini-pretzels, salted or salt-free, as desired
2 tablespoons tub margarine, melted
1 tablespoon packed brown sugar
1/2 teaspoon cinnamon
1 cup dried fruit bits or raisins

1. Preheat oven to 325°F.
2. In a large resealable plastic bag or plastic container with a cover, combine the oat squares and pretzels.
3. In a small microwavable bowl, melt the margarine, then add the brown sugar and cinnamon. Mix well, then pour over the cereal mixture.
4. Seal the bag or container and shake gently until the mixture is well coated. Transfer to a baking sheet.
5. Bake uncovered for 15 to 20 minutes, stirring once or twice.
6. Let cool, then add the dried fruit.
7. Store in an airtight container or smaller single-serving bags.

Yield: 10 servings

Nutrition Information: Total calories: 2,000
Calories per serving: 200

Nutrients	Grams
Carbohydrate	40
Protein	5
Fat	2

Recipe courtesy of the American Heart Association (www.deliciousdecisions.com)

SPICED WALNUTS

Walnuts (and other nuts) are a health-protective addition to your daily diet, helping to reduce the risk of heart disease. Nuts are also a satisfying snack, and when eaten in a portion that fits within your calorie budget, can provide sustained energy and curb the cookie monster.

This recipe offers a spicy alternative to plain nuts. If you are not a curry fan, you can delete the curry powder and add a Mexican blend (1/2 teaspoon each garlic powder and cumin, 1/8 teaspoon cayenne pepper, as well as the sugar and salt).

1 egg white, slightly beaten
1 teaspoon curry powder
1 teaspoon cumin
1/2 teaspoon salt
1 teaspoon sugar
2 cups walnut halves and pieces

1. Preheat oven to 350°F.
2. In a medium bowl, mix egg white with spices. Stir in the walnuts and coat thoroughly.
3. Spread on a nonstick baking sheet. Bake for 15 to 18 minutes or until dry and crisp. Cool completely before serving.

Yield: 8 servings

Nutrition Information: Total calories: 1,750
Calories per serving (1/4 cup): 220

Nutrients	Grams
Carbohydrate	4
Protein	6
Fat	20

PEANUT BUTTER BANANA ROLL-UP

This snack is popular with the family of Anne Fletcher, RD, author of *Sober for Good*. Kids of all ages enjoy it not only for an afternoon energy booster but also for a simple breakfast or dinner.

1 10-inch flour tortilla, white or whole wheat
2 tablespoons peanut butter
1/2 medium banana, sliced into coins
1 tablespoon raisins

1. Warm tortilla in the microwave oven for 20 to 30 seconds or until soft.
2. Spread with peanut butter to within 1/2 inch of the edges.
3. Place the banana coins in the middle of the tortilla, sprinkle with raisins, and roll it up like a burrito.

Yield: 2 servings for a snack; 1 serving for a quick breakfast or supper

Nutrition Information: Total calories: 500 (whole recipe)

Nutrients	Grams
Carbohydrate	70
Protein	12
Fat	19

Adapted from Fletcher, A., *Sober for Good* (http://annemfletcher.com)

APPLE CRISP

When making apple crisp, I prefer to leave the peels on the apples for added fiber and nutrients. The small amount of spices allows for a nice apple flavor to shine through the "crisp." For a crisp topping, the margarine or butter should be thoroughly worked into the flour, coating each granule.

6 cups sliced apples, preferably half Granny Smith, half MacIntosh
1/4 cup sugar
1/2 cup flour
1/3 to 1/2 cup sugar, preferably half white, half packed brown sugar
1/4 teaspoon cinnamon
3 to 4 tablespoons margarine or butter, cold from the refrigerator

Optional: 3/4 cup chopped almonds or pecans; 1/4 teaspoon nutmeg; 1/4 teaspoon salt

1. Core, slice, and place the apples in an 8" × 8" baking pan. Coat with 1/4 cup sugar.
2. Heat oven to 375°F.
3. In a medium bowl, mix together the flour, sugar, and cinnamon (and nutmeg and salt). Add the margarine or butter, pinching it into the flour with your fingers until it looks like crumbly wet sand. Add nuts, as desired.
4. Distribute the topping evenly over the apples.
5. Bake for 40 minutes. If you want a crisper topping, turn the oven up to 400°F for the last five minutes.

Yield: 6 servings

Nutrition Information: Total calories: 1,560
Calories per serving: 260

Nutrients	Grams
Carbohydrate	50
Protein	1
Fat	6

PEACH CRUMBLE

As opposed to a "crisp," a crumble uses oats in the topping. This recipe works well with most canned fruits (pears, cherries) as well as 1 1/2 to 2 pounds (6 cups) of other fresh fruits (blueberries, apples) of your choice. If using tart fruit, you might want to sprinkle 1/4 cup sugar into the fruit.

1/4 cup flour, preferably half white, half whole-wheat
1/2 cup sugar, preferably half packed brown, half white
1 teaspoon cinnamon
1/4 cup margarine or butter
1 cup rolled oats or muesli with dried fruits and nuts
2 16-ounce cans sliced peaches, drained

Optional: 1/2 cup chopped nuts; 1/2 cup raisins; 1/4 teaspoon salt

1. In a medium bowl, combine the flour, sugar, and cinnamon.
2. Add the margarine or butter, pinching it with your fingers until the mixture is crumbly.
3. Add the oatmeal (and nuts and raisins) and mix well.
4. Place the peaches in an 8" × 8" square baking dish. Cut them into 1/2-inch pieces. Sprinkle the topping mixture over the fruit. Bake at 375°F for about 30-40 minutes, until the topping is browned.

Yield: 6 servings

Nutrition Information: Total calories: 1,300
Calories per serving: 215

Nutrients	Grams
Carbohydrate	32
Protein	3
Fat	8

PEAR UPSIDE-DOWN GINGERBREAD CAKE

Desserts can have nutritional value and still be fun to eat. This cake is one example: the pears sneak in some fruit, and the molasses a tiny bit of iron. Enjoy warm from the oven, with a small dollop of whipped cream.

1 teaspoon margarine
2 tablespoons sugar
2 fresh pears, peeled and diced or the equivalent in canned pears
1/2 cup brown sugar
1/2 cup molasses
1/4 cup oil, preferably canola
1 egg
2 teaspoons ground ginger
1/2 teaspoon salt
1 1/2 cups flour
1 teaspoon baking soda dissolved in 1/2 cup hot water

1. Using your fingers, rub the bottom of an 8" × 8" baking pan with the teaspoon of margarine. Sprinkle with 2 tablespoons of sugar.

2. Dice the pears and spread them on the bottom of the baking pan. (Use enough pears to cover the bottom. If you are creative, you can make a pretty design.)

3. In a medium bowl, mix together the brown sugar, molasses, oil, egg, ginger, and salt. Beat well.

4. Blend in the flour, then add the water with the baking soda.

5. Pour the batter over the pears and bake at 350°F for 30 to 40 minutes, or until you can touch the top of the cake with your fingertip and the cake bounces back without leaving a mark.

6. Remove from the oven and let the cake stand for 5 minutes. Loosen around the edges with a knife. Turn the cake out of the pan onto a plate or cooling rack.

Yield: 12 servings

Nutrition Information: Total calories: 2,400
Calories per serving: 200

Nutrients	Grams
Carbohydrate	38
Protein	3
Fat	4

CARROT CAKE

Sports nutritionist Jenny Hegmann, RD, suggests, if you are destined to eat cake, at least have one filled with fruit, vegetables, and nuts! This carrot cake recipe fills that bill. Unlike most carrot cakes that are extremely high in fat, Jenny's recipe offers a lower fat option—with a heart-healthful fat at that, canola oil.

1 1/2 cups sugar
3/4 cup oil, preferably canola
3 eggs or 6 egg whites
2 cups grated carrot, lightly packed
1 cup crushed canned pineapple with juice
2 teaspoons vanilla extract
1 teaspoon salt
1 teaspoon cinnamon
1 teaspoon baking powder
1/2 teaspoon baking soda
2 1/2 cups flour
Optional: 1 cup chopped walnuts; 1 cup raisins

Frosting:
4 ounces low-fat cream cheese, at room temperature
1/2 pound (2 1/2 cups) confectioners' sugar, sifted
1 teaspoon vanilla extract or 2 teaspoons grated orange peel
1 to 2 tablespoons milk or orange juice

1. Treat a 9" × 13" baking pan with cooking spray or line it with waxed paper.
2. Grate the carrots, then preheat the oven to 350°F.
3. In a medium mixing bowl, beat together the sugar and oil, then the eggs.
4. Add the grated carrot, pineapple and its juice, and 2 teaspoons of vanilla. Mix well.
5. Add the salt, baking powder, and baking soda (and cinnamon and nuts if desired). Gently blend in the flour, being careful not to overbeat.
5. Pour the batter into the prepared pan. Bake for 35 to 40 minutes. Cool completely before frosting.

6. In a small mixing bowl, beat the cream cheese and confectioners sugar. Add 1 teaspoon of vanilla and milk (or orange juice and grated orange peel), and beat until smooth, creamy, and the desired consistency.

7. Spread the frosting on the cake.

Yield: 24 pieces

Nutrition Information:

Total calories plain cake: 4,200
Calories per serving: 175

Nutrients	Grams
Carbohydrate	26
Protein	2
Fat	7

Nutrition Information:

Total calories with frosting: 5,500
Calories per serving: 230

Nutrients	Grams
Carbohydrate	37
Protein	3
Fat	8

CHOCOLATE LUSH

What I like best about this brownie pudding is it's a low-fat yet tasty treat for those who want a chocolate fix. It forms its own sauce during baking. If you need to rationalize eating chocolate, remember it does contain some health-protective phytochemicals!

1 cup flour
3/4 cup sugar
2 tablespoons unsweetened dry cocoa
2 teaspoons baking powder
1 teaspoon salt
1/2 cup milk
2 tablespoons oil, preferably canola
2 teaspoons vanilla
3/4 cup brown sugar
1/4 cup unsweetened dry cocoa
1-3/4 cups hot water

Optional: 1/2 cup chopped nuts.

1. Preheat the oven to 350°.
2. In a medium bowl, stir together the flour, white sugar, 2 tablespoons cocoa, baking powder, and salt; add the milk, oil, and vanilla (and nuts). Mix until smooth.
3. Pour into an 8" × 8" square pan that is nonstick, lightly oiled, or treated with cooking spray.
4. Combine the brown sugar, 1/4 cup cocoa, and hot water. Gently pour this mixture on top of the batter in the pan.
5. Bake at 350°F for 40 minutes, or until lightly browned and bubbly.

Yield: 9 servings

Nutrition Information: Total calories: 2,100
Calories per serving: 230

Nutrients	Grams
Carbohydrate	46
Protein	3
Fat	4

Appendix A

RECOMMENDED READING

This list provides additional reading for many of the topics discussed in this book. Some of the books are classics; some are new releases. A few titles are primarily for professionals, but most are appropriate for the public. You can look for the books in your local library or bookstore. Alternatively, many are available through the following sources of reliable nutrition materials:

Nutrition Counseling and Education Services (NCES)
1904 East 123rd Street, Olathe, KS 66061-5886
877-623-7266, on the Web: www.ncescatalog.com

Gurze Eating Disorders Resource Catalogue
PO Box 2238, Carlsbad, CA 92018
800-756-7533, on the Web: www.bulimia.com

Adult Children of Alcoholics

Garner, A., and J. Woititz. 1990. *Lifeskills for Adult Children*. Deerfield Beach, FL: Health Communications.

Woititz, J. 2002.*The Complete Adult Children of Alcoholics Sourcebook: Adult Children at Home, at Work and In Love*. Deerfield Beach, FL: Health Communications.

Body Image

Cash, T. 1997. *Body Image Workbook: An 8-Step Program for Learning to Like Your Looks*. Oakland, CA: New Harbinger.

Freedman, R. 2002. *BodyLove: Learning to Like Our Looks and Ourselves*. Carlsbad, CA: Gurze Books.

Hirschmann, J., and C. Munter. 1995. *When Women Stop Hating Their Bodies*. New York: Ballantine.

Johnson, C. 2001 *Self-Esteem Comes in All Sizes: How to Be Happy and Healthy at Your Natural Weight*. Carlsbad, CA: Gurze Books.

Maine, M. 2000. *Body Wars: Making Peace with Women's Bodies*. Carlsbad, CA: Gurze Books.

Pope, H., K. Phillips, and R. Olivardia. 2000. *The Adonis Complex: The Secret Crisis of Male Body Obsession.* New York: The Free Press.

Calories

Netzer, C. 2000. *The Complete Book of Food Counts.* New York: Dell.

Pennington, J. 1998. *Bowes & Church's Food Values of Portions Commonly Used, 17th Edition.* Philadelphia: Lippincott.

Cancer

Dyer, D. 2002. *The Dietitian's Cancer Story: Information and Inspiration for Recovery and Healing.* Ann Arbor, MI: Swan Press

Weihofen, D., and C. Marino. 2002. *The Cancer Survival Cookbook: 200 Quick and Easy Recipes with Helpful Eating Tips.* New York: John Wiley.

Children

Friedman, S. 2001. *When Girls Feel Fat: Helping Girls Through Adolescence.* Toronto: HarperCollins.

Jennings, D., and S.N. Steen. 1995. *Play Hard, Eat Right: A Parent's Guide to Sports Nutrition.* Minneapolis: Chronimed.

Levine, J., and L. Bine. 2001. *Helping Your Child Lose Weight the Healthy Way.* New York: Citadel Press.

Litt, A. 2000. *The College Student's Guide to Eating Well on Campus.* Bethesda, MD: Tulip Hill Press.

Satter, E. 1999. *Secrets of Feeding a Healthy Family.* Madison, WI: Keley Press.

Satter, E. 2000. *Child of Mine: Feeding With Love and Good Sense.* Palo Alto, CA: Bull.

Ward, E. 2002. *Healthy Foods, Healthy Kids: A Complete Guide to Nutrition for Children From Birth to Six Years Old.* Avon, MA: Adams Media.

Cookbooks (See also Vegetarian)

American Heart Association. 2000. *AHA Meals in Minutes Cookbook: Over 200 All New Quick and Easy Low-Fat Recipes.* New York: Crown.

Bittman, M. 1998. *How to Cook Everything: Simple Recipes for Great Food.* New York: Macmillan.

Foco, Z. 1998. *Lickety-Split Meals.* Walled Lake, MI: ZHI.

Pivanka, E., and B. Berry. 2002. *5 a Day: The Better Health Cookbook.* Emmaus, PA: Rodale.

Ponichtera, B. 1995. *Quick and Healthy Recipes and Ideas.* The Dalles, OR: Scale-Down.

Diabetes

American Diabetes Association. 1999. *The American Diabetes Association's Ultimate Home Guide to Diabetes.* Alexandria, VA: American Diabetes Association.

Colberg, S. 2000. *The Diabetic Athlete.* Champaign, IL: Human Kinetics

Eating Disorders

Hirschmann, J., and C. Munter. 1989. *Overcoming Overeating: Living Free in a World of Food.* New York: Fawcett/Columbine.

Hirschmann, J., and C. Munter. 1995. *When Women Stop Hating Their Bodies: Freeing Yourself From Food & Weight Problems.* New York: Ballantine.

LoBue, A., and M. Marcus. 1999. *The Don't Diet, Live-It! Workbook: Healing Food, Weight and Body Issues.* Carlsbad, CA: Gurze.

Normandi, C.E., and L. Roark. 1999. *It's Not About Food: End Your Obsession With Food and Weight.* New York: Penguin Putnam.

Otis, C., and R. Goldingay. 2000. *The Athletic Woman's Survival Guide: How to Win the Battle Against Eating Disorders, Amenorrhea and Osteoporosis.* Champaign, IL: Human Kinetics.

Pope, H. 2000. *The Adonis Complex: The Secret Crisis of Male Body Obsession.* New York: The Free Press.

Roth, G. 1986. *Breaking Free From Compulsive Eating.* New York: Signet.

Roth, G. 1992. *When Food Is Love.* New York: Penguin.

Siegel, M., J. Brisman, and M. Weinshel. 1997. *Surviving an Eating Disorder: Perspectives and Strategies for Family and Friends.* New York: HarperPerennial.

Eating Disorders (Primarily for Professionals)

American Dietetic Association. 2001. "Nutrition Intervention in the Treatment of Anorexia Nervosa, Bulimia Nervosa and Eating Disorders Not Otherwise Specified." *Journal of the American Dietetic Association* 101: 810-819.

Costin, C. 2000. *Eating Disorders Sourcebook: A Comprehensive Guide to the Causes, Treatment and Prevention of Eating Disorders.* Los Angeles: Lowell House.

Katrina, K., N. King, and D. Hayes. 1996. *Moving Away From Diets: New Ways to Heal Eating Problems and Exercise Resistance.* Lake Dallas, TX: Helm.

Thompson, R., and R. Trattner Sherman. 1993. *Helping Athletes With Eating Disorders.* Champaign, IL: Human Kinetics.

Woolsey, M. 2002. *Eating Disorders: A Clinical Guide to Counseling and Treatment.* Chicago: American Dietetic Association.

Ergogenic Aids

Bahrke, M., and C. Yesalis. 2002. *Performance Enhancing Substances in Sport and Exercise.* Champaign, IL: Human Kinetics.

Exercise Addiction

Prussin, E. 1992 *Hooked on Exercise: How to Understand and Manage Exercise Addiction.* New York: Simon & Schuster.

Exercise Physiology

McArdle, W., F. Katch, and V. Katch. 2001. *Exercise Physiology: Energy, Nutrition and Human Performance.* Philadelphia: Lippincott, Williams and Wilkins.

Wilmore, J., and D. Costill. 1999. *Physiology of Sport and Exercise.* Champaign, IL: Human Kinetics.

General Nutrition

Duyff, R. 2002. *The American Dietetic Association's Complete Food & Nutrition Guide,* Second Edition. New York: John Wiley & Sons.

Heber, D. 2002. *What Color Is Your Diet?: The 7 Colors of Health.* New York: Regan Books.

Margen, S. 2002. *Wellness Foods A to Z: An Indispensable Guide for Health-Conscious Food Lovers.* New York: Rebus.

Tribole, E. 2000. *Stealth Health: How to Sneak Nutrition Painlessly Into Your Diet.* New York: Penguin.

Willett, W. 2001. *Eat, Drink and Be Healthy: The Harvard Medical School Guide to Healthy Eating.* New York: Simon & Schuster.

Good Health

Nelson, M., and J. Knipe. 2002. *Strong Women Eat Well.* New York: Berkley Publishing Group.

Webb, D., and E. Ward. 1999. *Super Nutrition After 50.* Lincolnshire, IL: Publications International Ltd.

Herbs

Foster, S., and V. Tyler. 1999. *Tyler's Honest Herbal.* Binghamton, NY: Hawarth.

Menopause

Laux, M., and C. Conrad. 1998. *Natural Women, Natural Menopause.* New York: HarperCollins.

Love, S., and K. Lindsey. 1998. *Dr. Susan Love's Hormone Book: Making Informed Choices About Menopause.* New York: Random House.

Nelson, M., and S. Wernick. 2001. *Strong Women, Strong Bones: Everything You Need to Know to Prevent, Treat, and Beat Osteoporosis.* New York: Perigree.

Newsletters

Environmental Nutrition
PO Box 420235, Palm Coast, FL 32142-0235
800-829-5384, on the Web: www.environmentalnutrition.com

Georgia Tech Sports Medicine & Performance Newsletter
PO Box 420235, Palm Coast, FL 32142-0235
800-783-4903

Tufts University Diet and Nutrition Letter
PO Box 57857, Boulder, CO 80322-7857
800-274-7581, on the Web: www.healthletter.tufts.edu

University of California at Berkeley Wellness Letter
Subscription Department, PO Box 420148, Palm Coast, FL 32142
386-447-6328, on the Web: www.berkeleywellness.com

Pregnancy

Erick, M. 1993. *No More Morning Sickness: A Survival Guide for Pregnant Women.* New York: Penguin.

Luke, B., and T. Eberlein. 1999. *When You Are Expecting Twins, Triplets or Quads.* New York: HarperPerennial.

Swinney, B. 2000. *Eating Expectantly: The Essential Eating Guide and Cookbook for Pregnancy.* New York: Simon & Schuster

Waterhouse, D. 2002. *Outsmarting the Female Fat Cell—After Pregnancy: Every Woman's Guide to Shaping Up, Slimming Down, and Staying Sane After the Baby.* New York: Hyperion.

Self-Improvement

Prochaska, J., J. Norcross, and C. DiClemente. 1994. *Changing for Good.* New York: Morrow, William & Co.

Sports Nutrition

Applegate, L. 2001. *Eat Smart, Play Hard.* Emmaus, PA: Rodale.

Benardot, D. 2000. *Nutrition for Serious Athletes.* Champaign IL: Human Kinetics.

Clark, N. 2002. *Nancy Clark's Food Guide for Marathoners: Tips for Everyday Champions.* Newton, MA: Sports Nutrition.

Coleman, E., and S. Nelson Steen. 2000. *Ultimate Sports Nutrition.* Palo Alto, CA: Bull.

Dorfman, L. 2000. *The Vegetarian Sports Nutrition Guidebook.* New York: Wiley & Sons.

Eberle, S. 2000. *Endurance Sports Nutrition.* Champaign, IL: Human Kinetics

Kleiner, S.M., and M. Greenwood-Robinson. 1998. *Power Eating.* Champaign, IL: Human Kinetics

Rosenbloom, K., ed. 2000. *Sports Nutrition: A Guide for Professionals Working With Active People.* Chicago: American Dietetic Association.

Vegetarian (See also Sports Nutrition)

Havala, S. 2001. *Being Vegetarian for Dummies.* New York: John Wiley.

Krizmanic, J. 2000. *The Teen's Vegetarian Cookbook.* New York: Viking Press.

Lappe, F.M. 2002. *Hope's Edge: The Next Diet for a Small Planet.* New York: Jeremy P. Tarcher.

Melina, V., B. Davis, and V. Harrison. 1995. *Becoming Vegetarian: The Complete Guide to Adopting a Healthy Vegetarian Diet.* Summertown, TN: Book Publishing Company.

Weight Control

Fletcher, A. 1998. *Eating Thin for Life: Food Secrets & Recipes From People Who Have Lost Weight & Kept It Off.* Boston: Houghton Mifflin.

Fletcher, A. 2001 *Thin for Life.* Boston: Houghton Mifflin.

Kirby, J. 1998. *Dieting for Dummies.* New York: John Wiley.

Kostas, G. 2001. *The Cooper Clinic Solution to the Diet Revolution.* Dallas: Good Health Press.

Tribole, E., and E. Resch. 1995. *Intuitive Eating: A Recovery Book for the Chronic Dieter.* New York: St. Martin's Press.

Appendix B

FOR MORE INFORMATION

The following list offers you numerous Web sites and newsletters as additional resources for quality nutrition, sports nutrition, and health information. The list reflects information gathered in September 2002. It is by no means complete; many other excellent resources and Web sites are available. For a more comprehensive list of nutrition-related Web sites, go to www.navigator.tufts.edu, the Tufts University Nutrition Navigator, which offers reviews and rankings of the quality of nutrition information. For a site with answers to any and all of your nutrition questions, go to www.nutrition.gov.

Because I am frequently asked how to become a sports nutritionist, I have included at the end of this appendix some information on starting down that road. Health professionals who want sports nutrition teaching materials can find handouts and slides on my Web site, www.nancyclarkrd.com.

Aging

www.healthandage.com

An exceptional resource to help you or your aging parents find answers to the nutrition, fitness, and health questions and concerns of older people. People with failing eyesight can even select a large type size to allow them to read the information more easily.

Alcohol

www.ncadd.org

The National Council on Alcoholism and Drug Dependence

www.smartrecovery.org, www.AddictionAlternatives.com, www.alcoholics-anonymous.org, www.secularsobriety.org, www.unhooked.com, www.moderation.org

All these Web sites offer helpful resources for people who want to stop drinking and for their loved ones.

Body Image (see also Eating Disorders)

www.bodypositive.com

Dedicated to boosting body image at any weight, this site offers over 200 ways to love the body you have, message boards, and helpful affirmations.

www.about-face.org

This Web site promotes positive self-esteem in women of all ages through a spirited approach to media education.

Clothing

www.raceready.com

This site has running shorts and other exercise apparel with pockets for holding sports foods.

Cancer (See also Healthy Eating)

www.cancer.org

The American Cancer Society's site has answers to all your questions about prevention and treatment, as well as how to maintain an exercise program during treatment.

www.aicr.org

The American Institute for Cancer Research offers dietary information about eating for a healthier life, including information on the New American Plate.

www.CancerRD.com

Diana Dyer, MS, RD, a three-time cancer survivor, offers nutrition information and inspiration for people with cancer who want to optimize their diets.

Children and Nutrition

www.nutritionexplorations.com

This site offers nutrition education activities for kids, as well as information for parents, teachers, and school food service staff about ways to improve children's eating practices.

www.kidnetic.com

This site was designed to promote healthful eating and physical activity among kids and parents.

Complementary and Alternative Medicine (See also Herbs, Medicinal)

www.nccam.nih.gov

National Center for Complementary and Alternative Medicine

http://dietary-supplements.info.nih.gov

The Office of Dietary Supplements offers information about alternative medicine, herbs, and dietary supplements.

Diabetes

www.ndep.nih.gov

The National Diabetes Education Program, part of the National Institute of Diabetes, Digestive and Kidney Disease (NIDDK) offers abundant information on how to improve diabetes care.

www.diabetes.org

The American Diabetes Association offers abundant information and resources for diabetes care.

www.hopewarshaw.com

Hope Warshaw is a respected diabetes educator, registered dietitian, and author.

Dietary Analysis and Nutrition Assessment

www.usda.gov/cnpp

Created by the USDA's Center for Nutrition Policy and Promotion, this Web site offers an interactive healthy eating index. You can assess 25 nutrients in your diet and see how your food choices stack up against the Food Guide Pyramid.

http://hin.nhlbi.nih.gov/menuplanner/menu.cgi

This menu planner lets you select a calorie level and plan meals with portions of the correct size.

www.nat.uiuc.edu

The Nutrition Analysis Tool offers both an energy calculator (to determine your calorie needs) and a way to assess your diet.

Eating Disorders

www.nationaleatingdisorders.org

The National Eating Disorders Association offers information about eating disorders and body image, and provides a referral network and educational materials for schools.

www.bulimia.com

This Web site offers information about eating disorders and a bookstore with more than 200 titles on eating disorders.

www.somethingfishy.org

Inspired by a woman who recovered from anorexia, this site offers a wellspring of hope and inspiration, as well as a referral network.

Exercise (See also Weight Management)

www.acsm.org *(click on Health and Fitness Information)*

The American College of Sports Medicine is the largest group of sports-medicine and sports-science professionals.

www.fitlinxx.com

This site offers a plethora of exercise advice for beginner and experienced exercisers alike.

www.justmove.org

This site, sponsored by the American Heart Association, offers exercise guidance to improve the fitness and health of people who want to start an exercise program.

www.wellcoach.com

Associated with the American College of Sports Medicine, this site offers personal coaching for your exercise program for a fee.

Food Information

www.ific.org

The International Food Information Council offers information about all aspects of food.

Food Labels

www.cfsan.fda.gov/~dms/foodlab.html

Sponsored by the USDA Center for Food Safety and Applied Nutrition, this site offers a comprehensive guide to understanding food labels. The entire site abounds with nutrition information.

Healthy Eating

www.americanheart.org *(click on Healthy Lifestyle, then Diet & Nutrition)*

Sponsored by the American Heart Association, this site allows you to search for nutrition information about your food of interest (soy, fish, eggs, and so on) to determine how they can fit into a heart-healthy food plan.

www.nal.usda.gov/fnic *(click on Consumer Corner, then Nutrition Over the Lifecycle)*

The National Agricultural Library's Food and Nutrition Information Center features dietary guidelines for infants, children, teens, adults, and seniors, and offers abundant links to other sites with information about health and nutrition.

www.aboutproduce.com

Sponsored by the Produce Marketing Association and the Produce for Better Health Foundation, this Web site offers comprehensive information on fruits, vegetables, health, and nutrition, including recipes, nutritional content, and answers to frequently asked questions.

www.5aday.gov

The National Cancer Institute's Web site offers practical advice for eating better to reduce your risk of cancer.

www.aboutseafood.com

Sponsored by the National Fisheries Institute, this site offers recipes and information about fish.

www.mayoclinic.com *(click on Healthy Living)*

The Mayo Clinic offers information on nutrition, fitness, sports nutrition, and sports medicine—and even recipes.

Herbs, Medicinal (See also Complementary and Alternative Medicine)

www.amfoundation.org *(click on HerbMed)*

The nonprofit Alterative Medicine Foundation, Inc. provides a consumer-friendly, scientific database regarding the use of herbs for health.

Hoaxes

www.quackwatch.com

This site offers an excellent guide to health fraud and quackery, and enhances your ability to make intelligent decisions regarding sports supplements and herbs.

www.healthfactsandfears.com

Sponsored by the American Council on Science and Health, this site provides answers to a multitude of nutrition and health concerns.

Hypertension and the DASH Diet

www.nhlbi.nih.gov *(click on Health Information, then Heart and Vascular Disease)*

Sponsored by the National Heart, Lung, and Blood Institute of the National Institutes of Health, this site offers abundant information on how to control high blood pressure.

Medical Information

www.WebMD.com

This site offers the latest medical information and helpful nutrition information.

www.medem.com *(click on Library Entry)*

Sponsored by the nation's medical societies, this site provides a full range of patient information.

Menopause

www.menopause.org

Sponsored by the North American Menopause Society, this site is devoted to promoting women's health through menopause and beyond.

www.power-surge.com

This site has been praised as a powerfully effective support group for perimenopausal women.

Pregnancy

www.morningsickness.net

This site is by Miriam Erick, RD, an expert in prenatal nutrition and morning sickness.

www.drbarbaraluke.com

This site is by Dr. Barbara Luke, RD, a nutrition expert for women expecting twins, triplets, and quads.

Recipes (See also Vegetarian Nutrition)

www.nal.usda.gov/fnic *(click on Consumer Corner)*

The National Agricultural Library's Food and Nutrition Information Center offers an extensive list of links to sites that have healthful recipes, including abundant information about meal planning, shopping, food, and cooking.

www.mealsforyou.com

You can search for recipes according to calories, nutrition concerns (allergies, diabetes), preparation time, and more. Recipes are available to suit any need!

www.foodfit.com

This site offers an array of healthful recipes, cooking classes, information on family fitness, calorie expenditure, and nutrition information.

Sports Nutrition

www.ais.org.au *(click on Sports Science and Sports Medicine, then on Nutrition)*

The Australian Institute of Sport invests in the development of Olympic-caliber athletes and coaches. Their Web site offers excellent sports nutrition information, including advice about sports supplements.

www.nutrifit.org *(click on Nutrition Information)*

This is the professional Web site of the American Dietetic Association's practice group of Sports, Cardiovascular and Wellness Nutritionists (SCAN).

http://umass.edu/cnshp *(click on Newsletter)*

The Center for Nutrition in Sports & Human Performance at the University of Massachusetts sponsors this site.

www.gssiweb.com

The mission of the Gatorade Sports Science Institute is to share knowledge on sports nutrition and exercise science. The site offers an excellent and extensive resource for both professionals and the public.

www.ncaa.org *(go to the Index, click on N, and then Nutrition and Performance)*

Sponsored by the National Collegiate Athletic Association (NCAA), this site focuses on the sports nutrition concerns of student athletes.

www.nlm.nih.gov *(click on PubMed, then search on your topic of interest)*

The National Library of Medicine offers access to the latest research in medical and scientific journals.

Stress Management and Relaxation

www.meditationcenter.com

This Worldwide Online Meditation Center, designed for both novices and experienced meditators, includes different types of meditation rooms complete with audio for stress reduction, healing, and centering.

www.learningmeditation.com

This site includes a meditation room with audio and meditations to help you heal food issues.

Supplements (See also Herbs, Medicinal and Sports Nutrition)

www.nal.usda.gov/fnic *(click on Dietary Supplements)*

The National Agricultural Library's Food and Nutrition Information Center offers abundant information on the safe use of supplements as well as links to sites and sources with credible information.

http://ods.od.nih.gov/databases/ibids.html

Sponsored by the International Bibliographic Information of Dietary Supplements Database (IBIDS), this site contains published, peer-reviewed scientific literature on dietary supplements, including vitamins, minerals, and herbs. The site is a joint effort between the NIH's Office of Dietary Supplements and the National Agricultural Library's Food and Nutrition Information Center.

www.oznet.ksu.edu/nutrition/supplements.htm

Sponsored by the nutrition department at Kansas State University, this educational Web site provides journal references and online links to information about popular athletic supplements.

www.iahsaa.org *(click on Wellness)*

The Iowa High School Association has excellent information on creatine and androstenedione.

www.drugabuse.gov

The National Institute of Drug Abuse offers a program on the dangers of steroids.

www.supplementwatch.com

This site contains up-to-date scientific information about dietary supplements. Some of the information is free; some requires payment of an access fee.

www.ConsumerLab.com

ConsumerLab provides the results of dietary supplement testing for quality and purity.

Vegetarian Nutrition

www.vrg.org

This site is sponsored by the Vegetarian Resource Group, a nonprofit organization dedicated to educating the public on vegetarianism and the interrelated issues of nutrition, ecology, ethics, and world hunger.

www.vegweb.com

Sponsored by Veggies Unite! this Web site was designed to create an Internet vegetarian community. It offers 4,300 recipes, discussion boards, articles, book reviews, health information, and even veggie poetry.

www.vegancooking.com

This Web site provides simple recipes that taste great and contain ingredients that you can find in your local grocery or health-food store. The site also sells cookbooks.

Weight Management

www.thedietchannel.com

The site offers a free eight-week weight-loss program.

www.caloriescount.com, www.cyberdiet.com, www.dietwatch.com, www.ediets.com, www. miavita.com, www.nutrio.com, www.shapeup.org

For a fee, any of the above sites offer a personalized diet and exercise program, chat rooms, and support.

www.DietRiot.com

For a fee, this "final link to diet freedom" focuses on the nondiet path to no more dieting. It includes support groups, exercise, recipes, and humor.

How to Become a Sports Nutritionist

Every week I receive letters from people who have read my books or articles and want to know where they can go to school to learn more about nutrition and exercise. Some even want to become sports nutritionists. Here's what I tell them.

- To date, relatively few institutions have a sports-nutrition major, but many of the larger state universities do have departments in both nutrition and exercise science. You can often combine the two programs to create a major that suits your needs.

  For a list of academic programs in nutrition accredited and approved by the American Dietetic Association, visit their Web site (www.eatright.org) or write or call them:

  American Dietetic Association
  120 S. Riverside Plaza, Suite 2000
  Chicago, IL 60606
  312-899-0040

  For a list of academic programs in exercise science, you can visit the Web site of the American College of Sports Medicine (www.acsm.org) or write or call them:

  American College of Sports Medicine
  PO Box 1440
  Indianapolis, IN 46206-1440
  317-637-9200

  If you just want to further your personal knowledge, you can take one or two classes in nutrition or exercise science without committing to four years of advanced education. I recommend the full program, however, to people who want to develop a career in sports nutrition.

  If you want to become a sports nutritionist, you need not have a double major in nutrition and exercise science. Rather, you can major in nutrition and take two or three elective courses in exercise science. For example, my master's degree at Boston University is in nutrition, but I took several courses in exercise physiology.

- If you want to do nutrition counseling, you should become a registered dietitian (RD). This means that you will be recognized by the American Dietetic Association, the largest organization of nutrition professionals in the nation. Career doors will open up to you. Some people take short certificate courses, but these cannot match the education you receive in four years of undergraduate schooling, plus an internship and perhaps a master's degree in nutrition. Getting proper education and credentials is an important professional responsibility.

By becoming a registered dietitian, you will also be eligible to join SCAN, the special interest group of the American Dietetic Association that handles the nutritional aspects of sports, cardiovascular disease, wellness, and eating disorders. SCAN members are the leading sports nutritionists.

- Although your career goals may be to work with athletes and other active, healthy people, I strongly recommend that students and new graduates work first in a clinical setting, such as a hospital, to learn more about how to handle heart disease, diabetes, cancer, and many of the ailments of aging. This knowledge will help you keep people well and enhance your work experience. I strongly believe that one or two years of clinical work is a good investment in your career. I have no regrets about the time I spent working in hospitals. Sports nutrition is not an entry-level position.

- Most sports nutritionists practice what they preach and are familiar with the nutritional needs of a variety of sports. I've found that my personal interests in hiking, camping, bike touring, running, and marathoning have enriched the knowledge I can offer my clients. Being involved in sports adds to your credibility.

- Get involved as a volunteer for Little League, youth soccer, the YMCA, or any sport that interests you. Work on nutrition and fitness programs sponsored by the dietetic association or council on physical fitness in your state. Write articles for the local newspaper or the newsletter of your local bicycle or running club. By developing networks that will help you meet other local sports nutritionists and sports-medicine professionals, you might open doors that eventually lead to paid work.

- Although sports nutrition should be an integral part of most training programs, when it comes to finding a job you are still unlikely to see many "Sports Nutritionist Wanted" notices. Some places for you to try to create a job include health clubs, YMCAs, corporate wellness programs, sports-medicine practices, high schools, and college and university athletic departments. Be creative!

Most people knock on several doors before finding a welcoming venue. Or they make their own jobs using their personal contacts. For example, some registered dietitians who are mothers of teenage athletes have started sports-nutrition classes targeted to other parents, coaches, and students. Some RDs who love tennis, ballet, or gymnastics have become known as the sports nutritionist for their sport. Many who work out at a health club have started to work with the members of the club. You can create your dream job, and with lots of hard work and time, you'll achieve your goals. Be patient. No one becomes a sports nutritionist overnight.

Appendix C

SELECTED REFERENCES

Ackermark, C., I. Jacobs, M. Rasmussan, and J. Karlsson. 1996. Diet and muscle glycogen concentration in relation to physical performance in Swedish elite ice hockey players. *Int J Sports Nutr and Exerc Metab* 6 (3):272-284.

Ainslie, P., I. Campbell, K. Frayn, S. Humphreys, D. MacLaren, T. Reilly, and K. Westerterp. 2002. Energy balance, metabolism, hydration, and performance during strenuous hill walking: The effect of age. *J Appl Physiol* 93 (2):714-723.

Alford, B.A., A. Blankenship, and D.R. Hagen. 1990. The effects of variations in carbohydrates, protein, and fat content of the diet upon weight loss, blood values, and nutrient intakes of adult obese women. *J Amer Diet Assoc* 90:534-540.

American College of Sports Medicine Position Stand. 1998. The recommended quantity and quality of exercise for developing and maintaining cardiorespiratory and muscular fitness, and flexibility in healthy adults. *Med Sci Sports Exerc* 30 (6):975-991.

American College of Sports Medicine, American Dietetic Association, and Dietians of Canada. 2000. Joint Position Statement Nutrition and Athletic Performance. *Med Sci Sports Exerc* 32 (12):2130-2145.

American Psychiatric Association. 2000. *Diagnostic and statistical manual of mental disorders.* 4th ed. Washington, DC: American Psychiatric Association.

Armstrong, L. 2002. Caffeine, body fluid-electrolyte balance, and exercise performance. *Int J Sports Nutr and Exerc Metab* 12:189-206.

Bailey, W., D. Jacobsen, and J. Donnelly. 2002. Changes in total daily energy expenditure as a result of 16-months of aerobic training: The Midwest Exercise Trial. *Am J Clin Nutr* 75 (2S):363S (abstract P78).

Barr, S. 1999. Vegetarianism and menstrual cycle disturbances: Is there an association? *Am J Clin Nutr* 70 (suppl):549S-545S.

Barr, S., K.C. Janelle, and J.C. Prior. 1995. Energy intakes are higher during the luteal phase of ovulatory menstrual cycles. *Am J Clin Nutr* 61:39-43.

Beals, K., and M. Manore. 2000. Behavioral, psychological, and physical characteristics of female athletes with subclinical eating disorders. *Int J Sports Nutr and Exerc Metab* 10 (2):128-143.

Beals, K., and M. Manore. 2002. Disorders of the female athlete triad among collegiate athletes. *Int J Sports Nutr and Exerc Metab* 12:281-293.

Bell, D.G. and T.M. McLellan. 2002. Endurance execise 1, 3 and 6 h after caffeine ingestion on caffeine users and nonusers. *J Appl Physiol* 2002:93 (4): 1227-1234.

Bergstrom, J., L. Hermansen, E. Hultman, et al. 1967. Diet, muscle glycogen, and physical performance. *Acta Physiol Scand* 71:140-150.

Bernadot, D., (ed.) and Sports and Cardiovascular Nutritionists. 1992. *Sports nutrition:A guide for the professional working with active people.* 2d ed. Chicago: American Dietetic Association.

Blackburn, G. 2001. The public health implications of the Dietary Approaches to Stop Hypertension Trial. *Am J Clin Nutr* 74:1-2.

Bouchard, C. 1990. Heredity and the path to overweight and obesity. *Med Sci Sports Exerc* 23 (3):285-291.

Brouns, F., W. Saris, and N. Rehrer. 1987. Abdominal complaints and gastrointestinal function during long lasting exercise. *Intl J Sports Med* 8:175-189.

Brown, B.G., X.Q. Zhao, A. Chiat, et al. 2001. Simvastatin and niacin, antioxidant vitamins, or the combination for the prevention of coronary disease. *N Eng J Med* 345:1583-1592.

Burke, L.M., A. Classen, J.A. Hawley, and T.D. Noakes. 1998. Carbohydrate intake during prolonged cycling minimizes effect of glycemic index of preexercise meal. *J Appl Physiol* 85 (6):2220-2226.

Cable A., D. Neiman, M. Austin, E. Hogen, and A. Utter. 2002. Validity of leg-to-leg bioelectrical impedance measurement in males. *J Sports Med Phys Fitness* 41 (3): 411-414.

Casa D., L. Armstrong, S. Montain, B. Rich, R. Reiff, W. Roberts, and J Stone. 2000. National Athletic Trainers' Association position statement: Fluid replacement for athletes. *J Athletic Training* 35 (2):212-224.

Clark, N., M. Nelson, and W. Evans. 1988. Nutrition education for elite women runners. *Phys Sportsmed* 16:124-135.

Coggan, A. and E. Coyle. 1987. Reversal of fatigue during prolonged exercise by carbohydrate infusion or ingestion. *J Appl Physiol* 63:2388-2395.

Costill, D., R. Bowers, G. Branam, et al. 1971. Muscle glycogen utilization during prolonged exercise on successive days. *J Appl Physiol* 31:834-838.

Costill, D.L., D.S. King, R. Thomas, and M. Hargreaves. 1985. Effects of reduced training on muscular power in swimmers. *Phys Sportsmed* 13 (2):94-101.

Costill, D.L., W. Sherman, W. Fink, C. Maresh, M. Witten, and J Miller. 1981. The role of dietary carbohydrate in muscle glycogen resynthesis after strenuous exercise. *Am J Clin Nutr* 34:1831-1836.

Costill, D.L., R. Thomas, R.A. Robergs, D. Pascoe, C. Lambert, S. Barr, and W. Fink. 1991. Adaptations to swimming training: Influence of training volume. *Med Sci Sports Exerc* 23 (3):371-377.

Couzin, J. 2002. Nutrition research: IOM panel weighs in on diet and health. *Science* 297(5588):1399-1409.

Coyle, E.F., M. Hagberg, B. Hurley, W. Martin, A. Ehsani, and J Holoszy. 1983. Carbohydrate feeding during prolonged strenuous exercise can delay fatigue. *J Appl Physiol* 55 (1):230-235.

Coyle, E.F. and S.J. Montain. 1992. Benefits of fluid replacement with carbohydrates during exercise. *Med Sci Sports Exerc* 24 (suppl):324-330.

Dawson, D., C. Henry, C. Goodman, I. Gillam, J. Beilby, S. Ching, V. Fabian, D. Dasig, P. Morling, and B. Kakulus. 2002. Effect of C and E supplementation on biochemical and ultrastructural indices of muscle damage after a 21 km run. *Int J Sports Med* 23 (1):10-15.

Demura, S., S. Yamaji, F. Goshi, and Y. Nagasawa. 2002. The influence of transient change of total body water on relative body fats based on three bioelectrical impedance analyses methods. Comparison between before and after exercise with sweat loss, and after drinking. *J Sports Med Phys Fitness* 42 (1): 38-44.

Deutz, R., D. Benardot, D. Martin, and M. Cody. 2000. Relationship between energy deficits and body composition in elite female gymnasts and runners. *Med Sci Sports Exerc* 32 (3):659-668.

Dueck, C., K. Matt, M. Manore, and J. Skinner. 1996. Treatment of athletic amenorrhea with a diet and training intervention program. *Int J Sport Nutr and Exer Metab* 6 (1):24-40.

Expert Panel on Detection, Evaluation and Treatment of High Blood Cholesterol in Adults. 2001. Executive summary of the third report of the National Cholesterol Education Program Expert Panel on detection, evaluation, and treatment of high cholesterol in adults. *JAMA* 285:2486-2497.

Fairchild, T., S. Fletcher, P. Steele, C. Goodman, B. Dawson, and P. Fournier. 2002. Rapid carbohydrate loading after a short bout of near maximal-intensity exercise. *Med Sci Sports Exerc* 34 (6):980-986.

Fairfield, K., and R. Fletcher. 2002. Vitamins for chronic disease prevention in adults. *JAMA* 287 (23):3116-3126.

Fields, D., M. Goran, and M. McCrory. 2002. Body-composition assessment via air-displacement plethysmography in adults and children: A review. *Am J Clin Nutr* 75:453-467.

Garner, D. 1998. The effects of starvation on behavior: Implications for dieting and eating disorders. *Healthy Weight Journal* 12 (5):68-72.

Geleijnse, J., L. Launer, D. van der Kuip, A. Hofman, and J. Witteman. 2002. Inverse association of tea and flavinoid intakes with incident myocardial infarction: The Rotterdam Study. *Am J Clin Nutr* 75:880-886.

Gibson, A., V. Heyward, and C. Mermier. 2000. Predictive accuracy of Omron Body Logic Analyzer in estimating relative body fat of adults. *Int J Sports Nutr and Exerc Metab* 10:216-227.

Ginsberg, H.N., et al. 1995. Increases in dietary cholesterol are associated with modest increases in both LDL and HDL cholesterol in healthy young women. *Arteriosclerosis, Thromb, and Vasc Biol* 15:169-178.

Godard, M., D. Williamson, and S. Trappe. 2002. Oral amino-acid provision does not affect muscle strength or size gains in older men. *Med Sci Sports Exerc* 34 (7): 1126-1131.

Hawley, J.A. 2002. Effect of increased fat availability on metabolism and exercise capacity. *Med Sci Sports Exerc* 34 (9):1485-1491.

Hickner, R., C. Horswill, J. Welker, J. Scott, J. Roemmich, and D. Costill. 1991. Test development for the study of physical performance in wrestlers following weight loss. *Intl J Sports Med* 12 (6):557-562.

Hill, J.O., W. McArdle, J. Snook, and J. Wilmore. 1992. *Commonly asked questions regarding nutrition and exercise: What does the scientific literature suggest?* Vol. 9 of *Sports science exchange*. Chicago: Gatorade Sports Science Institute.

Hooper, S.L., L.T. Mackinnon, A. Howard, R. Gordon, and A. Bachmann. 1995. Markers for monitoring overtraining and recovery. *Med Sci Sports Exerc* 27 (1): 106-112.

Horowitz, J.F. and E.F. Coyle. 1993. Metabolic responses to preexercise meals containing various carbohydrates and fat. *Am J Clin Nutr* 58:235-241.

Houmard, J.A., D.L. Costill, J.B. Mitchell, S.H. Park, R.C. Hickner, and J.N. Roemmich. 1990. Reduced training maintains performance in distance runners. *Intl J Sports Med* 11 (1):46-52.

Hu, F., L. Bronner, W. Willett, M. Stampher, K. Rexrode, C. Albert, D. Hunter, and J. Manson. 2002. Fish and omega-three fatty acid intake and risk of coronary heart disease in women. *JAMA* 287:1807-1814.

Institute of Medicine. 2002. *Dietary reference intakes for energy, carbohydrate, fiber, fat, fatty acids, cholesterol, protein and amino acids.* Food and Nutrition Board. Washington, DC: National Academy Press.

Ivy, J. 2001. Dietary strategies to promote glycogen synthesis after exercise. *Can J Appl Physiol* 26 (suppl):S236-245.

Ivy, J., H. Goforth, B. Damon, T. McCauley, E. Parsons, and T. Price. 2002. Early postexercise muscle glycogen recovery is enhanced with a carbohydrate-protein supplement. *J Appl Physiol* 93 (4):1337-1344.

Janssen, G., C. Graef, and W. Saris. 1989. Food intake and body composition in novice athletes during a training period to run a marathon. *Int J Sports Med* 10: S17-21.

Kaiserauer, S., A. Snyder, M. Sleeper, and J. Zierath. 1989. Nutritional, physiological, and menstrual status of distance runners. *Med Sci Sports Exerc* 21 (2):120-125.

Kant, A., R. Ballard-Barbash, and A. Schatzkin. 1995. Evening eating and its relation to self-reported weight and nutrient intake in women, CSFII 1985-1986. *J Am College Nutr* 14 (8):358-363.

Keys, A., J. Brozek, A. Henschel, et al. 1950. *The biology of human starvation* Vols. I and II. Minneapolis: University of Minnesota Press.

Kilduff, L., P. Vidakovic, G. Cooney, R. Twycross-Lewis, P. Amuna, M. Parker, L. Paul, and Y. Pitsiladis. 2002. Effects of creatine on isometric bench-press performance in resistance-trained humans. *Med Sci Sports Exerc* 34 (7):1176-1183.

Kirk, E.P., J. Donnelly, and D. Jacobsen. 2002. Time course and gender effects in aerobic capacity and body composition for overweight individuals: Midwest Exercise Trial (MET). *Med Sci Sports Exerc* 34 (5S):S120 (abstract).

Kirwan, J.P., D. Cyr-Campbell, W.W. Campbell, J. Schreiber, and W. Evans. 2001. Effects of moderate and high glycemic index meals on metabolism and exercise performance. *Metabolism* 50 (7):849-855.

Knowler, W.C., E. Barrett-Conner, S.E. Fowler, R.F. Hamman, J.M. Lachin, E.A. Walker, and D.M. Nathan. 2002. Reduction in the incidence of type II diabetes with lifestyle intervention or metformin. *N Eng J Med* 346:393-403.

Kris-Etherton, P., W. Harris, and L. Appel. 2002. American Heart Association Scientific Statement: Fish consumption, fish oil, omega-3 fatty acids, and cardiovascular disease. *Circ* 106:2747-2757.

Kris-Etherton, P., G. Zhao, A.E. Binkoski, S.M. Coval, and T.D. Etherton. 2001. The effects of nuts on coronary heart disease. *Nutr Rev* 59 (4):103-111.

Kritchevsky, S., and D. Kritchevsky. 2000. Egg consumption and coronary heart disease: An epidemiologic overview. *J Am Coll. Nutr* 19 (5 suppl):549S-555S.

Leibel, R.L., M. Rosenbaum, and J. Hirsch. 1995. Changes in energy expenditure resulting from altered body weight. *N Engl J Med* 332:621-628.

Lemon, P. 1995. Do athletes need more protein and amino acids? *Intl J Sport Nutr* 5 (suppl):S39-S61.

Levine J., N. Eberhardt, and M. Jensen. 1999. Role of non-exercise activity thermogenesis in resistance to fat gain in humans. *Science* 282 (5399):212-214.

Loucks, A.B. 2001. Physical health of the female athlete: Observations, effects, and causes of reproductive disorders. *Can J Appl Physiol* 26 (suppl):S176-185.

Luscombe, N., P. Clifton, M. Noakes, B. Parker, and G. Wittert. 2002. The effects of energy-restricted diets containing increased protein on weight loss, resting energy expenditure and the thermic effect of feeding in type 2 diabetes. *Diabetes Care* 25:652-657.

Lutter, J. and S. Cushman. 1982. Running while pregnant. *J Melpomene Institute* 1 (1):2-4.

Malinow, M.R., M.D. Duell, D.L. Hess, et al. 1998. Reduction of plasma homocysteine levels by breakfast cereal fortified with folic acid in patients with coronary heart disease. *N Eng J Med* 338 (15):1009-1015.

Marchioli, R., C. Schweiger, G. Levantesi, L. Tavassi, and F. Valagussa. 2001. Antioxidant vitamins and prevention of cardiovascular disease: Epidemiological and clinical trial data. *Lipids* 36 (suppl):S53-63.

Mason, W.L., G. McConell, and M. Hargreaves. 1993. Carbohydrate ingestion during exercise: Liquid vs. solid feedings. *Med Sci Sports Exerc* 25 (8):966-969.

McManus, K. et al. 2001. A randomized controlled trial of a moderate fat, low-energy diet compared with a low-fat, low energy diet for weight loss in overweight adults. *Int J Obes Relat Metab Disord* 25:1503-1511.

Nativ, A. 2000. Stress fractures and bone health in track and field athletes. *J Sci Med Sport* 3 (3):268-279.

Nelson, M., M. Fiatarone, C. Morganti, I. Trice, R. Greenberg, and W. Evans. 1994. Effects of high-intensity strength training on multiple risk factors for osteoporosis fractures. *JAMA* 272 (24):1909-1914.

Nelson, M., E. Fisher, P. Catsos, et al. 1986. Diet and bone status in amenorrheic runners. *Am J Clin Nutr* 43:910-916.

Nieman, D., D. Henson, S. McAnulty, L. McAnulty, et al. 2002. Influence of vitamin C supplementation on oxidative and immune changes after an ultramarathon. *J Appl Physiol* 92 (5):1070-1077.

O'Dea, J. and P. Rawstorne. 2001. Male adolescents identify their weight gain practices, reasons for desired weight gain, and sources of weight gain information. *J Amer Diet Assoc* 101 (1):105-107.

Olivardia, R. 2002. Body image obsession in men. *Healthy Weight Journal* 16 (4): 59-63.

Pasman, W., M. van Baak, A. Jeukendrup, and A. de Haan. 1995. The effects of different dosages of caffeine on endurance performance time. *Intl J Sports Med* 16:225-230.

Pereira, M., D. Jacobs, J. Pins, S. Raatz, M. Gross, J. Slavin, and E. Seaquist. 2002. Effect of whole grains on insulin sensitivity in overweight hyperinsulinemic adults. *Am J Clin Nutr* 75:848-855.

Pereira, M., D. Jacobs, L. Van Horn, M. Slattery, A. Kartashov, and D. Ludwig. 2002. Dairy consumption, obesity and the insulin resistance syndrome in young adults. *JAMA* 287 (16):2081-2089.

Phillips, P., B. Rolls, J. Ledingham, et al. 1984. Reduced thirst after water deprivation in healthy elderly men. *N Engl J Med* 311:753-759.

Rasmussen, B., K. Tipton, S. Miller, S. Wolf, S. Owens-Stavoll, B. Petrini, and R. Wolfe. 2000. An oral essential amino acid-carbohydrate supplement enhances muscle protein anabolism after resistance exercise. *J Appl Physiol* 88:386-392.

Rauch, L.H.G., I. Rodger, G. Wilson, J. Belonje, S. Dennis, T. Noakes, and J. Hawley. 1995. The effects of carbohydrate loading on muscle glycogen content and cycling performance. *Intl J Sports Nutr* 5 (1):25-35.

Reuters News. 2001. Runners beware: Too much water can be dangerous. Ultramarathon World [Online], December 1. Available: www.ultramarathonworld.com/uw%5Farchive/n01de01a.html.

Sanborn, C.F. et al. 2000. Disordered eating and the female athlete triad. *Clin Sports Med* 19 (2):199-213.

Schabort, E., A. Bosch, S. Welton, and T. Noakes. 1999. The effect of a preexercise meal on time to fatigue during prolonged cycling exercise. *Med Sci Sports Exerc* 31 (3):464-471.

Schlundt, D.G., J.O. Hill, T. Sbrocco, J. Pope-Cordle, and T. Sharp. 1992. The role of breakfast in the treatment of obesity: A randomized clinical trial. *Am J Clin Nutr* 55 (3):645-651.

Sellmeyer, D., M. Schloetter, and A. Sebastian. 2002. Potassium citrate prevents increased urine calcium secretion and bone resorption induced by a high sodium chloride diet. *J Clin Endocrinol Metab* 87 (5):2008-12.

Sesso H., R. Pfaffenbarger, and I. Lee. 2000. Physical activity and coronary heart disease in men: The Harvard Alumni Health Study. *Circ* 102 (9):975-980.

Sherman, W., G. Brodowicz, D. Wright, W. Allen, J. Simonsen, and A. Dernbach. 1989. Effects of 4 h preexercise carbohydrate feedings on cycling performance. *Med Sci Sports Exerc* 21 (5):598-604.

Sherman, W., D. Costill, W. Fink, and J. Miller. 1981. Effect of exercise-diet manipulation on muscle glycogen and its subsequent utilization during performance. *Intl J Sports Med* 2:114-118.

Sherman, W., M. Pedan, and D. Wright. 1991. Carbohydrate feedings 1 hour before exercise improves cycling performance. *Am J Clin Nutr* 54:866-870.

Sherriffs, S. and R. Maughan. 1997. Restoration of fluid balance after exercise-induced dehydration: Effects of alcohol consumption. *J Appl Physiol* 83 (40):1152-1158.

Sims, E. 1976. Experimental obesity, dietary induced thermogenesis, and their clinical implications. *Clin Endo Metab* 5:377-395.

Sims, E. and E. Danforth. 1987. Expenditure and storage of energy in man. *J Clin Invest* 79:1-7.

Siris, E.S., P.D. Miller, E. Barrett-Connor, et al. 2001. Identification and fracture outcomes of undiagnosed low bone mineral density in postmenopausal women: results of the National Osteoporosis Risk Assessment. *JAMA* 286 (22):2815-2822.

Staten, M. 1991. The effect of exercise on food intake in men and women. *Am J Clin Nutr* 53:27-31.

Terjung R.L., P. Clarkson, R. Eichner, P.L. Greenhaff, P.J. Hespel, et al. 2000. American College of Sports Medicine Roundtable. The physiological and health effects of oral creatine supplements. *Med Sci Sports Exerc* 32 (3):706-717.

Thompson, J., M. Manore, J. Skinner, E. Ravussin, and M. Spraul. 1995. Daily energy expenditure in male athletes with differing energy intakes. *Med Sci Sports Exerc* 27 (3):347-354.

Torres, I.C., L. Mira, C.P. Ornelas, and A. Melim. 2000. Study of the effects of dietary fish intake on serum lipids and lipoproteins in two populations with different dietary habits. *Br J Nutr* 83 (4):371-379.

Tremblay, A., J. Despres, C. Leblanc, et al. 1990. Effect of intensity of physical activity on body fatness and fat distribution. *Am J Clin Nutr* 51:153-157.

Varner, L. 1995. Dual diagnosis: Patients with eating and substance-related disorders. *J Am Diet Association* 95 (2):224-225.

Weaver, C.M., D. Teegarden, R.M. Lyle, G.P. McCabe, et al. 2001. Impact of exercise on bone health and contraindication of oral contraceptive use in young women. *Med Sci Sports Exerc* 33:873-880.

Wee, S.L., C. Williams, S. Gray, and J. Horabin. 1999. Influence of low and high glycemic index meals on endurance running capacity. *Med Sci Sports Exerc* 31 (3):393-399.

Westerterp, K., G. Meijer, E. Janssen, W. Saris, and F. Ten Hoor. 1992. Long term effects of physical activity on energy balance and body composition. *Br J Med* 68 (1):21-30.

Wilmore, J., K. Wambsgans, M. Brenner, C. Broeder, I. Paijmans, J. Volpe, and K. Wilmore. 1992. Is there energy conservation in amenorrheic compared with eumenorrheic distance runners? *J Appl Physiol* 72 (1):15-22.

Wing, R.R., K.A. Matthews, L.H. Kuller, E.N. Meilahn, and P.L. Plantinga. 1991. Weight gain at the time of menopause. *Arch Intern Men* 151 (1):97-102.

Woolsey, M. 2001. *Eating disorders: A clinical guide to counseling and treatment.* Chicago: American Dietetic Association, 2001.

Wyatt, H.R., G.K. Grunwald, C.L. Mosca, M.L. Klem, R.R. Wing, and J.O. Hill. 2002. Long-term weight loss and breakfast in subjects in the National Weight Control Registry. *Obes Research* 10 (2):78-82.

Yoshioka, M., E. Doucet, S. St-Pierre, N. Almeras, D. Richard, A. Labrie, J. Despres, C. Bouchard, and A. Tremblay. 2001. Impact of high-intensity exercise on energy expenditure, lipid oxidation and body fatness. *Int J Obes Relat Metab Disord* 25 (3):332-339.

Zachweija, J. 2002. Protein: Power or puffery? [Online]. Gatorade Sports Science Institute-Sports Science Center. Available: www.gssiweb.com/reflib/refs/338/Protein_in_Sports_Drinks.cfm?pid=38 [July 2002].

Zarkadas, P., J. Carter, and E. Banister. 1994. Taper increases performance and aerobic power in triathletes. *Med Sci Sports Exerc* 26 (suppl):Abstract 194.

Zelasko, C. 1995. Exercise for weight loss: What are the facts? *J Am Diet Assoc* 95 (12):1414-1417.

INDEX

Note: The italicized *f* and *t* following page numbers refer to figures and tables, respectively.

A

activities, nonfood, 227-228
addiction, foods. *See* eating disorders; coffee; cravings
adipose tissue, 182. *See also* body fat
aerobic exercise, 184, 188, 223*t*
age, 106, 117
AIDS, 177
alcohol beverages, 199, 233; abuse of, 132, 250-251, 250*t*; coffee and, 68, 131; diuretic effect of, 131; exercise, recovery and, 128*t*, 129*t*, 130-132; fat and, 131; stomach absorption of, 131; in weight-gain diet, 209; women v. men use of, 132. *See also* beer
alfalfa sprouts, 73*t*
allergies, 25, 27
allylic sulfide, 41*t*
almonds, 18*t*, 35, 40*t*, 165*t*
—recipe with: chicken salad with almonds and mandarin oranges, 318
amenorrhea, 48-49, 252, 253, 262; complexity of, 254-255; diet for resolving, 255-257; vegetarians and, 168-169
American College of Sports Medicine, 229
American Dietetic Association, 220, 237, 260, 261
American Heart Association, 31, 32, 33, 35, 335, 365
American Psychiatric Association, 253, 254
amino acids, 6, 13, 29, 93, 144*f*; muscle building/repair with, 127-128, 175; protein and, 175; supplements of, 175-177; vegetarians and, 173-174, 175
anemia, iron-deficiency, 246; coffee, tea and, 172; iron deficiency, 13, 58, 59, 65, 171; vegetarian, 171-172. *See also* iron
animal. *See* meats
anorexia, 177, 190, 197, 199, 245, 259; case study of, 252-253; description of, 242, 253; prevalence of, 243; signs/symptoms of, 257-258
antacids, 45
antioxidants: for cancer prevention, 39-40, 42; for heart disease prevention, 36-38; in salads/vegetables, 42, 72; in supplement vitamins, 36-38, 42
appetite: exercise killing, 236; morning, 255-256
appetizers, 79
apple, 207*f*, 368; nutritional value of, 8*t*, 10*t*, 50*t*, 72, 92*t*, 142*t*, 156*t*
apple crisp, 368
apple juice, 9, 10*t*, 67, 142*t*
apple-shaped body, 189
apricots, 10*t*, 41*t*, 92*t*, 142*t*, 156*t*, 158, 270*t*
arginine, 175
Armstrong, Larry, 102
arteriosclerosis. *See* heart disease
arthritis, 30, 172
ascorbic acid. *See* vitamin C
asparagus, 12*t*, 38*t*
athletes: compulsive, 242, 257; endurance, 115-116, 121, 143, 145-149, 153, 162, 171, 249; nutrition game plan of, 122-123; teenage, 163, 171, 203, 239. *See also* specific kinds of athletes
avocado, 38*t*, 74*t*

B

bagels, 35, 158, 168; nutritional value of, 7-8, 129*t*, 142, 156*f*; as snack, 91, 108
baked goods, 44*t*
baked vegetables, 305
baking, of fish, 328, 330
baking soda, 45
balanced diet, 210-212. *See also* variety, in diet

balsamic dressing, 75
banana, 55, 64; calories in, 207*f*; carbohydrates and, 72, 140, 142*t*, 156*t*, 158; nutritional value of, 8*t*, 9, 10*t*, 50*t*, 92*t*; as recovery food, 128*t*; starch, sugar and, 139
—recipes with: banana bread, 276
bars: energy, 38*t*, 93-94, 94*t*, 364; protein, 142*t*, 175-177, 214
bean curd. *See* tofu
Beano, 15
beans, dried (legumes), 85; fiber in, 49-51, 50*t*; health benefit of, 38, 38*t*, 41*t*; iron in, 170*t*; nutritional value of, 5*t*, 13*t*, 18, 72; as protein source, 14-15, 15*t*, 16, 165*t*, 173, 174-175; serving suggestions for, 346; types of, 345-346; vegetarians and, 167-169; in weight-gain diet, 208; zinc in, 170*t*
—recipes with: chicken black bean soup, 319; country pasta with turkey sausage and white beans, 322; hummus roll-ups, 352; Mexican baked chicken with pinto beans, 325; Mexican tortilla lasagna, 351; minestrone soup, 348; pasta with white bean soup with sundried tomatoes, 349; quick and easy chili, 350; southwestern rice and bean salad, 297
beans, green, 12*t*, 73*t*, 156*t*, 207*f*
beef: cholesterol in, 29, 30*t*; fats in, 337; heart disease and, 29-30; lean, 29-30, 167, 256; nutritional value of, 5*t*, 170*t*, 337; as protein source, 4, 14, 15*t*, 16, 167; reduced servings in, 80; salt replacements with, 45
—recipes with: enchilada casserole, 339; sweet and spicy orange beef, 341; warm taco salad, 340
beer, 128*t*, 129*t*, 131. *See also* alcohol beverages
beets, 12*t*, 15*t*, 72, 73*f*
Benecol, 34
Bergstrom, Dr. J., 150
berry jams, 23
beta-carotene: cancer prevention and, 41*t*, 43, 74*f*; heart disease prevention and, 36-37; sources of, 10-12, 43, 74*f*
beverages: caffeine in, 67-68; carbohydrates in, 157*t*; suggestions for, 355. *See also* alcoholic beverages; fluids; liquid food; water
—recipes for: Diana's soy shake, 358; fruit smoothie, 357; homemade sports drink, 356; protein shake, 359; thick and frosty milkshake, 360
bicycling, 146-147, 223*t*
binge eating, 242, 245, 247, 254, 260. *See also* bulimia
bioelectrical impedance, 196, 199-200. *See also* body fat
birth control pill, 48
blender meals, 175-177
blood glucose (sugar), 24, 46-47, 101, 107, 108, 114, 127, 143*t*, 150, 220; carbohydrates and, 140. *See* high blood pressure
blueberries, 10*t*
blueberry oatmeal muffins, 277
Bod Pod Body Composition System, 196, 197
body building. *See* weightlifting
body dysmorphic disorder (BDD), 191
body fat: average, 181, 182; calorie deficient to lose, 183, 187; dietary fat v., 244; exercise and, 183-187, 236; function of, 182-183; genetics effect on, 194, 195, 196, 201, 204, 239, 245, 255; individual patterns of, 198; measurement of, 195-201, 200*t*, 247; muscles into, 185-186; not spot reducing of, 185; percentage of fat and, 182*t*; steps to successful loss of, 225-230; variability in, 198, 200*t*; women and, 182-183, 182*t*, 185, 187-188, 237, 244, 254-255. *See also* cellulite
body image, 182*t*, 188-18189, 237; dissatisfaction with, 190-191

body type: acceptance of, 191-193, 201; description of, 182*t*, 189-190; genetics effect on, 186, 188-189, 213, 239, 245; sports and, 194

body weight: average/normal, 194-195, 213; measuring of, 193-194

bok choy, 12, 12*t*, 18*t*, 20

bones: amenorrhea and, 257; broken, 20; caffeine and, 68; osteoporosis and, 16, 18, 47-49, 58, 68; stress fracture, 168, 246, 262

bonking, 150-152

Boston Market, 84, 87*t*

bowl movements, 49, 51, 103, 123-124, 148. *See also* constipation; diarrhea; fiber

bran, 7, 49, 50*t*, 60*t*, 61, 142*t*, 148, 156*t*, 171*t*, 207*f*. *See also* oat bran

breads, 142*t*; baking time for, 274; baking tips for, 273-274; carbohydrates in, 156*t*; enriched, 171, 171*t*; fiber in, 49-51, 50*t*, 155; as protein source, 15*t*; sodium content in, 44*t*, 129*t*; unbuttered, 80; in weight-gain diet, 208; white, 141, 142*t*; whole grain, 7*t*, 8, 38*t*, 46, 50*t*, 56, 64, 72, 85, 142*t*, 148

—recipe for: banana bread, 276

breakfast: calories in, 57, 64, 99, 226; coffee as alternative to, 66; for dieters, 56-58; with endurance exercise, 148*t*, 149, 153; skipping, 53-56, 70, 97, 237; suggestions for, 17, 54, 57-65, 148*t*, 209*t*, 212*t*. *See also* breads; breakfast cereals, cooked; breakfast cereals, ready-to-eat; muffins

—recipes for: oatmeal pancakes, 285; wheat germ and cottage cheese pancakes, 286

breakfast cereals, cooked: carbohydrates in, 156*t*; fiber in, 33-34, 49-51, 50*t*; folate acid and, 38*t*; heart disease prevention and, 33-34; as protein source, 15*t*; in weight-gain diet, 207*f*. *See also* oat bran

—recipes with: Jenny's favorite oatmeal, 282

breakfast cereals, ready-to-eat: alternatives to, 63-65; calcium in, 58, 59, 60*t*-61*t*; carbohydrates in, 156*t*; cholesterol in, 58; fat in, 58, 60*t*-61*t*, 63; fiber in, 49-51, 50*t*, 58, 60*t*-61*t*, 61, 155; folic acid in, 59, 61; iron in, 58-59, 60*t*-61*t*, 171*t*; natural, 59; nutritional value of, 17, 18*t*, 58-59, 60*t*-61*t*, 61-62; as protein source, 15*t*; as snack, 90; sodium content in, 44*t*, 60*t*-61*t*, 129*t*; sugar in, 58, 60*t*-61*t*, 61-63; in weight-gain diet, 207*f*; whole-grain, 7, 7*t*; in zinc, 171*t*

—recipes with: cereal-to-go, 281; cold cereal with hot fruit, 280; honey nut granola, 284; swiss muesli, 283

Brenda's Greek salad, 309

broccoli, 12; calcium in, 18*t*; cancer prevention and, 39, 41*t*, 42; diarrhea and, 123; folate in, 38*t*; nutritional value of, 11, 11*t*, 12*t*, 18*t*, 20, 73*t*, 156*t*, 170*t*

—recipe for: sesame pasta with broccoli, 296

broiling, of fish, 80, 328

brown rice, 171, 289

brussel sprouts, 12, 12*t*, 50*t*

bulimia, 245; case study of, 249-251; description of, 242, 254; prevalence of, 243; signs/symptoms of, 257, 258, 259

bulking up. *See* weight gain

Burger King, 83*t*, 86*t*

butter, 44*t*, 72, 80, 82; sodium in, 44*t*

C

cabbage, green, 12, 12*t*, 41*t*, 73*t*

caffeine: alternatives to, 67, 68; in beverages, 67-68; diuretic effect of, 102; before exercise, 101-103; fat release stimulated with, 102; GI problems and, 107; iron absorption and, 65; physical effect of, 67; soft drinks, coffee and, 68, 103*t*; sources of, 103*t*; withdrawal from, 67

calcium, 162, 175; amenorrhea and, 256-257; boosting intake of, 17; in cereals, 59, 60*t*-61*t*; choices for, 19-20; high blood pressure prevention and, 45, 46; intake recommended for, 19*t*, 77; muscle cramping and, 120; osteoporosis prevention and, 48, 49; pregnancy and, 51;

RDA of, 26*t*; requirements of, 16-18, 48-49; in salads, 74; sources of, 18*t*, 19-20, 22, 58; as supplement, 17

calories: body fat lost by deficiency of, 183, 187; for breakfast, 57, 64, 99, 226; carbohydrates and, 7, 147; cereal, sugar and, 62-63; at coffee houses, 66*t*; consumption of, 6, 21; daily need and plan for, 248, 268; evenly divided between meals, 70, 248; excessive, as fattening, 6, 154-155; exercise and, 99, 100, 101, 108, 114, 115, 135, 223*t*; exercise, energy bars and, 93, 94*t*; fast foods and, 82, 83*t*, 84, 86*t*-88*t*; from fats, 22, 22*t*, 35-36, 43, 72, 232-233, 256; limited, 162; for lunch, 71, 72; muscles correlated to, 184; obesity and, 237; restriction of, 25; in salad/salad dressing, 72, 74-75, 75*t*; in snacks, 91*f*, 93; for weight gain, 204, 206-209, 207*f*, 209*t*-210*t*, 211-212, 212*t*; weight lost and counting, 221-222, 223*t*, 224-225, 226, 239, 246, 255

cancer, 177; fat (obesity) and, 39, 42-43; prevention of, 8, 30; protective diet against, 12, 22, 41*t*, 43, 63, 74*f*, 220; protective (antioxidant) nutrients for, 39-40, 40*t*, 42

candy, 91*f*, 142*t*, 240; craving of, 103-105; with sorbitol, 123. *See also* chocolate

canned food, 8*t*, 11, 30*t*, 45, 92*t*, 156*t*, 207*f*, 231

canola oil, 32, 33, 34, 37, 40*t*, 304

cantaloupe, 9, 10*t*, 59, 92*t*

capsaicin, 41*t*

carbohydrates: alcohol beverages and little, 130; blood sugar and, 140; bonking and, 150-152; with breakfast, 148*t*, 149, 152; calories and, 7, 147, 155, 157; in cereals, 58; in common foods, 155, 156*t*-157*t*, 158; complex, 139, 140; counting, 158-159; daily load for, 144, 145, 147, 153, 158-159, 210, 230-231, 268; digestible, 108; dinner rich with, 77, 79, 80, 82, 83*t*-84*t*; endurance exercise and, 145-149; energy from, 161, 166; exercise and, 56, 99, 101, 107-108, 114, 122, 135, 144; exercise, energy bars and, 93, 94*t*; fats replaced with, 75, 147; fiber and, 148; glycemic-index and, 140-142, 142*t*; insulin and, 230, 231; muscles and, 150-153, 161, 199, 205, 214; not fattening, 154-155; performance influenced by intake of, 144-145; powders, 127; premenstrual cravings for, 96; protein and, 127, 147, 150-151, 233; rapid (heavy) loading of, 146-147; recovery and exercise, 126-127, 135; recovery from daily training with, 153-154, 153*f*; in salads, 72; selection and variety of, 149; simple, 137-138, 140; in soft drinks, 125, 139; solid or liquid, 114; sources of, 4, 6, 7, 8, 15, 23; in sports drinks, 125, 127, 139; stored, 143; tapering in training and reducing of, 146; in vegetables, 139; for weight gain, 205-206, 210-211

carotenoids, 39

carrots: cancer prevention and, 12, 41*t*, 42, 74*f*; nutritional value of, 11, 12*t*, 15*t*, 50*t*, 72-73, 73*t*, 74*f*, 142*t*, 156*t*

—recipes with: carrot cake, 317-372; carrot raisin muffins, 276; carrot-raisin salad, 310

cast-iron skillets, 172

cauliflower, 12, 12*t*, 41*t*, 72-73, 73*t*

celery, 11, 12*t*

cells, temperature of, 116

cellulite, 186-187. *See also* body fat

cereals. *See* breakfast cereals, cooked; breakfast cereals, ready-to-eat

cereal-to-go, 281

Cheerios, 38*t*

cheese, 170*t*; as calcium source, 17, 18*t*, 20; cholesterol and, 30*t*; feta, 332; low-fat, 20, 44*t*; as protein source, 15*t*, 165*t*; saturated fat in, 172; sodium content in, 44*t*, 45, 129*t*

—recipes with: easy lasagna, 294; egg-stuffed baked potato, 299; gourmet lasagna, 295; Greek shrimp with feta and tomatoes, 332; wheat germ and cottage cheese pancakes, 286

cherries, 10*t*

chewing gum, 123

chicken: cholesterol and, 30*t*; cooking tips for, 312-313; as example of muscle fiber types, 311; nutritional value of, 311-312; preparation of, 80, 82; as protein source, 13*t*, 14, 15*t*, 165*t*; salt replacements with, 45; sodium content in, 44*t*, 129*t*
—recipes with, 339; chicken and oriental noodles in peanut sauce, 317; chicken black bean soup, 319; chicken salad with almonds and mandarin oranges, 318; chicken with pasta and spinach, 316; Mexican baked chicken with pinto beans, 325; oven-fried chicken, 314; sautéed chicken with mushrooms and onions, 315
chickpeas, 38*t*, 50*t*, 72, 74, 74*f*, 80, 82, 142*t*, 175
children, 117, 237
chili, 324, 340, 345; quick and easy chile, 350
chili peppers, 41*t*
Chinese food, 81, 341
chips, 45, 91*f*
chlorogenic acid, 41*t*
chocolate, 97, 142*t*, 227
chocolate lush, 373
cholesterol, blood (serum): desirable, 29; (soluble) fiber and, 50-51; foods with no, 14, 345; genetics and, 28, 29, 33; HDL (high-density lipoprotein, good), 28-29, 32, 173; heart disease and, 28-29; LDL (low-density lipoprotein, bad), 28-29, 32, 33, 34, 173; ratio of HDL to total, 29; saturated fats influence on, 28, 29, 33
cholesterol, dietary: in beef, 29, 30*t*; in cereals, 58, 274; in dairy products, 30*t*, 58; in eggs, 32-33; in fish, 29, 30*t*; reducing, 32, 33, 34, 35
chromium, 93
chronic fatigue. *See* fatigue
coffee: abstention from, 65; addiction to, 67; alcohol and, 68, 131; as alternative to breakfast, 66; anemia and, 172; caffeine sources in, 68, 103*t*; decaffeinated, 67; espresso v., 67; health issues and, 65; house calories/fats, 66*t*; pregnancy and, 52, 68; soft drinks, caffeine and, 68; whiteners in, 17, 65-66. *See also* caffeine
cola, 103*t*, 128*t*, 129*t*, 142*t*. *See also* soft drinks
cold cereal, with hot fruit, 280
collard (greens), 12, 18*t*, 40*t*
colorful pasta salad, 293
commercial fluid replacers, 125
complete protein, 173
condiments, 45
congeners, 130
constipation, 8, 61, 123, 148. *See also* bowel movements; fiber
convenience foods, carbohydrates in, 157*t*
cooking: efficiently, 268; metric conversions in, 269; microwave, 270, 306, 328; tips, 76-78
copper, 37
corn, 12*t*, 15*t*, 50*t*, 72, 73*t*, 123, 140, 142*t*, 156*t*, 207*f*
corn oil, 34
cottage cheese: as calcium source, 18*t*, 74; cholesterol in, 30*t*; as protein source, 15*t*, 73, 165*t*
—recipes with: wheat germ and cottage cheese pancakes, 286
cotton mouth, 20
country pasta with turkey sausage and white beans, 322
crackers, 6, 8, 34, 45, 91, 108, 119, 129, 129*t*, 142*t*
cramping, 215; muscle, 119, 120-121, 129; in stomach, 25, 105, 124
cranberry juice, 9, 10*t*, 127, 128*t*, 142*t*
cravings: chocolate, 97, 227; four meals reduces, 70; pre-dinner and avoidance of, 95-96; pregnancy and, 52; premenstrual, 96; prevention of, 97-98; for salt, 44, 130; snacks and, 95-98
C-reactive protein (CRP) test, 29
Cream of Wheat, 33, 142*t*, 156*t*, 171*t*
creatine, 214-215
croutons, 72
cucumbers, 11, 12*t*, 73*t*
cured foods, 45

D
dairy products: choices of, 19-20; iron in, 170*t*; low-fat, 16, 17, 19-20, 30*t*, 121; nutritional value of, 5*t*, 15*t*, 16-21, 256; as protein source, 15*t*; serving sizes of, 19*t*; zinc in, 170*t*. *See also* cottage cheese; milk; yogurt
dancing, 223*t*
DASH (Dietary Approaches to Stop Hypertension) diet, 45-46
dates, 10*t*, 276-270*t*
deficiency, vitamin, 24-25
dehydration: energy loss, fatigue and, 56, 118; GI problems and, 107; muscle, 116, 120; prevention of, 116, 122, 125-126; urination and, 166. *See also* fluids; sweating; water
depletion, of glycogen, 145, 150-151, 153
depression, 133
desserts, 4; carbohydrates in, 157*t*; low-fat, 81; in weight-gain diet, 209 desserts. *See also* snack foods
—recipes with: apple crisp, 368; carrot cake, 371-372; chocolate lush, 373; oatmeal cookies, 363; peach crumble, 369; pear upside-down gingerbread cake, 370
diabetes, 172; glycemic index for, 140; prevention of, 6, 35, 46-47. *See also* hypoglycemia
Diana's soy shake, 358
diarrhea, 98, 105-106, 123-124. *See also* bowl movements
diet(s): amenorrhea, 255-257; blowing out of, 222, 224; breakfast, weight loss and, 56-58; carbohydrate loaded, 145-149, 148*t*, 150-151, 152, 158, 206; DASH, 45-46; exercise, health and, 28; fad, 230-232; high protein/fat, 108, 150-151, 164, 176, 206, 231; high-protein, low carbohydrate, 233; low-fat, 35-36, 79-81, 159; low-salt, 44-45; lunch and, 71-72; moderation in, 4; not working, 239; protein, 167-168, 233; shaping of, 5-6; sports, 122-123; variety in, 4, 58-59, 63, 78; vegetarian, 15-16, 15*t*, 25, 162, 172-175, 174*t*; weight gain, 204, 206-209, 209*t*-210*t*, 210-212, 212*t*. *See also* weight-reduction diet
Dietary Approaches to Stop Hypertension. *See* DASH diet
dietitian, registered (RD), 25, 178, 220, 243, 244
digestion (gastrointestinal system), 93-94, 100, 101, 104, 105, 107-109, 118; steps of, 144*f*
dinner, 69; carbohydrate-rich, 77, 79, 80, 82, 83*t*-84*t*, 84-85, 148*t*, 152; as dining-out meal, 78-81; fast food, 81-85, 83*t*-84*t*, 86*t*-88*t*; at home, 75-78; lunch and, 71, 76; reducing size of, 85; suggestions, 77-78, 82, 83*t*-84*t*, 84-85, 148*t*, 152, 210*t*, 212*t*
disaccharides, 137-138, 138*f*. *See also* sugar
disorientation, 119
diuretics, 102, 131
Double-Duty Exercise Program, 231-232
Dr. Atkin's Diet Revolution, 231
dressings, for salads. *See* salad dressing
Dunkin' Donuts, 66*t*, 83*t*, 87*t*
dysmorphia, 191

E
easy lasagna, 294
eating: binge, 242, 245, 247, 254; during extensive exercise, 113-116; favorite foods, 227; GI problems and, 106-107; guidelines for, 3-4; moods influencing, 133, 218, 226, 227-228, 235; at night, 235-236; properly, 218-220; slowly, 226-227; timing of, 54-56, 69, 101, 108, 149 eating. *See also* diet; digestion; fast foods; liquid foods; snacking
eating disorders, 241; amenorrhea and, 254-257; basis of, 246-247; case studies of, 247-253; helping someone with, 257-262; hunger, food fuel and, 244-246, 251, 255; prevalence of, 242-243; prevention of, 262; professional resources for, 260; red-flag traits with, 250*t*, 251; subclinical, 243-244 eating disorders. *See also* anorexia; bulimia
Eating Disorders Awareness and Prevention Program (EDAP), 192
Echinacea, 110
ectomorph, 189
eggs: cholesterol, heart disease and, 32-33; designer, 33; folate in, 38*t*; iron and zinc in, 170*t*; as protein source,

14-15, 15*t*, 165*t*; salt replacements with, 45; sodium content in, 44
—recipes for: egg-stuffed baked potato, 299
electrical impedance. *See* bioelectrical impedance
electrolytes: imbalance, 119, 120, 246; recovery, 128-130
enchilada casserole, 339
endomorph, 189
endurance athletes, 115-116, 121, 143, 145-149, 153, 162, 171, 249
energy, 6, 161, 162, 166
energy bars, 38*t*, 142*t*, 177*t*; calories, carbohydrates and, 93, 94*t*; digestibility of, 93-94; exercise and, 93; fat content of, 94; peanutty energy bars, 364; standard food v., 94, 94*t*. *See also* protein, powders and bars
energy enhancers, 110, 232; coffee as, 65-68
enriched foods, 38*t*, 58-59, 61, 149, 171, 171*t*
entrees, carbohydrates in, 157*t*
ephedra, 110, 232
ephedrine, 232
espresso, 67
estrogen, 48, 49, 96, 256
exercise: addict, 248-249; appetite killed by, 236; appointments scheduled for, 229-230; body fat and, 183-187, 236; caffeine before, 101-103; calories and, 99, 100, 101, 108, 114, 115, 135; carbohydrates and, 56, 99, 101, 107-108, 114, 122, 135, 144; cardiovascular disease influenced by, 229; compulsive, 242, 257; diabetes, weight-reduction and, 47; diet, health and, 28; digestion before, 100, 101, 104; energy bar snack and, 93, 94*t*; in the heat, 119; high-fat protein and, 108, 176; intensity of, 100, 106, 109, 123; osteoporosis prevention and, 48; oxidative damage from, 133; pre-competition food intake and, 106; pre-exercise snack and, 98, 107-110; recreational, 125; snack before afternoon, 100; snack before morning, 99; for strengthening muscles, 176, 184, 188, 213; sugar before, 104-105, 108; supplements and, 110-111; timing of food with, 101; vitamin intake and, 24; weight loss and, 236-237. *See also* aerobic exercise; low-intensity, fat-burning exercise
exercise, extensive, 184, 185, 242, 243; alcohol recovery after, 130-132; all-day events and sustenance needed in, 121-124; carbohydrate daily load for, 144, 145; carbohydrates recovery after, 126-127, 135; eating during, 113-116; electrolytes recovery after, 128-130; fluid recovery after, 125-126, 135; fluids during, 116-120, 135; potassium recovery after, 128, 128*t*; protein recovery after, 127-128; recovering from, 124-136, 184; rest time and, 134, 135, 151-152, 154; sodium recovery after, 128-130, 129*t*; vitamins recovery after, 133; weighing after, 193

F

fad dieting, 230-232
fast foods, 4; alternatives within, 82, 83*t*-84*t*; calories and fat in, 82, 86*t*-88*t*; carbohydrates in, 157*t*; dinner of, 81-85, 83*t*-84*t*, 86*t*-88*t*; health issues for, 30*t*, 46; nutritional value of, 21, 22*t*
fast-twitch muscle fibers, 311
fat(s): alcohol beverages and, 131; amenorrhea and, 256; body fat v., 244; burning body, 98; caffeine stimulating release of, 102; calories from, 22, 22*t*, 35-36, 43, 72, 232-233, 256; cancer and, 39, 42-43, 63; carbohydrates and, 75, 147; in cereals, 58, 60*t*-61*t*, 63; choices of, 22; cholesterol and, 28, 29, 33, 34; at coffee houses, 66*t*; in crackers, 8; energy bars and, 94; excess fat creating, 234; fast foods and, 82, 86*t*-88*t*; free (non), 234-235, 243; GI problems and high, 106; hard v. soft, 34; high blood pressure and, 43, 63, 74*t*; low, 16, 17, 19-20, 30*t*, 35-36, 159, 234, 243; low saturated, 34; low v. no, 35-36; monounsaturated, 22, 35, 71; night eating and, 235-236; nutritional value of, 5*t*, 22; partially hydrogenated saturated, 34; polyunsaturated, 30-31, 31*t*, 34; proportion for, 35-36, 268; protein, high, 108, 150-151, 166, 167, 176, 206, 231; in salad dressing, 74-75, 75*t*; saturated, 28,

29, 33, 34, 172; serving sizes for, 22*t*; in snacks, 91*f*; trans, 28, 34; unsaturated, 22, 34; in weight-gain diet, 211, 211*t*. *See also* body fat; fatty acids
Fat-Burning Thermogenic Program, 232
fatigue, 5, 124, 240; hyperhydration and, 119; hypoglycemia and, 90, 101, 108; iron deficiency and, 170*t*; recovery, exercise and, 133-134
fatty acids, 144*f*
favorite foods, 227
fecal weight, 49, 51
fiber: in bread and cereals, 49-51, 50*t*, 58, 61, 155; with endurance exercise, 148; in fruits and vegetables, 50*t*; GI problems and, 107; health benefits of, 33-34, 35, 40, 45, 61; insoluble, 49; in legumes, 49-51, 50*t*; myth, 51; soluble, 33-34, 49-50; sources of, 6, 8, 11, 23, 49-50, 50*t*, 74*f*. *See also* bran; breads; grains and starches
figs, 10*t*
fish: broiling of, 80, 328; buying of, 327; as calcium source, 17, 18*t*; cancer prevention and, 40, 41*t*, 43; cholesterol and fats in, 29, 30*t*; cooking tips for, 327-328; heart disease benefits from, 40; iron and zinc in, 170*t*; nutritional value of, 16; oil, 30-31; omega-3 fatty acids in, 30-31, 31*t*, 41*t*, 43; preparation of, 80; as protein source, 13*t*, 14, 15*t*, 165*t*, 177*t*; salt replacements with, 45; smoked, 45; sodium content in, 44*t*
—recipes with: crunchy oven-baked fish sticks, 329; fish and spinach bake, 330; fish in foil Mexican style, 334
flavonoids, 41*t*, 66
flax—recipes with: molasses muffins with flax and dates, 276
flaxseed oils, 32, 41*t*
flour, enriched, 38*t*, 171
fluids, 118*f*; body, water and, 118*f*; capacity and need of, 117-119; cramping and, 120; drinking too much, 119; during endurance exercise, 149; during exercise, 109-110, 135; during extensive exercise, 116-120, 135; lost with sweating, 114, 115, 125-126; pre-exercise, 107, 109; recovery, 125-126, 135; replacement of, 114, 116-117; thirst mechanism of, 117. *See also* beverages; dehydration; soups; sports drinks; water
folate (folic acid), 9; in cereals, 59, 61; heart disease prevention and, 35, 38, 38*t*, 59, 61; pregnancy, birth defects and, 51, 59; RDA and, 26*t*; sources of, 74*f*
Food and Drug Administration, 111
food cravings. *See* cravings
Food guide pyramid: diet reflected in, 4-5, 23, 78, 210, 218, 268; illustration of, 5*f*; planning good nutrition with, 6-26, 78
food storage, 76-77, 77*t*, 271
free radicals, 39-40
freezing: fruit, 357; proper method of, 76, 270-271; of tofu, 346-347
french fries, oven, 298
fried chicken, oven, 314
frozen foods, 45, 76, 91
frozen yogurt, 17, 20, 21
fructose, 138, 142*t*
fruit: breakfast and, 58, 59, 64; cancer prevention and, 41*t*; canned, 8*t*; carbohydrates in, 72, 156*t*; choices of, 9-10, 10*t*; citrus, 8*t*, 9, 10*t*, 39, 41*t*, 52; color of, 13*t*, 39; dried, 10, 10*t*, 35; fiber in, 50*t*; freezing, 357; iron in, 170*t*; nutritional value of, 5*t*, 8*t*; potassium content of, 9, 10*t*; serving size for, 8*t*; snacks, 91, 92*t*; sugar, starch and, 139; in weight-gain diet, 207*f*; zinc in, 170*t*
—recipes with: cold cereal with hot fruit, 280; Diana's soy shake, 358; fruit smoothie, 357; homemade sports drink, 356; stir-fry pork with fruit, 343
fruit juice, 6, 8*t*, 18, 18*t*, 56, 58, 59, 64, 91*t*, 92*t*, 125, 127, 142*t*, 239; iron and zinc in, 170*t*; potassium content of, 9, 10*t*, 46; as recovery food, 127, 128*t*, 129*t*; sodium content in, 44*t*; in weight gain diet, 207*f*. *See also* names of specific fruit juices

G

galatose, 138

garlic, 40, 41*t*

gastric juices, 98, 105

gastrointestinal (GI) problems, 106-107, 123-124, 145

Gatorade, 129*t*, 130, 142*t*

gender, 106

genetics: body fat, body type and, 186, 188-189, 194, 195, 196, 201, 204, 213, 239, 245, 255; cholesterol, heart disease and, 28, 29, 33, 51; iron deficiency and, 172

genistein, 41*t*

ginseng, 110

GI. *See* gastrointestinal (GI) problems

glaze. *See* sauces

glucose, 127, 142*t*, 162; stored, 143-145. *See also* blood glucose (sugar)

glucose polymers, 138, 139

glycemic index, 140-142, 142*t*; high, 140-141, 142*t*; low, 33, 142*t*, 220

glycogen, 56, 98, 99, 126-127, 134; depletion, 145, 150-151, 153; high levels of, 147; liver, 139, 143*t*, 150; muscle, 139, 143-145, 143*t*, 147, 150-151, 162, 184; sources of, 150-151

gourmet lasagna, 295

grains and starches: carbohydrates in, 142*t*, 157*t*; choices of, 7-8; iron in, 171, 171*t*; nutritional value of, 5*t*, 6-7, 23; potassium in, 46; processed/refined, 6; as protein source, 15*t*, 174-175; serving size for, 7*t*; zinc in, 171*t*. *See also* breads; breakfast cereals, cooked, breakfast cereals, ready-to-eat; pasta; potatoes and sweet potatoes; rice; starches; whole grains

granola, 59, 156*t*, 158, 207*f*; fats in, 63; recipes for, 284

grapefruit, 9, 10*t*, 59, 92*f*, 142*t*

grapefruit juice, 10*t*

grapes, 10*t*

Greek salad, Brenda's, 309

Greek shrimp with feta and tomatoes, 332

ground turkey mix for spaghetti sauce or chili, 324

gum, sugar-free, 123

Gurze Books, 261

H

ham: canned lean, 30*t*; leanest cuts of, 338

hamburger, 13, 165*t*; turkey meatballs or turkey burgers, 323

headaches, 119. *See also* dehydration

heart disease: beef and, 29-30; cholesterol influence on, 28-29, 30*t*; cooking oil's health benefits for, 34; eggs and, 32-33; exercise and, 229; fiber benefits for, 33-34, 61; fish's health benefits for, 30-32, 31*t*; genetics and, 28, 29, 33; nut and peanut butter's benefits for, 14, 34-35, 71; oatmeal's health benefits for, 33-34; prevention of, 6, 14, 22, 30-38, 65, 66, 220; supplement's health benefits for, 36-38. *See also* cholesterol

heat, 116, 119. *See also* dehydration; fluids

herbs, 45, 75*t*

high blood pressure (hypertension): causes of, 43; DASH diet against, 45-46; measuring, 43; prevention of, 8, 9, 12, 16, 30, 44-46, 59, 61

Hippocrates, 51

holistic health, 43

homocysteine, 29, 38

honey, 138, 140, 142*t*

honeydew melon, 10*t*, 92*t*

honey-glazed pork chops, 342

honey nut granola, 284

hormones, 48, 96, 188; GI problems and, 107

hot cereals. *See* breakfast cereals, cooked

hot tubs, 131

hourglass shaped body, 190

hummus, 16, 50, 165*t*, 345

hummus roll-ups, 352

hunger, 244-246, 255; scale, 251

hydration. *See* fluids

hyperhydration, 119

hypertension. *See* high blood pressure

hypoglycemia (low blood sugar): fatigue and, 90, 101, 108; poor performance with, 150; prevention of, 110, 116; snacks for, 98; sugar's effect on, 104-105

hyponatremia (low blood sodium), 119

I

ice cream, 17, 20, 21, 30*t*, 91*f*, 157-158

ice hockey, 144-145

incomplete protein, 173

indoles, 41*t*

injuries, 185-186, 215

insomnia, 133

Institute of Medicine, 229

insulin, 47, 104, 105, 127, 230, 231. *See also* hypoglycemia

International Olympic Committee, 102

intestines, 144*f*

inverted-triangle shaped body, 190

iron: absorption of, 58, 59, 65; cooking pots, 172; deficiency, 13, 25, 162, 170*t*, 175; heme v. nonheme, 172; pregnancy and, 25, 51; RDA of, 26*t*; recommended intake of, 170*t*; sources of, 4, 22, 29, 58-59, 60*t*, 170*t*-171*t*; supplement, 59, 172

isoflavones, 41*t*

isothiocanates, 41*t*

J

jams, berry, 23

Jenny's favorite oatmeal, 282

juice. *See* fruit juice

junk food. *See* desserts; fast foods; snack foods

K

kale: calcium in, 18*t*, 20; cancer prevention and, 41*t*; nutritional value, 12, 12*t*

Kentucky Fried Chicken (KFC), 82, 86*t*

ketosis, 231

Keys, Ancel, 245

kidney beans, 13*t*, 38*t*, 49, 50*t*, 72, 123, 129, 142*t*, 165*t*

kidneys, 43, 221*t*

kiwi, 9, 10*t*, 39, 50*t*

kohlrabi, 12

L

labels, food, 62, 158, 159, 171

Lactaid milk, 20

lactase, 20

lactic acid, 118*f*, 124

lactose, 138; intolerance, 20, 25

large intestine, 144*f*

lasagna, recipes for: easy lasagna, 294; gourmet lasagna, 295

laxatives, 45, 242

lean, 29-30

leftovers, 71

legumes. *See* beans, dried (legumes)

lemon dressing, 318

lentils, 142*t*, 289; fiber in, 50*t*; folate in, 38*t*; as protein source, 15*t*, 16

lentil soup, 13*t*

lettuce, 12*t*, 38*t*, 50*t*, 72, 73*t*, 74*f*

lifestyle, 188, 223*f*, 260; calories and activities of, 223*f*; cancer prevention through, 43; rest time in, 134, 135, 151-152, 154, 228

lignans, 41*t*

liquid foods (beverages): pre-exercise and, 109

liver, 32, 144*f*, 221*t*; glycogen, 139, 143*t*

love/acceptance, 191-193, 246, 253, 256, 262

low blood sugar. *See* hypoglycemia

low-fat diet, 35-36, 79-81, 159

low-intensity, fat-burning exercise, 184

low salt diet, 44-45

low saturated fat, 34

lunch, 69; brown bagging of, 70-71; for dieters, 71-72; dinner and, 71, 76; suggestions, 17, 148*t*, 152, 210*t*, 212*t*; super salads for, 72-75, 73*t*; two times for, 70, 89, 90, 209, 210*t*
lutein, 41*t*
lycopene, 12, 74*f*

M

macular degeneration, 42
"magic food," 109
magnesium, 35, 45
ma huang, 110, 232
mango, 92*t*
marathon. *See* endurance athletes
margarine, 208; cholesterol and, 32, 34; sodium in, 44*t*
marinade. *See* sauces
mayonnaise, 82
McDonald's, 22*t*, 30*t*, 83*t*, 86*t*
meals: appropriate portions at, 219; every 2 to 4 hours, 23, 70, 224, 248; liquid, 109; snacks v., 95-96; timing of, 54-56, 69, 101, 108, 149
meat: cholesterol and fats in, 30*t*; healthful (low-fat), 166-167, 256; iron in, 170*t*; lean, 29-30, 167, 172-173, 256; nutritional value of, 5*t*, 13*t*; as protein source, 15*t*, 165*t*; selenium benefits from, 40; smoked, 45; sodium content in, 44*t*; in weight-gain diet, 208; zinc in, 170*t*. *See also* beef; hamburger; pork
meatless diet. *See* diet, vegetarian
meatless entrees. *See* beans, dried (legumes); cheese; eggs; fish; tofu
meditation, 228
Mediterranean shrimp and scallops with pasta, 333
menopause, 170*t*, 187-188
menstruation, 170*t*, 246; lack of (amenorrhea), 48, 252, 253, 254-257; premenstrual cravings and, 96
mental stamina, 150
mercury poisoning, 31, 32
mesomorph, 189
metabolism, 183; muscles and rate of, 187-188; resting rate (RMR) of, 221-222, 221*t*
Mexican baked chicken with pinto beans, 325
Mexican tortilla lasagna, 351
microwave cooking, 270, 306, 328
microwaved vegetables, 306
milk, 9, 58, 64; as calcium source, 17, 18*t*, 19-20; cholesterol and, 30*t*; lactose intolerance for, 20, 25; low-fat, 19, 44*t*, 49, 72, 74, 165*t*, 177*t*; myths, 19; nutritional value of, 15*t*, 16-17, 49, 142*t*, 170*t*, 256; as protein source, 15*t*, 165*t*; 173, 174, 177*t*; selenium benefits from, 40; sodium content in, 44*t*; in weight-gain diet, 207*f*. *See also* dairy products; milkshake
—recipes with: protein shake, 359; thick and frosty milkshake, 360
milkshake: homemade, 362; thick and frosty, 360
Mind/Body Medical Institute, 228
minerals, 6; deficiency of, 24-25; recommended intake of, 24-25, 26*t*; sources of, 10; supplements of, 24-25, 133. *See also* calcium; iron; zinc
minestrone soup, 348
moderation: in alcohol drinking, 131-132; in diet, 4
molasses, 22, 171*t*
molasses muffins, with flax and dates, 276
molds, 27
monosaccharides, 137-138, 138*f*
mouth, 144*f*
muffins, 64, 91, 108, 128, 148, 156*t*, 158
—recipes for: blueberry oatmeal muffins, 276; carrot raisin muffins, 276; molasses muffins with flax and dates, 276
muscle(s): into body fat, 185-186; building/repairing, 13, 126, 127-128; calories correlated to, 184; carbohydrates and, 150-153, 161, 199, 205, 214; cramping, 119, 120-121, 129; creatine and, 214-215; damage, 133; energy

for, 6; exercise for, 176, 184; fiber types, 311; glycogen, 139, 143-145, 143*t*, 147, 150-151, 162, 184; heat of, 116; metabolic rate driving, 187-188; oxidative damage of, 13, 126, 127-128, 133; protein and, 153, 161, 176, 205; strengthening, 176, 184, 188, 213; tone of, 186; trained v. untrained, 143; weight, 195
muscle dysmorphia, 191
mushrooms, 11, 12*t*, 73*t*, 315
mustard greens, 12, 18*t*

N

National Agricultural Library's Food and Nutrition Information Center, 111
National Eating Disorders Association, 260
National Research Council, 42
natural foods, 59
nausea, 119, 215
niacin, 35; RDA of, 26*t*
noodles. *See* pasta
nursing women, caffeine and, 68
nutrient losses: in cooking, 11, 46; in freezing, 11
nutrients: describing, 5-7; processed foods and, 6
nutrition, post-exercise. *See* recovery foods
nutrition, pre-event. *See* pre-event foods
nutrition rainbow, 13*t*, 22
nuts: in cereals, 284; health, disease prevention from, 34-35, 40; as protein source, 167, 168; snacks, 92
—recipes with: honey nut granola, 284

O

oat bran, 33-34, 49-51, 50*t*, 63
oatmeal: health benefits of, 33-34, 38*t*, 49-51, 51*t*, 156*t*, 274; ideas for, 274; nutritional value of, 7, 15*t*, 142*t*; as snack, 90. *See also* Breakfast cereals, cooked
—recipes with: blueberry oatmeal muffins, 277; Jenny's favorite oatmeal, 282; oatmeal cookies, 363; oatmeal pancakes, 285
obesity. *See* overweight
oils: canola, 32, 33, 34, 37, 40*t*, 304; choices of, 22, 32; corn, 34; fats compared to, 22; fish, 30-31; nutritional value of, 32; olive, 22, 32, 34, 37, 40, 40*t*, 74*f*, 75, 75*t*, 304; safflower, 34, 40*t*; sesame, 304; sunflower, 34
olive oil. *See* oils, olive
omega-3 fatty acids, 30-31, 31*t*, 33, 41*t*, 43
Omron, 199, 200
onions, 12*t*, 41*t*, 123, 315
orange juice: calcium fortified, 18, 18*t*; nutritional value of, 6, 8*t*, 10*t*, 58, 59, 91*t*, 92*t*, 142*t*; as recovery food, 128*t*, 129*t*
oranges, 9, 10*t*, 59, 72, 156*t*; carotenoids in, 39; fiber in, 50*t*; folate in, 38*t*
—recipes with: chicken salad with almonds and mandarin oranges, 318; sweet and spicy orange beef, 341
oriental dressing, 318
ornithine, 175
osteoporosis, 18, 47, 68, 197; prevention of, 16, 48-49, 58
oven-baked fish sticks, crunchy, 329
oven french fries, 298
oven-fried chicken, 314
overeating, 186, 235-236. *See also* binge eating; bulimia; overweight
overtraining, 133-134, 152
overweight, 27, 39, 42-43, 44-45, 47, 184, 195, 204, 226, 237. *See also* weight-reduction diet

P

pancakes, recipes for: oatmeal pancakes, 285; wheat germ and cottage cheese pancakes, 286
papaya, 92*t*
pasta, 80-81, 145, 171*t*; carbohydrates in, 72, 140, 142*t*, 157*t*; cooking tips for, 287-289; fiber in, 50*t*; as protein source, 15*t*; serving suggestions for, 288-289; sodium in, 128, 129*t*; varieties of, 78, 287; vegetable, 78; whole grain, 7*t*, 78

—recipes for: chicken and oriental noodles in peanut sauce, 317; chicken with pasta and spinach, 316; colorful pasta salad, 293; country pasta with turkey sausage and white beans, 322; easy lasagna, 294; gourmet lasagna, 295; Mediterranean shrimp and scallops with pasta, 333; pasta with white bean soup with sundried tomatoes, 349; salmon pasta salad, 335; sesame pasta with broccoli, 296; shrimp fettuccine, 331; tofu lo mein, 353

pasta with white bean soup with sundried tomatoes, 349

peach crumble, 369

peaches, 10t, 41t, 92t, 142t

peanut butter, 13t, 55, 168, 361; fiber in, 50t; health and disease prevention from, 14, 34-35, 38t, 71; as protein source, 14, 15t, 16, 165t, 177t

—recipes with: peanut butter banana roll-up, 367; peanutty energy bars, 364

peanuts, 40t, 41t, 44, 154

—recipes with: chicken and oriental noodles in peanut sauce, 317

pears, 10t, 50t, 92t, 142t

pear-shaped body, 189

pear upside-down gingerbread cake, 370

peas, green, 12t, 15t, 38t, 41t, 50t, 72, 74t, 142t, 156t, 170f

peppers, green, 11, 12t, 39, 74t

peppers, red, 73, 74t

perimenopausal, 187

perspiration. See sweat

phosphorous, 16

phytochemicals, 40, 41t, 72, 172

pineapple, 10t, 41t

pineapple juice, 9, 10t, 128t

pizza, 64, 155; nutritional aspects of, 18t, 23, 84t, 86t; thick crust, 85

plant protein, 15t

poaching, of fish, 328

polymers, glucose, 138, 139

polyunsaturated fats, 30-31, 31t, 34

popcorn, 8, 34, 50t, 90

pork, 30t; fat in, 30t; leanest cuts of, 337; as protein source, 165t

—recipes with: honey-glazed pork chops, 342; stir-fry pork with fruit, 343

potassium: cramping and, 120-121; health benefits of, 9; high blood pressure prevention and, 45, 46; intake increased for, 46; recovery, 128, 128t; sources of, 6, 8, 9, 10, 10t, 11, 12t, 16, 22, 73, 74f

potato chips, 129t

potatoes and sweet potatoes: cancer prevention and, 42; carbohydrates and, 72, 80, 140, 142t; cooking tips for, 290-291; fiber in, 50t; nutritional value of, 12t, 15t, 46, 142t; as protein source, 12t; as recovery food, 128t, 140; serving suggestions for, 291-292; snacks, 92; with toppings, 84-85; in weight-gain diet, 208-209

—recipes for: egg-stuffed baked potato, 299; oven french fries, 298

poultry. See chicken; turkey

PowerAde, 129t, 130, 142t

PowerBar, 38t, 142t, 177t

pre-event foods, 89-111

pregnancy, 31; body fat and, 182-183; caffeine/coffee and, 52, 68; folic acid and, 25, 51, 59; iron and, 25, 51; nutrition during, 51-52; weight gain during, 51, 52f; weight loss after, 240

pretzels, 91, 91f, 119, 128, 129, 129t, 154

processed foods, 11, 148; loss of nutrients in, 6

prostate cancer, 40

protein, 144f, 178; amenorrhea and, 256; amino acids and, 175; for building muscle, 153; calculating, needs, 164-165, 210, 268; carbohydrates and, 127, 147, 150-151, 233; choices of, 14-16; comparing, content, 15t; complementary, over day, 174-175; complete, 173; consumed

like calories, 162; daily requirement of, 13-14, 13t, 210; deficiency, 25, 162; defining, needs, 162-164; excess, 13, 162, 165-166; GI problems and high, 106; high-fat, 108, 150-151, 166, 167, 176, 206, 231; iron in, 170t; little, 162; muscles and, 153, 161, 176, 205; powders and bars, 142t, 175-177, 214; pre-exercise and, 128; pregnancy and, 51; RDA of, 163t; recovery, 127-128; seafood and, 13t, 14, 15t, 165t, 177t; serving size for, 13t; sources of, 4, 15t, 19-20, 73-74; supplements, 164, 175-177, 214; vegetarian sources for, 74, 167-175, 345-346; in weight-gain diet, 210-212

protein alternatives. See supplements, protein; vegetarians

protein shake, 359

prunes, 10t, 50t, 170t

psychology, food and, 133, 150, 218, 226, 227-228, 235

Q

quick service breakfasts, 64

quinones, 41t

R

raisins, 10t, 50t, 55, 72, 92t, 128t, 142t, 156t, 158, 170t

—recipes with: carrot raisin muffins, 276; carrot-raisin salad, 310

raspberries, 92t

RDA. See Recommended Dietary Allowances (RDAs)

recipes: cooking efficiently with, 268-269; freezing foods and, 270-271; microwave cooking of, 270, 306, 328; nutritional information in, 267-268; spicing in, 269-270

Recommended Dietary Allowance (RDA), 25, 26t

recovery foods, 54-56, 124-135, 140, 153, 183. See also rest time

reducing diet. See weight-reduction diet

refined foods. See processed foods

restaurants, 78; fast-food, 81-85, 86t-88t; low-fat/healthful, 79-81; selecting, 79

rest time, 134, 135, 151-152, 154, 228

riboflavin (Vitamin B-2), 175; deficiency in, 25; sources of, 16

rice: carbohydrates and, 72, 140, 142t; cooking tips for, 289-290; fiber in, 50t; as protein source, 15t; serving suggestions for, 290; white, 142t; whole-grain, 7t, 81, 142t, 171t

—recipes with: southwestern rice and bean salad, 297

rosemary, 41t

running, 100, 105, 114-116, 121, 133, 143, 153, 171, 185, 190

S

safety, in food storage, 271

safflower oil. See oils

salad dressing: balsamic, 75; calcium in, 17; calories in, 72, 74-75, 75t; fats in, 74-75, 75t, 80; lemon, 318; oriental, 308, 318; sweet and spicy dressing, 307

salads, 11t, 46; carbohydrates in, 72; nutritional values in, 72-74, 73t, 80, 84, 84t; potassium in, 73; suggestions in, 72-74; vegetable ranking in, 73t, 74; vitamins in, 73; in weight-gain diet, 208

—recipes for: Brenda's Greek salad, 309; carrot-raisin, 310; chicken salad with almonds and mandarin oranges, 318; salmon pasta salad, 335; southwestern rice and bean salad, 297; spinach salad with oriental dressing, 308; spinach salad with sweet and spicy dressing, 307; warm taco salad, 340

salmon, 17, 18t, 31, 31t

—recipes with: salmon pasta salad, 335

salt, 129t; in canned food, 11, 45; content in foods, 44-45, 44t; cravings for, 44; DASH diet and, 45-46; eaten in heat, 119; high blood pressure and, 43-46; recommended intact for, 44; reducing intact of, 11, 44-45; in sweat, 44, 46, 274

sandwiches, 92, 208

sardines, 17, 18t, 31t

saturated fats, 28, 29, 33, 34, 172

sauces: hoisin (peanut), 317; honey glaze, 342; marinade, 320; sweet and spicy, 307; tomato, 11-12, 11*t*, 12*t*, 156*t*, 289

sautéed chicken with mushrooms and onions, 315

scallops, recipes with: Mediterranean shrimp and scallops with pasta, 333

seafood. *See* fish; salmon; sardines; scallops; shrimp; tuna

seasonings, 45, 74, 75

seeds, 175; sesame, 18, 296; sunflower, 40*t*, 74*f*

selenium, 40

self-esteem, 191-193, 246, 253, 260, 262

seltzers, 45

senior citizens, 117

serum cholesterol. *See* cholesterol, blood (serum)

serving sizes, 7

sesame pasta with broccoli, 296

sesame seeds, 18, 304. *See also* tahini (sesame paste)

sexual abuse, 192

shakes, recipes for: Diana's soy shake, 358; protein shake, 359; thick and frosty milkshake, 360

shopping, food, 76

shrimp, recipes with: Greek shrimp with feta and tomatoes, 332; Mediterranean shrimp and scallops with pasta, 333; shrimp fettuccine, 331

skinfold calipers, 196, 198-199, 200

slow-twitch muscle fibers, 311

sluggishness, 98

small intestine, 144*f*

smoked foods, 45

smoking, 43; coffee and, 65

smoothies, 55, 56, 91, 357. *See also* shakes

snack attacks, 95-98

snack foods, 4, 148*t*; candy, 91*f*; carbohydrates in, 157*t*; energy and protein bar, 38*t*, 92-94, 94*t*, 142*t*, 175-177, 214, 364; fruitful, 92*t*; nutritional value of, 361; suggestions for, 361-362; in weight-gain diet, 209. *See also* candy; desserts

—recipes with: peanut butter banana roll-up, 367; peanutty energy bars, 364; spiced walnuts, 366; sugar and spice trail mix, 365

snacking, 100; before afternoon exercise, 100; fast, 90-92; meals v., 95-96; before morning exercise, 99; pre-exercise/pre-competition, guidelines, 98, 107-110; timing for, 101, 108; wise and useful, 89-90, 92-94, 111

sodium, 125; blood levels of, 117, 119; in cereals, 44*t*, 60*t*-61*t*; cramping and, 121; osteoporosis prevention and, 48; recovery, 128-130, 129*t*; reducing, 11; in vegetables, 11, 12. *See also* salt

soft drinks: caffeine in, 68, 103*t*; calories in, 91*f*, 239; carbohydrates in, 125, 139; as recovery food, 128*t*, 129*t*. *See also* cola

Something Fishy Web Site on Eating Disorders, 261

sorbitol, 123

soups, 80, 85, 129, 129*t*, 207*f*, 208, 289

—recipes for: chicken black bean soup, 319; minestrone soup, 348; pasta with white bean soup with sundried tomatoes, 349

southwestern rice and bean salad, 297

soybean curd. *See* tofu

soy milk: as calcium source, 18, 18*t*, 19; cancer prevention and, 41*t*; heart health and, 32; as protein source, 14-15, 15*t*

soy nuts, 32

spaghetti. *See* pasta

spices, 269-270; for salt replacement, 45

spinach: absorption limitation of, 20; cancer prevention and, 40*t*, 41*t*; fiber in, 50*t*; folate in, 38*t*; iron and zinc in, 170*t*; nutritional value of, 11, 11*t*, 12*t*, 20, 72, 73*t*, 74*f*

—recipes with: chicken with pasta and spinach, 316; fish and spinach bake, 330; spinach salad with oriental dressing, 308; spinach salad with sweet and spicy dressing, 307

sports competition: fluid during, 113-120; food before, 106-107, 109-110, 145

sports drinks, 114, 122, 129*t*, 130, 142*t*, 239; carbohydrates in, 125, 127, 139; electrolytes in, 129*t*, 130; polymers sweetening of, 138, 139; potassium in, 128*t*; as recovery food, 129*t*, 130; sodium containing, 119; sodium content in, 129*t*, 130. *See* energy bars

sports drinks, homemade, 356

sports nutritionist, 122, 124

squash, summer. *See* zucchini

squash, winter, 12*t*, 15*t*; cancer prevention and, 12, 41*t*

Starbucks, 66*t*, 88*t*

starches, 139; carbohydrates and, 157*t*; sugar and, 139. *See also* breads; carbohydrates, complex; grains and starches; pasta; potatoes and sweet potatoes; rice

starvation, 244-246, 251, 260

steamed vegetables, 303

stir-fried vegetables, 304

stir-fry pork with fruit, 343

stomach, 114, 185; alcohol absorption into, 131; cramping, 25, 105, 124. *See also* digestion (gastrointestinal system)

strawberries, 9, 10*t*, 23, 41*t*, 59, 92*t*, 142*t*

stress, 43, 78, 106, 218, 228, 240, 247

sucrose, 138. *See also* sugar

sugar: calories from, 22, 22*t*; in cereals, 58, 60*t*-61*t*, 61-63; choices of, 22-23; diabetes and, 47; fluids in stomach influenced by, 114; frozen yogurt and, 21; GI problems and, 107; limiting value of, 138; nutritional value of, 22-23, 142*t*; pre-exercise consumption of, 104-105, 108; reduced amounts of, in recipes, 273; serving sizes of, 22*t*; simple, 137-138; starches and, 139; substitutes for, in recipes, 274; types of, 137-138

sugar-free gum, 123

sulfate/ferous gluconate, 172

sunflower oil. *See* oils

sunflower seeds, 40*t*, 74*f*

supplements, 231; amino acid, 175-177; antioxidant, 36-38, 42; beta-carotene, 136-137; calcium, 17; chelated, 37; creatine, 214-215; heart disease and benefits from, 36-38; iron, 59, 172; natural v. synthetic vitamins as, 37; protein, 164, 175-177, 214; recovery not helped by vitamin, 133; for snack/quick fix, 110-111; vegetarian, 175, 177; vitamin/mineral, 24-25, 133

supply, cupboard, 76-77, 77*t*

support crew, 115

support groups, 257-262

Surviving an Eating Disorder: A Survival Guide for Parents and Friends (Siegal and Brisman), 260

sweating, 125; fluids lost with, 114, 115, 125-126, 239; iron and, 171; measuring, 115, 116, 126; physiology of, 116, 117, 118*f*, 129; potassium loss from, 121; replacement of fluids after, 239; salt and, 44, 46, 274; women's v. men's, 116; zinc and, 170*t*

sweet and spicy orange beef, 341

sweet potatoes. *See* potatoes and sweet potatoes

sweets. *See* desserts; snack foods; sugar

swimming, 106, 146, 152

swiss muesli, 283

T

table sugar, 138. *See also* sugar

taco salad, warm, 340

tahini (sesame paste), 296, 352

Take Control, 34

tangerines, 92*t*

Tanita scale, 199, 200

tea, 66, 67, 103*t*, 172

teenagers, 163, 171, 203, 239

terpenes, 41*t*

thiamin, 24, 35; RDA of, 26*t*

timing: of exercise with food, 101; meals of, 54-56, 69, 101, 108, 149

tofu: as calcium source, 17, 18t, 74, 346; cancer prevention and, 41t; cholesterol benefits from, 32, 173; nutritional value of, 17, 32, 74, 168, 170t, 346-347; as protein source, 15-16, 15t, 32, 74, 165t, 173
—recipes with: Diana's soy shake, 358; protein shake, 359; tofu burritos, 354; tofu lo mein, 353
tomatoes: nutritional value of, 11-12, 11t, 12t, 72-73, 73t, 74f, 80, 129t tomatoes. *See also* sauces, tomato
—recipes with, 334; Greek shrimp with feta and tomatoes, 332; pasta with white bean soup with sundried tomatoes, 349
trail mix, sugar and spice, 365
training: gastrointestinal (GI) problems, 106-107; quality v. quantity, 134; recovery from daily, 153-154, 153f; tapering of, and carbo-loading, 146; untrained individuals and, 163
treats, excessive, 4
tuna, 13t, 15t, 30t, 31, 31t, 40, 165t, 170t, 177t
turkey, 71, 170t; as protein source, 13t, 14
—recipes with, 339, 340; country pasta with turkey sausage and white beans, 322; ground turkey mix for spaghetti sauce or chili, 324; turkey meatballs or turkey burgers, 323; turkey piccata, 321; turkey teriyaki, 320
twins, 204

U

ulcers, 65
Ultra Slim-Fast, 231
underwater weighing, 196-197
underweight. *See* weight gain; diet
urine and urination: frequency, 166; function of, 118f; sweat loss and color of, 117, 126. *See also* alcoholic beverages; diuretics
U.S. Department of Agriculture (USDA) Food pyramid. *See* Food guide pyramid
U.S. Pharmacopoeia, 37

V

variety: in diet, 4, 58-59, 63, 78; in snacks, 90. *See also* balanced diet; diet
vegetables, 81; cancer prevention and, 12, 39, 41t, 43; canned, 11; carbohydrates in, 72, 139, 156t; choices of, 11-12, 12t; color of, 11, 13t, 17, 20, 38, 72, 74f; cooking effect on, 11, 46; cooking tips for, 301, 303-306; cruciferous, 12; fiber in, 11, 50t; fresh v. frozen v. canned, 11, 75; green, 11, 13t, 17, 20, 38, 138t; heart disease prevention and, 38, 38t; iron in, 170t; nutritional value of, 5t, 10-12, 12t, 17, 46, 72-74; potassium content in, 11, 12t, 72; as protein source, 15t, 165t; ranking of, in salads, 73t, 74; serving size for, 11t; sodium content in, 11, 12, 44t; starch, sugar and, 139; starchy, 15; vitamins in, 72; in weight-gain diet, 208; zinc in, 170t. *See also* names of specific vegetables
—recipes with: baked vegetables, 305; microwaved vegetables, 306; steamed vegetables, 303; stir-fried vegetables, 304
vegetarians, 345-346; anemia and, 171-172; beans utilized by, 167; combining proteins, over day for, 174-175; diet, 15-16, 15t, 25, 162, 172-175, 174t; meals, 168t, 174t; protein and, 74, 167-175, 345-346; supplements for, 175, 177; women, 168-169, 256
vinegar, 75, 75t
vitamin A: function of, 24; RDA of, 26t; sources of, 9, 10-11, 10t, 12t
vitamin B: sources of, 6, 9, 14. *See also* riboflavin
vitamin B-1. *See* thiamin
vitamin B-6: heart disease prevention and, 38, 38t; RDA of, 26t
vitamin B-12, 175; deficiency, 25; heart disease prevention and, 38, 38t; RDA of, 26t
vitamin C (ascorbic acid): cancer prevention and, 39, 43; heart disease prevention and, 36-37; iron absorption and, 58, 59; RDA of, 26t; recovery and, 133; sources of, 4, 6, 8, 9, 10, 10t, 11, 12t, 72-73, 73t, 74f
vitamin D, 16, 24; deficiency of, 25; RDA of, 26t
vitamin E, 33, 74f; cancer prevention and, 40, 40t; heart disease prevention and, 36-37; RDA of, 26t; recovery and, 133
vitamin K: RDA of, 26t
vitamins: antioxidant, 36-38; deficiency, 24-25; function of, 24; natural v. synthetic, 37; recommended intake, 24-25, 26t; recovery, 133; sources of, 10; supplements of, 24-25, 36-38. *See also* beta-carotene

W

walking, 143, 223t
walnuts, 22, 32, 35; spiced, 366
water, 149, 239; the body, nutrients and, 118f; carbohydrates holding, 233; cramping and, 120; drinking, 125-126; foods with, 125. *See also* fluids
watermelon, 10t, 92t, 142t
weather, 116, 119
weight gain, 22, 63, 176, 204; balancing of, 210-212; calories needed for, 204, 206-209, 207f, 209t-210t; carbohydrates for, 205-206, 210-211; diet, 206-209, 209t-210t, 212t; fidgeting influence on, 204; lean physique and, 213-215; muscles, protein and, 205-206; preventing of, 16, 183; protein powders, drinks, creatine and, 214-215; regular meals for, 205-206; variance in, 204
weightlifting, 162, 214
weight limits, 238-239
weight loss: calorie counting for, 221-222, 223t, 224-225, 226, 239, 246, 255; calories' deficiency for, 183, 187, 222; eating properly for, 218-220; exercise and, 236-237; maintaining, 183; myths and truths of, 232-237; after pregnancy, 240; supportive of, 262-263; women's v. men's, 185, 217
weight-reduction diet, 94, 231; appropriate portions for, 219; avoiding temptation (out of sight) with, 227; breakfast and, 56-58, 61; diabetes, exercise and, 47; exercise appointments scheduled with, 229-230; high-protein, low-carbohydrate diet for, 233; low glycemic index food for, 220; mental attitude with, 230; nonfood activities important to, 227-228; realistic plan for, 228-229; salt reduction, high blood pressure and, 44-45; steps to successful, 225-230; weight limits and, 238-239; without starvation, 217-218, 222; writing down records of, 225-226
weight. *See* body weight
Wendy's, 83t-84t, 85
wheat germ, 40t, 171t
—recipe with: wheat germ and cottage cheese pancakes, 286
whole grain, 7t; breads, 7t, 8, 38t, 46, 56, 64, 72, 85, 148; cereals using, 7; crackers using, 8; nutritional value of, 46; selenium benefits from, 40; substitution, 273
wholesomeness foods, need for, 4, 27
win with nutrition, 122-123
wrestling, 238-239

Y

yoga, 223t
yogurt, 55, 158; as calcium source, 17, 18t, 20; frozen, 17, 20, 21; low-fat, 20, 44t, 49, 75; nutritional value of, 16-17, 21, 49, 91, 142t, f; as protein source, 15t, 165t; as recovery food, 128t, 129t; as snack, 91, 91f; sodium content in, 44t, 128, 129t
—recipe with: fruit smoothie, 357

Z

zinc, 37, 170t; deficiency, 25, 162, 175; RDA of, 26t; recommended intake of, 170t; sources of, 29, 170t-171t
Zone Diet, 230-231
zucchini (summer squash), 11, 12t, 156t

ABOUT THE AUTHOR

Nancy Clark, MS, RD, is the director of nutrition services at SportsMedicine Associates in Brookline, Massachusetts, one of the largest athletic injury clinics in the Boston area. A registered dietitian specializing in nutrition for sports and exercise, weight management, wellness, and the nutritional management of eating disorders, Clark counsels everyone from casual exercisers to competitive athletes. Her more famous clients include members of the Boston Red Sox and Boston Celtics as well as many elite and Olympic athletes. She is also the sports nutrition consultant to Boston College's sports medicine department and the Arthritis Foundation's Joint in Motion Marathon Training Program.

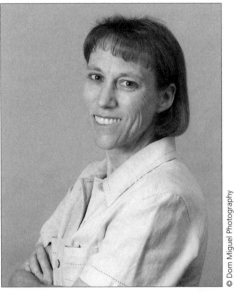

© Dom Miguel Photography

Clark is the nutrition columnist for *New England Runner*, *Adventure Cycling*, *Rugby*, and Active.com. She is a regular contributor to *Shape* and *Runner's World*, and she writes a monthly nutrition column titled "The Athlete's Kitchen," which appears in more than 100 sports and health publications and Web sites. In addition, Clark is the author of *Nancy Clark's Food Guide for Marathoners: Tips for Everyday Champions*. She has also developed teaching materials for health professionals; visit www.nancyclarkrd.com for more information.

An internationally-known lecturer, Clark has given presentations to such groups as the American Dietetic Association (ADA), the American College of Sports Medicine (ACSM), and the International Food Information Council. She has also led workshops for athletes at the Olympic Training Centers in Colorado Springs and Lake Placid. Clark received her undergraduate degree in nutrition from Simmons College in Boston and her master's degree in nutrition from Boston University. She completed her internship in dietetics at Massachusetts General Hospital. She is a fellow of the ADA, recipient of their 1995 Media Excellence Award, and an active member of ADA's practice group of nutrition entrepreneurs (NE) and sports nutritionists (SCAN) and a recipient of SCAN's 1992 Honor Award. In addition, Clark is a fellow of the ACSM and recipient of the 1994 Honor Award from ACSM's New England chapter.

An athlete herself, Clark has biked across America, run marathons, and trekked in the Himalayas. A regular bike commuter and member of the Greater Boston Track Club, she lives in Newton, Massachusetts, with her husband and two children.